*Cover: color-enhanced
cardiac angiogram.
Photograph by Howard Sochurek.*

*Inside front and back covers:
heart muscle.*

NURSE'S CLINICAL LIBRARY™

CARDIOVASCULAR DISORDERS

NURSING84 BOOKS™
SPRINGHOUSE CORPORATION
Springhouse, Pennsylvania

NURSING84 BOOKS™

Library of Congress Cataloging in Publication Data
Main entry under title:
Cardiovascular disorders.

(Clinical Library)
"Nursing84 Books."
Includes bibliographies and index.
1. Cardiovascular disease nursing. I. Series.
[DNLM: 1. Cardiovascular disease nursing. Nursing texts. WY 152.5 C26746]RC674.C363 1984 616.1 83-17004
ISBN 0-916730-56-5

CONTENTS

Contributors

At the time of publication, the contributors held the following positions:

Katherine Green Baker, RN, MN, Clinical Specialist, Center for Health Sciences, University of California, Los Angeles

Charlotte M. Dienhart, PhD, Assistant Professor of Anatomy and Associate Professor of Community Health, Emory University School of Medicine, Atlanta

Jeanne E. Doyle, RN, BS, Nurse Consultant, Peripheral Vascular Surgery, University Hospital, Boston

Kathleen Dracup, RN, DNS, CCRN, FAAN, Assistant Professor, School of Nursing, Center for Health Sciences, University of California, Los Angeles

Barbara Boyd Egoville, RN, MSN, Former Senior Instructor, Lankenau Hospital School of Nursing, Lankenau, Pa.

Mitzi Andrews Ekers, RN, BSN, Peripheral Vascular Consultant, Baltimore

Janis W. Fink, RN, MSN, Nursing Consultant and Staff Nurse, Shady Grove Adventist Hospital, Rockville, Md.

Terri Forshee, RN, MSN, CCRN, Visiting Lecturer, School of Nursing, Center for Health Sciences, University of California, Los Angeles

Anna Gawlinski, RN, MSN, CCRN, Clinical Nurse Specialist, University of California, Medical Center, Los Angeles

Jeanette C. Hartshorn, RN, BA, MN, CCRN, Independent Consultant, Hartshorn Enterprises, Charleston, S.C.

Martha N. Hill, RN, MSN, Assistant Professor, Johns Hopkins University, Baltimore

Doris Houser, RN, BSN, MA, Clinical Nursing Specialist, University of Iowa Hospitals and Clinics, Iowa City

Lauren Marie Isacson, RN, Instructor of Nursing Education, Jersey Shore Medical Center, Neptune, N.J.

Gail D'Onofrio Long, RN, MS, Critical-Care Clinical Specialist/Consultant and Medical Student, Boston University School of Medicine, Boston

Kathleen M. McCauley, RN, MSN, Cardiovascular Clinical Specialist, Hospital of the University of Pennsylvania; Clinical Instructor, University of Pennsylvania School of Nursing, Philadelphia

Carolyn G. Smith Marker, RN, MSN, CNA, Faculty Consultant and Former Assistant Director of Critical Care Areas, Anne Arundel General Hospital, Annapolis, Maryland

Leona G. Matheny, RN, BS, Life Support Educator, University of California at Davis Medical Center, Sacramento

Phyllis Pletz, MSN, Independent Educator/Consultant, Baltimore

Bhagwan Satiani, MB, BS, FACS, Program Director, Peripheral Vascular Surgery, Grant Hospital, Columbus, Ohio

Klaus J. Schulz, MD, Staff Cardiologist and Director, Pacemaker Evaluation Center, Jersey Shore Medical Center, Neptune, N.J.

Kristine Ann Scordo, RN, BSN, MS, Clinical Nurse Specialist in Cardiology, Bethesda Hospital, Cincinnati, Ohio

Janis B. Smith, RN, MSN, Instructor, University of Delaware College of Nursing, Newark

Arlene Strong, RN, MN, ANP, Cardiac Clinical Specialist and Adult Nurse Practitioner, Anticoagulant Clinic, Veterans Administration Medical Center, Portland, Ore.

Peggy L. Wagner, RN, MSN, CCRN, Cardiovascular Clinical Nurse Specialist, St. Michael Hospital, Milwaukee

Clinical Consultants

At the time of publication, the clinical consultants held the following positions:

Henry D. Berkowitz, MD, Associate Professor of Surgery and Chief, Peripheral Vascular Laboratory, University of Pennsylvania, Philadelphia

Franklin E. Chatham, MD, Cardiology Instructor, Johns Hopkins University School of Medicine, Baltimore

Edward K. Chung, MD, FACP, FACC, Professor of Medicine and Director of Heart Station, Thomas Jefferson University, Philadelphia

Leonard V. Crowley, MD, Clinical Assistant Professor, Department of Laboratory Medicine and Pathology and Department of Family Practice and Community Health, University of Minnesota Medical School, Minneapolis; Pathologist, St. Mary's Hospital, Minneapolis

David B. Freiman, AB, MD, Chairman, Radiology Department, Presbyterian–University of Pennsylvania Medical Center, Philadelphia

A-Hadi I. Hakki, MD, Assistant Professor of Surgery, Hahnemann University Hospital, Philadelphia

Morrison Hodges, MD, Professor of Medicine, University of Minnesota, Minneapolis

Herbert Y. Kressel, MD, Associate Professor of Radiology, Department of Radiology, Hospital of the University of Pennsylvania, Philadelphia

Peter G. Lavine, MD, Director, Coronary Care Unit, Crozer-Chester Medical Center, Chester, Pa.

William K. Levy, MD, Staff Cardiologist, Abington Memorial Hospital, Abington, Pa.

Elaine H. Niggemann, RN, MD, Department of Internal Medicine, University of Arizona Health Sciences Center, Tucson

Leonard J. Perloff, MD, Associate Professor of Surgery, University of Pennsylvania, Philadelphia

FOREWORD

New knowledge and new procedures for detecting and treating various cardiovascular disorders have profoundly changed cardiovascular nursing. When it applies to acute illness, cardiovascular nursing now takes place almost exclusively in the highly specialized cardiac care and surgical intensive care units.

But that's just part of it. The new emphasis on holistic and preventive care has expanded nursing involvement during early prodromal stages of cardiovascular illness and during chronic maintenance as well. Such involvement often takes place at sites away from the hospital where nurses must practice more independently than ever before. For example, nurses have become coordinators of cardiac rehabilitation programs. In this role, they work with exercise physiologists, cardiologists, and nutritionists. They define patient entrance criteria, set exercise protocols, and establish patient education programs. Similarly, nurses have entered collaborative practices with cardiac surgeons and cardiologists in outpatient clinics—notably those for patients with hypertension or pacemakers—in which they manage patient care under standardized protocols and conduct independent and collaborative research in cardiac-care settings. In the emergency department and all other hospital departments, nurses must be ready to handle sudden dysrhythmia, shock, or cardiac arrest, knowing which situations are likely to provoke cardiovascular complications or emergencies and how to handle them correctly.

To meet these challenging new responsibilities, nurses need to continuously expand and update their understanding of the cardiovascular system and its normal function, and the devastating effects of its dysfunction on interlocking vital systems. CARDIOVASCULAR DISORDERS, the first volume of a new reference series for nurses, will help you meet these new challenges. The first section, the introduction, reviews cardiovascular fundamentals. The chapters in this section review cardiovascular anatomy and physiology and the mechanisms of heart failure. They also contain complete information on cardiovascular assessment and diagnostic tests, including such advances as nuclear magnetic resonance (NMR) scanning and digital subtraction angiography.

The remaining three sections of this volume cover specific disorders of circulation, pump failure, cardiac musculature, and electroconduction. Each chapter contains three major sections. *Pathophysiology* covers the causes, fundamental mechanisms, and characteristic signs and symptoms of each disorder, and its effects on the cardiovascular system and vital organs. *Medical management* focuses on specific tests and other diagnostic methods used to detect each disorder, and discusses their characteristic findings. This part of each chapter also summarizes treatment, including new and traditional drug therapy, surgery, and supportive procedures. *Nursing management* provides detailed information for planning nursing care, presented according to the nursing process. For each disorder, the discussion includes a detailed patient history, characteristic assessment findings, and typical nursing diagnoses. Expanding on these diagnoses, it summarizes the goals of patient care, suggests nursing interventions needed to achieve them, and, finally, offers a guide to evaluation.

Throughout this volume, scores of useful anatomic drawings, illustrations, charts, and diagrams clarify and augment the text. Special graphic devices call attention to patient-teaching aids and emergency management of life-threatening complications, such as hypertensive crisis and acute pulmonary edema. Two appendices provide supplementary information on congenital heart defects and cardiovascular drugs.

Given nursing's expanding role in health care, nurses have a special need to keep their knowledge of cardiovascular disorders current and accurate. This volume—which offers such knowledge in both theoretical and practical forms—will be an excellent reference for nurses at all professional levels.

KATHLEEN A. DRACUP, RN, DNS, CCRN, FAAN
Assistant Professor, School of Nursing
University of California, Los Angeles

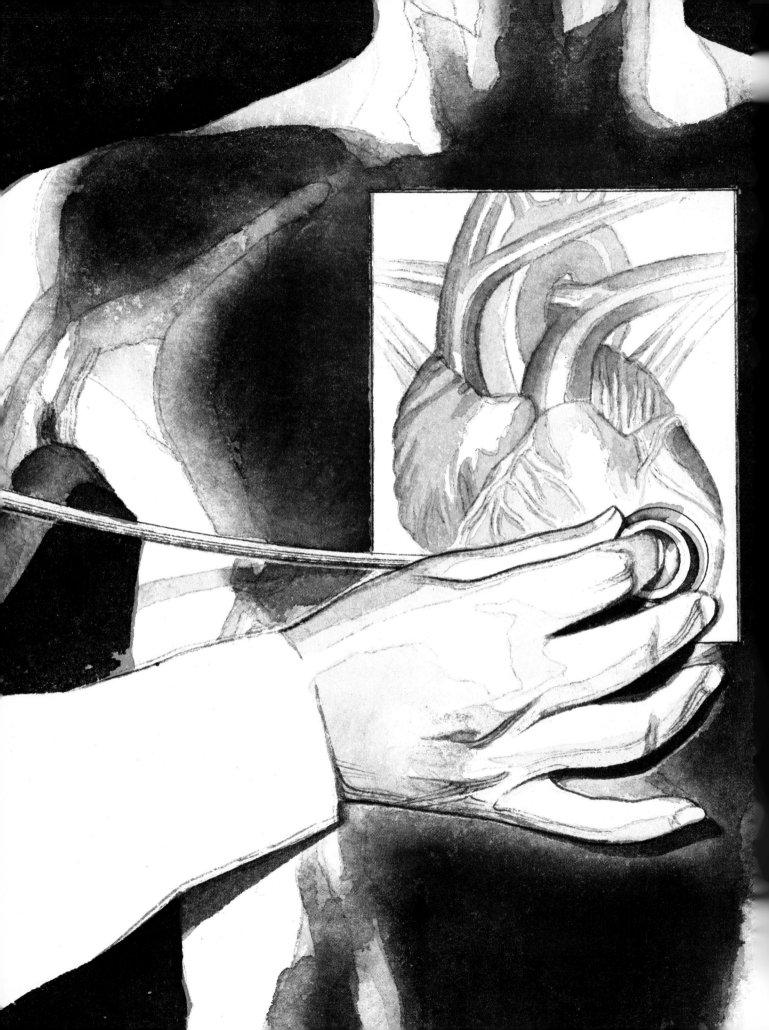

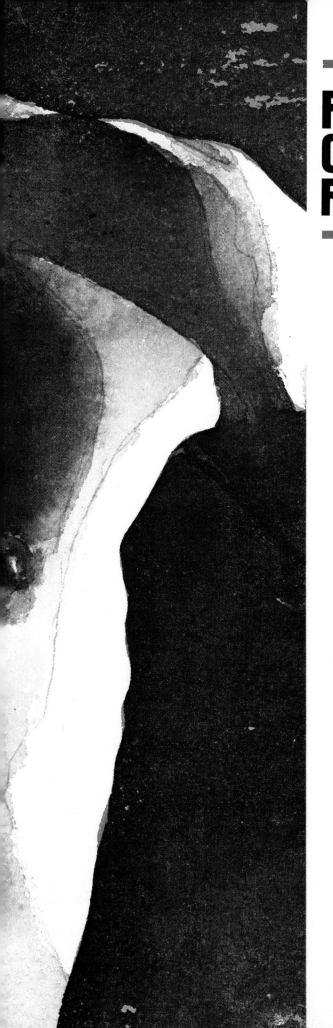

FUNDAMENTAL CARDIOVASCULAR FACTS

1 REVIEWING FUNDAMENTAL PRINCIPLES

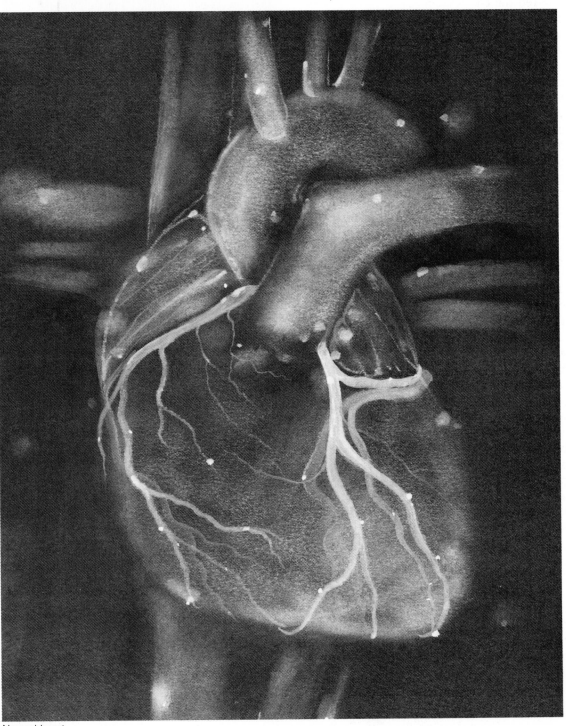

Normal heart

f patients with cardiovascular disorders are regularly a part of your nursing practice, you know that artificial hearts—for all their drama—are not the most important changes in this health-care field. Much less dramatic, but more pervasive in their potential impact, are the steadily accumulating improvements in prevention, diagnosis, and treatment. Especially during the last 10 years, these improvements have lowered the cardiovascular death rate, despite a steadily aging population. More people than ever before are living longer, many of them with various forms of cardiovascular disease.

What does this mean to you? Obviously, it means you'll have to deal with cardiovascular disorders more often—no matter where you practice nursing. You'll be expected to play a larger role in developing and promoting good health; in preventing and controlling disease; and in developing and implementing community health education programs. You'll be challenged to develop new teaching methods to reach the healthy population. And finally, as more sophisticated technologies and treatments emerge, you'll need expanded assessment and therapeutic management skills. All in all, the challenge of cardiovascular disease is enormous. Meeting it demands an expertise based on thorough understanding of this complex and vital system.

A formidable foe

Before reviewing cardiovascular structure, function, and pathology, let's consider the formidable challenge presented by the ravages of diseases in this system. You already know that this system is subject to a host of ills, but the magnitude of the problem becomes apparent when you realize that roughly 42 million Americans suffer some form of cardiovascular disease, and that many persons suffer from more than one of these disorders. This complex of illnesses is the leading cause of death in the United States. According to the National Center for Health Statistics, it caused nearly a million deaths in 1982.

The most prevalent cardiovascular diseases are hypertensive heart disease (37 million patients), coronary heart disease (4.5 million), rheumatic heart disease (2 million), and cerebrovascular accident (1.8 million). Health-care costs of cardiovascular diseases are expected to reach $57 billion in 1983, the American Heart Association estimates.

A major part of these huge costs stems from the advanced technology associated with di-

agnosis and treatment. Such advances include improved imaging techniques such as nuclear magnetic resonance; treatments such as percutaneous transluminal coronary angioplasty and streptokinase infusions to help restore circulation in an obstructed coronary artery; and mechanical ventricular assist devices that take over the work of a failing pump.

As the list of advances grows, so does your need to understand fundamental cardiovascular mechanisms. Without such understanding you can't make full and competent use of these new methods. In this chapter we'll briefly review cardiovascular structure and function, with an overview of pathophysiology associated with pump failure. In later chapters, we'll discuss the pathophysiology of specific disorders.

THE HEART AND VESSELS

The heart is the center of the circulatory system. In the normal adult, it keeps 10 pints of blood in constant circulation, pumping the equivalent of 2,100 gallons (about 7,949 liters) of fluid every day. Located in the mediastinum between the lungs, this hollow muscular organ is about the size of a man's clenched fist and weighs about 10.6 to 14.1 ounces (300 to 400 grams) in a normal adult. Roughly cone-shaped, the organ lies obliquely in the chest, with two thirds of its bulk to the left of the midline, one third to the right. Its position changes with each respiration, moving vertically during inspiration as the diaphragm descends, and horizontally during expiration as the diaphragm ascends. Details of the heart's internal structures are shown on page 10.

A vast network of arteries, arterioles, capillaries, venules, and veins—in all, about 60,000 miles (96,558 kilometers) of vessels—delivers blood to and from every functioning cell in the body. This network can be divided into two branches: *pulmonary circulation,* in which blood picks up new oxygen and liberates carbon dioxide as waste; and *systemic circulation,* including the coronary circulation, in which blood carries oxygen and nutrients to all active cells while transporting waste products to the kidneys, liver and skin for excretion. A detailed view of the coronary circulation appears on page 11.

HEMODYNAMIC REGULATION

Many physiological factors—blood flow, vascular resistance, and neurologic, hormonal, and physical regulators of blood pressure—

Inside the normal heart

The heart's internal structure consists of the pericardium, the 3 layers of the heart wall, 4 chambers, 11 openings, and 4 valves.

The *serous pericardium* is a sac which is invaginated by the heart; thus, the visceral pericardium becomes the outer layer of the heart wall, or epicardium. The parietal serous layer has an outer strengthening coat of dense fibrous tissue, the so-called fibrous pericardium. The potential pericardial space between the parietal and epicardial layers contains about 30 ml of pericardial fluid, but may hold up to 1 liter in trauma or disease. The heart wall (see enlargement) consists of three layers: an outer *epicardium;* a thick *myocardium,* which forms most of the

heart wall and consists of interlacing bundles of cardiac muscle fibers; and an inner *endocardium,* which is formed of a thin layer of endothelial tissue.

The *right atrium* lies in front and to the right of the *left atrium,* from which it is separated by the interatrial septum. It receives blood from the superior and inferior venae cavae. The *right ventricle* lies behind the sternum and forms the largest part of the sternocostal surface and inferior border of the heart. Its posterior wall is formed by the interventricular septum. The *left atrium,* smaller but with thicker walls than the right atrium, forms the uppermost part of the left border of the heart, extending to the left of and behind the right atrium. Its posterior aspect

forms most of the heart's base. The *left ventricle* forms the apex and most of the left border of the heart and its diaphragmatic surface.

The *tricuspid valve* guards the right atrioventricular orifice and consists of three triangular cusps or leaflets. Their free margins are attached by thin but strong *chordae tendineae* to the papillary muscles in the right ventricle. The *bicuspid* or *mitral valve* guards the left atrioventricular opening. It has two cusps, a large anterior and a smaller posterior. Their free margins are attached to papillary muscles by chordae tendineae in the left ventricle.

The two *semilunar valves* have three cusps and guard the orifices of the pulmonary artery and the aorta.

Heart wall

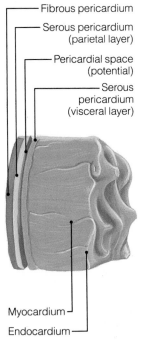

- Fibrous pericardium
- Serous pericardium (parietal layer)
- Pericardial space (potential)
- Serous pericardium (visceral layer)
- Myocardium
- Endocardium

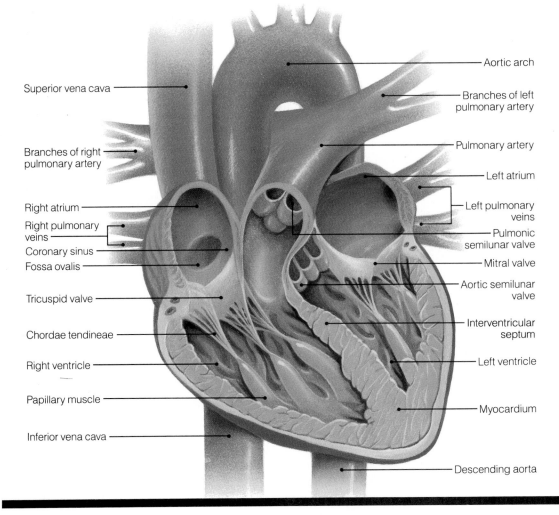

- Aortic arch
- Branches of left pulmonary artery
- Pulmonary artery
- Left atrium
- Left pulmonary veins
- Pulmonic semilunar valve
- Mitral valve
- Aortic semilunar valve
- Interventricular septum
- Left ventricle
- Myocardium
- Descending aorta

- Superior vena cava
- Branches of right pulmonary artery
- Right atrium
- Right pulmonary veins
- Coronary sinus
- Fossa ovalis
- Tricuspid valve
- Chordae tendineae
- Right ventricle
- Papillary muscle
- Inferior vena cava

The heart's blood supply

Although the heart passes blood to the rest of the body, it relies on two *coronary arteries* and their branches to supply itself with oxygenated blood, and on seven *cardiac veins* to remove oxygen-depleted blood. During left ventricular systole, blood is ejected into the aorta. During diastole, blood flows into the coronary ostia and is distributed through the coronary arteries to nourish the heart muscle.

The *right coronary artery* supplies blood to the right atrium (including the sinoatrial and atrioventricular nodes of the conduction system), part of the left atrium, and most of the right ventricle, and the inferior part of the left ventricle.

The *left coronary artery,* which splits into the anterior interventricular and circumflex arteries, supplies blood to the left atrium, most of the left ventricle, and most of the interventricular septum. Many collateral arteries connect the branches of the right and left coronary arteries, but those are usually clinically insignificant.

Variations in the pattern of arterial branching are common.

The *cardiac veins* lie superficial to the arteries. The largest vein, the *coronary sinus,* lies in the posterior part of the coronary sulcus and opens into the right atrium. Most of the major cardiac veins empty into the coronary sinus, except for the *anterior cardiac veins,* which empty into the right atrium.

Since coronary vessels must distribute blood quickly and under high pressure, their intimal layers are especially vulnerable to injury or accumulations of cholesterol and fats that cause atherosclerotic plaques. These plaques may later embolize, or occlude the vessel, or cause vasospasm. Plaques commonly form in the first few centimeters of the coronary arteries, when they cause ischemia and possible myocardial infarction.

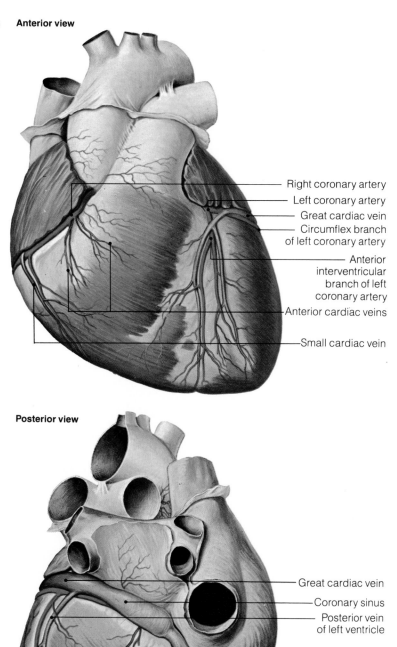

Anterior view

Right coronary artery
Left coronary artery
Great cardiac vein
Circumflex branch of left coronary artery
Anterior interventricular branch of left coronary artery
Anterior cardiac veins
Small cardiac vein

Posterior view

Great cardiac vein
Coronary sinus
Posterior vein of left ventricle
Small cardiac vein
Right coronary artery
Middle cardiac vein
Posterior interventricular branch of right coronary artery

Blood vessels: Form follows function

As blood courses through the vascular system, it travels through five distinct types of blood vessels: arteries, arterioles, capillaries, venules, and veins. In the aorta, vascular resistance to blood flow is almost nil, and mean arterial pressure remains almost constant at 100 mm Hg. But when blood reaches the arterioles, which have much smaller diameters, vascular resistance has increased enough to reduce mean blood pressure to 85 mm Hg. When the blood crosses the arterioles to the capillaries, vascular resistance causes the mean blood pressure to fall to 35 mm Hg. Such low pressure is essential for optimum exchange of nutrients and gases in the capillary bed.

Although blood pressure is only about 15 mm Hg when blood begins to return to the heart, it decreases still further despite a steady increase in venous diameter. Why? Because many veins are collapsed much of the time by pressure from the surrounding tissues.

Differences in blood pressure are reflected in vessel structure. Arteries have thick, muscular walls to accommodate the flow of blood at high speeds and pressures. Arterioles have thinner walls than arteries, and they can constrict or dilate as needed to control blood flow to the capillaries. The capillaries are microscopic vessels with walls composed of only a single layer of endothelial cells. Venules gather blood from the capillaries, but have thinner walls than arterioles. Similarly, veins have thinner walls than arteries, but have larger diameters because of the low blood pressures required for return of venous blood to the heart. Veins of the extremities and neck have valves that open in the direction of blood flow to prevent venous backflow.

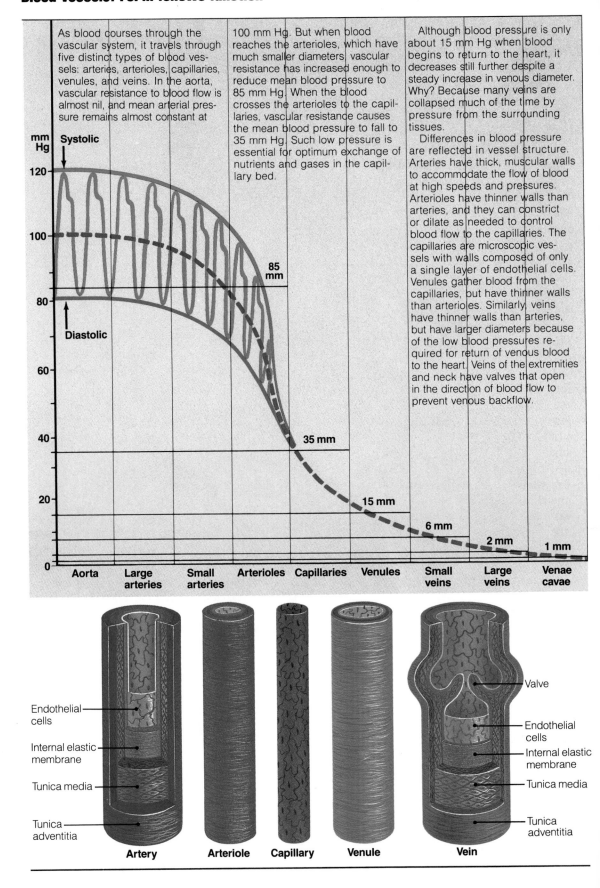

interact to allow the heart and blood vessels to function most efficiently. If you know how these factors operate to ensure optimum perfusion of all body cells, you'll be better able to assess your patient's clinical status and manage his care more effectively.

Blood flow

Blood flow is the amount of blood that passes an arbitrary point in the circulation in a given time. It can be used as a measure of cardiac output, since it's the amount of blood pumped by each ventricle per unit of time. The rate of blood flow is proportional to the difference in pressure between the two ends of a blood vessel; this pressure difference forces blood to flow from the high-pressure end to the low-pressure end. In a normal person at rest, blood flow is about 5,000 ml per minute.

Vascular resistance

Resistance depends on blood viscosity, length of the vessel and, most importantly, inside diameter of the vessel. Even though a short, wide vessel typically offers less resistance to blood flow than a long, narrow one, slight changes in inside diameter can significantly affect blood flow. (See *Blood vessels: Form follows function,* page 12.) Such changes allow the rate of blood flow to adjust automatically to changes in arterial pressure (autoregulation). For example, a sudden increase in arterial pressure widens a vessel's inside diameter, accelerating the rate of blood flow.

Vascular resistance can also be expressed as the hemodynamic equation $R = \Delta P/Q$, where R is the resistance, ΔP the pressure difference between the two ends of the blood vessel, and Q the rate of blood flow.

Blood pressure

Blood pressure is the pressure exerted on the blood vessels by the blood as it flows through them. Three pressure-regulating mechanisms —neural, hormonal, and physical—interact to ensure that enough blood is channeled to, or diverted from, the right part of the body at the right time.

Neural regulators include baroreceptors and chemoreceptors. Baroreceptors are nerve endings embedded in blood vessels that are sensitive to the stretching of vessel walls. They're most abundant in the walls of the internal carotid arteries—in the carotid sinuses just above the carotid bifurcation. They're less plentiful in the walls of the aortic arch and in most large arteries of the neck and

thorax. When the vessel walls stretch in response to increasing blood volume, baroreceptors signal the central nervous system to inhibit the vasoconstrictor center in the medulla and to stimulate the vagal center. This causes peripheral vasodilation, decreased heart rate, and less vigorous contractions, decreasing arterial blood pressure. Conversely, when baroreceptors detect decreased blood pressure, they induce peripheral vasoconstriction, increased heart rate, and more vigorous contractions. (See *How baroreceptors regulate blood pressure,* page 14.)

Although baroreceptors quickly respond to small changes in blood pressure, they fail to respond to higher pressure levels after one or more days. Thus, they lose their ability to control arterial pressure changes in the patient with chronic hypertension.

Chemoreceptors are nerve endings located in the walls of the carotid arteries, the aorta, and the medullary area of the brainstem. Responding to abnormally low levels of dissolved oxygen and carbon dioxide in the blood, these nerve endings stimulate sympathetic activity and inhibit parasympathetic activity to cause a reflex increase in arterial pressure.

Four *hormonal regulators* control arterial pressure: secretion of *norepinephrine* and *epinephrine* by the adrenal glands; secretion of *renin* by the juxtaglomerular cells of the kidneys, with subsequent formation of *angiotensin I and II;* secretion of *antidiuretic hormone* (also called *vasopressin*) by the hypothalamus; and secretion of hormonelike *prostaglandins* by various body tissues.

In the circulation, norepinephrine and epinephrine are released by the adrenal medullae and cause effects similar to direct sympathetic stimulation of the cardiovascular system: increased heart rate, blood pressure, automaticity, and contractility. These hormones achieve their effects by stimulating the sympathetic system's *alpha* and *beta receptors* throughout the vasculature. These receptors consist of specialized lipoprotein complexes in the cell membranes of blood vessel walls. Alpha stimulation causes vasoconstriction; beta stimulation, vasodilation.

Renin is released by the kidneys when blood pressure drops excessively. Persisting in the blood up to an hour, this enzyme acts on the plasma protein angiotensinogen to form the hormone angiotensin I. When blood containing this hormone reaches the lungs, an enzyme in the small vessels of the lungs catalyzes its conversion to angiotensin II. An-

How baroreceptors regulate blood pressure

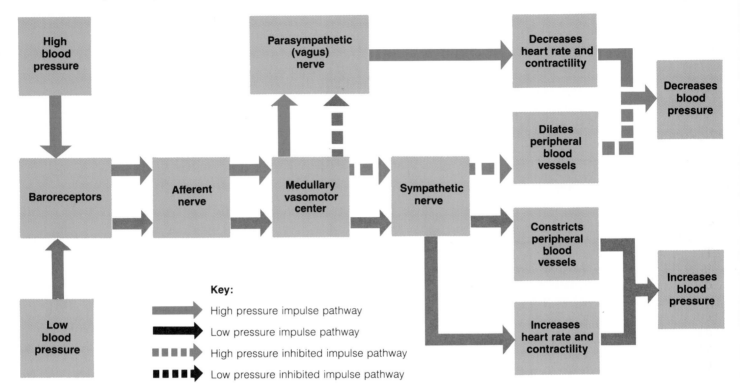

Key:
→ High pressure impulse pathway
→ Low pressure impulse pathway
▪▪▪▪▶ High pressure inhibited impulse pathway
▪▪▪▪▶ Low pressure inhibited impulse pathway

When baroreceptors in the carotid sinuses and aortic arch detect changes in arterial blood pressure, they stimulate the vasomotor center in the medulla, which constricts or dilates peripheral blood vessels, and stimulates or depresses heart rate and contractility. This mechanism is inactive at arterial pressures below 60 mm Hg, and most active at 150 to 180 mm Hg.

giotensin II strongly constricts arterioles, raising arterial pressure, and moderately constricts veins, promoting venous return to the heart and providing additional blood to pump against the increased pressure. Exerting a direct effect on the kidneys, angiotensin II decreases excretion of salt and water. It also causes the adrenal cortex to secrete aldosterone, further decreasing salt and water excretion. This reduced fluid loss tends to increase blood volume and raise blood pressure.

The hypothalamus responds to decreased blood pressure by secreting *antidiuretic hormone,* which, like angiotensin, is a vasoconstrictor. It acts on the renal tubules to promote water retention, which in turn increases plasma volume and thus increases peripheral resistance and blood pressure.

Various prostaglandins, hormonelike substances found in many body tissues, are thought to be involved in blood pressure regulation. In general, prostaglandins A and E dilate arteries and veins, while prostaglandin F constricts veins.

Two *physical regulators—vascular stress-relaxation* and *capillary fluid shift*—regulate blood pressure. Unlike neural or hormonal mechanisms, these slower mechanisms take an hour or more to exert their full effects.

Stress-relaxation allows a blood vessel to compensate for sudden shifts in volume and

pressure by adjusting its diameter without prolonging a change in its diameter and tension. A rapid increase in blood volume and pressure distends a blood vessel but causes only a transient increase in tension. Similarly, a sharp decrease in volume and pressure shortens the vessel but causes only a transient decrease in tension.

Capillary fluid shift is a compensatory mechanism that regulates fluid exchange across capillary membranes in response to changes in arterial pressure. With a sharp increase in arterial pressure, capillary hydrostatic pressure increases, causing more fluid to shift into the interstitial spaces. As a result, less fluid is circulating, and blood pressure decreases. With a sharp decrease in blood pressure, capillary hydrostatic pressure falls, causing an increase in circulating volume and a corresponding increase in blood pressure.

CARDIAC CONDUCTION SYSTEM

Cardiac conduction results from the workings of the extrinsic and intrinsic systems. The *extrinsic conduction system* consists of the afferent and efferent nerve fibers of the autonomic nervous system, which controls the heart's contractility. Consequently, the heart can respond to the body's changing physiologic needs by changing the rate and force of its contractions.

The sympathetic fibers of the middle, superior, and inferior cardiac nerves and the parasympathetic fibers in branches of the vagus nerve combine to form the *cardiac plexi,* located near the aortic arch. From these plexi, nerve fibers accompany the right and left coronary arteries into the heart. Most of these fibers end in the sinoatrial (SA) node, the remainder in the atrioventricular (AV) node.

Stimulation of the sympathetic fibers supplying the SA and AV nodes and all heart chambers increases heart rate and contractility. Stimulation of the parasympathetic fibers supplying the SA node and the atria decreases heart rate and contractility. When stimulated, the sympathetic fibers that supply the coronary arteries dilate these arteries.

The heart's *intrinsic conduction system* consists of the SA and AV nodes, postulated internodal tracts, the atrioventricular (AV) bundle, bundle branches, and the Purkinje fibers. The intrinsic system initiates the heartbeat and coordinates chamber contraction. The conducting fibers, like other cardiac muscle fibers, possess dark-staining junctional complexes called intercalated disks. These disks have low electrical resistance and conjoin individual cardiac cells in such a way that the cells act electrically as a unit when stimulated. Because of these disks, any stimulated cardiac muscle fiber sends an electrical impulse across the entire cardiac muscle mass, producing an all-or-nothing response.

Cardiac muscle: Four characteristics

The physiological characteristics of cardiac muscle are excitability, automaticity, conductivity, and contractility.

Excitability is a cell's capacity to respond to an electrochemical stimulus. Like most other body cells, cardiac muscle cells have a *resting membrane potential;* that is, the outer surface of the resting cell membrane bears a positive electrical charge, and the inner surface of the membrane bears a negative charge. During the resting stage, cardiac muscle cells are *polarized*—the number of positive charges on the outside of each cell equals the number of negative charges on the inside. Electrical stimulation makes the cell membrane permeable to the flow of sodium, potassium, and calcium ions (see *Cardiac depolarization-repolarization,* page 16).

Cardiac muscle cells also possess a compensatory mechanism that makes them *refractory* to restimulation during the action potential—the rapid pulselike change in

Fast track: The internal conduction system

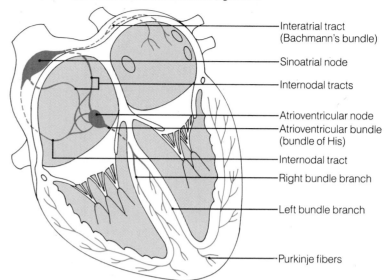

The SA node and the AV node, together with the atrioventricular bundle and Purkinje fibers, constitute the intrinsic conduction system of the heart. These specialized fibers can initiate a contraction, but the SA node usually paces the heart. A system of conduction pathways, or *internodal tracts,* has been postulated to connect the SA and AV nodes, but their existence is controversial.

membrane potential accomplished by exchange of sodium and potassium ions. The refractory period is absolute during systole, when cardiac muscle does not respond to *any* stimulus. This prevents tetanic contractions that could lead to circulatory failure. When this absolute refractory period ends, cardiac muscle gradually recovers its excitability; recovery, known as the *relative refractory period,* occurs early in diastole.

Automaticity is a cell's capacity to reach threshold potential and generate action potential without external stimulation. The cells of the SA node have a lower resting membrane potential (−55 to −60 millivolts)—and, therefore, a greater degree of automaticity—than the surrounding muscle tissue (−85 to −95 millivolts). Consequently, the SA node can spontaneously generate action potentials, allowing the heart to function independently of the autonomic nervous system.

Conductivity is a cell's ability to transmit electrical impulses. For example, the SA node generates rhythmic impulses at a rate of 60 to 100 beats/minute. Transmission of these impulses to the AV node, though, is delayed by a compensatory mechanism called *decremental conduction,* which allows the ventricles to fill adequately before they contract.

When functioning as a pacer, the AV node transmits electrical impulses at an intrinsic

Power for the cardiac cycle

The stylized cardiac muscle cell at right is undergoing one complete cycle of polarization-repolarization in response to a stimulus from the cardiac conduction system. At top, the cell is at rest, just before diastole. The concentration of sodium ions is greater outside the cell than inside it, while potassium concentration is greater inside than outside. A stimulus from the sinoatrial node briefly reverses this ionic status, causing depolarization (left). Sodium ions move from the outside to the inside of the cell until the charges on the inner and outer surfaces are reversed and the cell membrane is fully depolarized (bottom). Immediately, potassium ions begin to flow from inside the cell to outside, and the cell repolarizes (far right). The cell returns to its resting state through the action of an ion-transport mechanism called the *sodium-potassium pump,* which is fueled by energy from adenosine triphosphate as it's changed to adenosine diphosphate by the enzyme adenosine-triphosphatase.

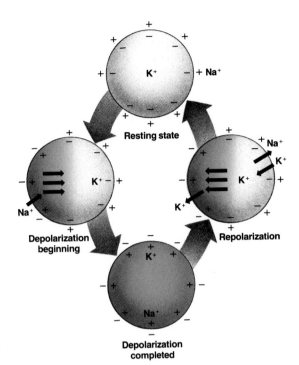

Resting state

Depolarization beginning

Depolarization completed

Repolarization

rate of 40 to 60 beats/minute to the AV bundle. The AV bundle itself divides into right and left branches that extend downward into the interventricular septum, where they join with the network of Purkinje fibers. These fibers penetrate both right and left ventricular masses and rapidly conduct impulses to the ventricular myocardium, where they terminate. These fibers may also act as pacemakers in severe conduction disturbances, such as complete heart block. The intrinsic rate of the Purkinje network is less than 40 beats/minute.

Contractility is the ability of cardiac muscle fibers to shorten when stimulated. The force of the contraction depends on oxygen supply and demand, electrolyte balance (especially of calcium), drug effects, and disease. The heart can deliver equal volumes of blood each minute, even when the right and left ventricles deliver very different volumes of blood per stroke. This results from the contractile qualities of cardiac muscle, which are described by *Starling's law.* This law states that the force of a contraction depends on the length of the muscle fibers of the heart walls. Thus, if right ventricular output exceeds left ventricular output, the fibers of the left ventricle lengthen at end diastole to increase the force of contraction.

Calcium also plays an important role in cardiac muscle contractions: intracellular calcium ions (Ca^{++}) trigger the sliding action of the actin and myosin filaments that cause cardiac muscle contractions. But before such

contractions can take place, a cardiac muscle cell must take in additional Ca^{++} ions through its cell walls from the extracellular space. The increased Ca^{++} levels enhance contractility. Conversely, decreased Ca^{++} levels reduce contractility. Capitalizing on this effect, calcium-blocker drugs, which reduce cellular permeability to Ca^{++} ions, are used to reduce myocardial oxygen demand in patients with angina and dysrhythmias.

THE CARDIAC CYCLE

Aided by the heart's conduction system, each electrical impulse from the SA node spreads through the myocardium, activating the atria and ventricles. Each complete heartbeat, or cardiac cycle, consists of two parts: contraction (depolarization) or systole, and relaxation (repolarization) or diastole. A cardiac cycle occurs about once every 0.8 second, assuming a heart rate of 72 to 75 beats per minute. This short interval accommodates the complex sequence of events from ventricular systole to the end of diastole. (See page 17.)

In ventricular systole, which lasts 0.3 second, pressure builds in the ventricles, closing the atrioventricular valves and preventing the backflow of blood into the atria. When the ventricles contract, ventricular pressure rises sharply—to about 120 mm Hg in the left ventricle and about 26 mm Hg in the right ventricle. When this pressure exceeds pressures in the aorta and pulmonary artery, the *semilunar valves* open to eject blood into these two arteries. About half the blood is ejected during the first quarter of ventricular systole; most of the remaining blood is ejected during the next two quarters.

After ejection, ventricular diastole, lasting about 0.5 second, begins. Ventricular pressure then drops below that of the aorta and pulmonary artery, and the semilunar valves shut to prevent backflow into the ventricles.

During the latter part of ventricular systole, in which the atria have already filled with blood from the pulmonary veins and venae cavae, atrial pressure begins to rise. As ventricular pressure drops below atrial pressure, the atrioventricular valves open, and the ventricles fill rapidly with blood.

In late ventricular diastole, following the rapid filling of the ventricles and the beginning of atrial contraction, the atrioventricular valves remain open and atrial and ventricular pressures equalize. Then atrial diastole begins, the atrioventricular valves close, and another cardiac cycle begins.

Electrocardiography: Tracing the cardiac cycle

Electrocardiography graphically records the electrical potential generated during each cardiac cycle. This potential radiates from the heart in all directions and, on reaching the skin, is measured by electrodes connected to an amplifier and strip chart recorder.

Each wave of the EKG tracing corresponds to an event in the cardiac cycle. These waves have been arbitrarily labelled *P, QRS, and T*.

The *P wave* reflects depolarization of the atria, and normally originates in the sinoatrial node. The *PR interval* (normally 0.12 to 0.20 second) reflects the time elapsed from the onset of sinus activation to the onset of ventricular activation. The *QRS complex* (normally 0.06 to 0.10 second) indicates ventricular depolarization. The *ST segment* represents the plateau of the ventricular action potential, or the period between complete depolarization and the start of repolarization. The *T wave* is generated during ventricular repolarization.

Sounds of the cardiac cycle

Valve action during the cardiac cycle causes vibrations in the adjacent blood mass, heart walls, and major vessels around the heart. These vibrations are transmitted to the body surface, producing distinct heart sounds that are audible by auscultation and have major diagnostic value. These sounds are usually described phonetically as "lub dub."

The *first heart sound* ("lub," or S_1) is associated with closure of the tricuspid and mitral valves. Asynchronous closure of these valves commonly splits S_1 into two parts, usually heard at the heart's apex. The first part indicates mitral closure; the second, tricuspid closure. This splitting is clinically unimportant unless very pronounced, as in conduction system disturbances such as complete right or left bundle branch block. Systole occurs between S_1 and S_2.

The *second heart sound* ("dub," or S_2) is associated with closure of the aortic and pulmonic valves and is best heard at the base of the heart. During inspiration, physiologic splitting of S_2 occurs, since pulmonic valve closure is delayed by the large volume of blood returning to the right side of the heart. Diastole occurs between S_2 and S_1.

The *physiologic third heart sound* (S_3) is commonly audible in children and young adults, but not usually in adults over age 30. When present in older adults, it's called a

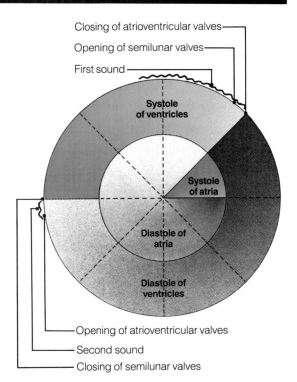

Closing of atrioventricular valves
Opening of semilunar valves
First sound

Systole of ventricles

Systole of atria

Diastole of atria

Diastole of ventricles

Opening of atrioventricular valves
Second sound
Closing of semilunar valves

The cardiac cycle
Progressing counterclockwise, this illustration shows the major events in a single cardiac cycle of systole and diastole. The outer circle represents movement of the ventricles; the inner circle, movement of the atria. Each cycle takes about 0.8 second to complete, assuming a heart rate of 75 beats per minute. Each segment of the circle represents 0.1 second.

"ventricular gallop," and is a classic sign of congestive heart failure. A low-pitched sound, S_3 occurs during the rapid ventricular filling phase of diastole, and is best heard at the apex when the patient is supine.

The *fourth heart sound* (S_4), or atrial gallop, is often heard in the elderly, patients with angina, and patients with previous myocardial infarction. It may result from vibrations caused by sudden forceful ejection of atrial blood into noncompliant ventricles, and is heard at the apex immediately before S_1.

HEMODYNAMIC MEASUREMENTS

Electrocardiography and auscultation are valuable diagnostic tools, but they provide only two ways of studying cardiac conduction and valvular disorders. Hemodynamics describes the behavior of the heart's chambers and valves as they interact with the blood during each cardiac cycle. Hemodynamic measurements include cardiac output, cardiac index, stroke volume, ejection fraction, and preload and afterload. Understanding these measurements will help you assess your patient's cardiac function.

Cardiac output is the volume of blood ejected by the left ventricle into the aorta in 1 minute. Since the blood transports oxygen and other substances to all body tissues, cardiac output is probably the *most important* circulatory measurement. Normal cardiac output for a young, healthy adult male averages about 5 liters per minute.

Understanding preload and afterload

Preload

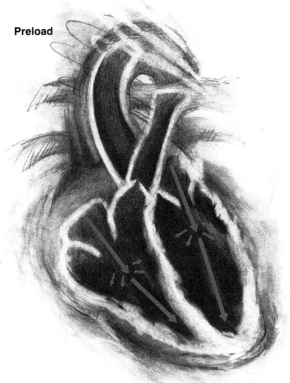

Afterload

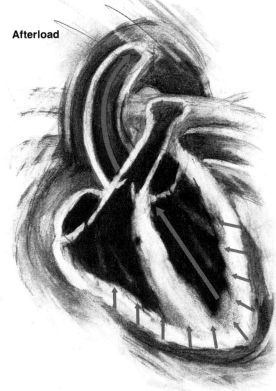

Understanding the concepts of preload and afterload can improve your assessment and management of the patient with heart failure.

Preload—a key factor in the heart's increased contractility—is a passive stretching force exerted on the ventricular muscle at end diastole. According to Starling's law, the more cardiac muscles are stretched in diastole, the more forcefully they contract in systole.

Afterload refers to the pressure the ventricular muscles must generate to overcome the higher pressure in the aorta. Normally, end-diastolic pressure in the left ventricle is 5 to 10 mm Hg; but in the aorta, it's 70 to 80 mm Hg. This difference means that the ventricle must develop enough pressure to force open the aortic valve. Drugs may sometimes be used to gradually reduce afterload, which increases stroke volume and cardiac output.

Since cardiac output increases in proportion to body size, it's important to have some means of comparing cardiac output in different-sized patients. To promote such comparisons, cardiac output is frequently expressed as the *cardiac index,* which is cardiac output per square meter of body surface area. For example, an adult weighing 70 kg (154 lb) has a body surface area of about 1.7 square meters (about 2 sq. yards) and will have a cardiac index of about 3 liters (about 0.8 gal) per minute.

Stroke volume refers to the output of each ventricle at every contraction, which in the normal heart is 60 to 70 ml. Multiplying the stroke volume by the heart rate tells you the cardiac output per minute. The amount of blood left in the ventricles following ejection is called *residual volume.*

Ejection fraction is the ratio of blood expelled from the ventricle in one contraction (systolic volume) to the ventricle's total capacity (end-diastolic volume). For example, if systolic volume is 80 ml and end-diastolic volume is 130 ml, the ventricle's ejection fraction is 61.5% ($80 \div 130 = 0.615$). The ejection fraction provides important information about stroke volume during periods of stress and increased cardiac output. At rest, the healthy heart normally has an ejection fraction of 60% to 70%, giving it a reserve of 30% to 40%. When the heart remains at rest, this reserve contributes to the next stroke volume; when cardiac output increases, this reserve helps the heart increase its ejection fraction to 80% or 90%.

The heart's ability to increase its ejection fraction depends on the hemodynamic effects of *preload* and *afterload,* which are, respectively, the ventricular filling pressure at end diastole, and the resistance against which the heart must pump to eject the blood into the aorta during systole. (See *Understanding preload and afterload,* page 18.)

MECHANISMS OF HEART FAILURE

Heart failure—the inability to pump enough blood to satisfy the body's normal metabolic needs—results from various disorders, such as severe coronary artery disease, coronary thrombosis, myocardial ischemia, conduction and congenital heart defects, and vascular abnormalities. Regardless of the cause, the sequence of events in heart failure is the same, depending on the effectiveness of compensatory mechanisms.

If blood flow to the myocardium is insufficient, contractility declines, and stroke volume and cardiac output fall. Also, left ventricular end-diastolic volume increases and the ejection fraction decreases. The initial acute decrease in cardiac output lasts only a few seconds before primary compensatory mechanisms respond.

Baroreceptors in the carotid sinuses and aortic arch sense diminished cardiac output and transmit afferent impulses to medullary centers; sympathetic stimulation then increases heart rate and contractility, as well as constriction of peripheral arterioles and the venous vasculature. These responses, along with Starling's mechanism, combine to raise cardiac output and stroke volume.

During the initial acute decrease in cardiac output, renal perfusion also decreases because of reduced renal blood flow. This activates slower-acting secondary compensatory mechanisms, such as the renin-angiotensin-aldosterone (RAA) feedback system, which increases renal reabsorption of sodium and water. This extracellular fluid retention increases blood flow to the heart. If mean arterial pressure can be maintained, a feedback mechanism shuts off RAA activity. These compensatory mechanisms are not achieved without compromising cardiac reserve.

Decompensated heart failure occurs when the myocardium is so severely damaged that normal compensatory mechanisms fail to support adequate cardiac output, arterial pressure, or renal perfusion. The RAA feedback system continues to operate; increased circulating blood volume further increases the workload of the heart and predisposes the

patient to acute pulmonary edema and death. Hypertrophy of the left ventricle, a response to prolonged myocardial tension, helps augment contractility. Decompensation may be slowed by cardiotonic drugs or diuretics. Cardiotonics such as digitalis may slow decompensation by forcing the heart to pump enough blood to perfuse the kidneys; diuretics may slow decompensation by reducing fluid retention.

Cardiogenic shock

If intrinsic compensatory mechanisms and extrinsic therapies fail, cardiac output may plummet so steeply that body tissues undergo acute anoxia. Death then follows from cardiogenic shock—circulatory shock that results from pump failure. (See Chapter 6 for management of this life-threatening emergency.)

Cardiogenic shock profoundly affects the kidneys, liver, and lungs, as well as the heart. Diminished blood supply to the kidneys leads to a reduced glomerular filtration rate, tubular necrosis, decreased osmolality, electrolyte imbalance, decreased urinary output, and acute renal failure. Diminished blood supply to the liver results in ischemia and necrosis of the central lobules; disrupted cell metabolism impairs the liver's normal abilities to detoxify substances in the blood, to deaminate amino acids, to form urea, and to convert glycogen to glucose (glyconeogenesis).

In the lungs, diminished blood supply leads to hypoxia, and respiratory alkalosis develops as the patient attempts to compensate by breathing rapidly and deeply. Diminished blood supply also decreases the capillaries' ability to exchange gases. Pulmonary edema results when: left atrial and pulmonary capillary wedge pressures rise too high; fluid escapes into the interstitial spaces, reducing lung compliance, and into the alveoli; and decreased PO_2 and increased PCO_2 make breathing more difficult. These life-threatening consequences of cardiogenic shock can be prevented or reversed only if the heart's pumping mechanism can be restored.

Expanding your knowledge base

Today, improvements in the prevention, diagnosis, and treatment of cardiovascular disorders are allowing many patients to live longer and more productive lives. As a result, it's become increasingly important to understand cardiovascular anatomy, physiology, and pathophysiology, to provide effective nursing care and patient teaching.

Points to remember

• The heart maintains continuous flow of blood, using a system of valves to prevent backflow. The heart itself receives blood through a network of coronary arteries.
• Blood flows through a network of arteries, veins, arterioles, capillaries, and venules. Blood flow and pressure is greatest in the larger vessels, and is least in the capillary beds.
• The cardiac cycle consists of diastole (relaxation) and systole (contraction). These two movements are precisely coordinated by the heart's conduction system, which involves rhythmic stimulation and polarization-repolarization of cardiac muscle cells.
• Neural, hormonal, and physical mechanisms act to control blood pressure. Neural mechanisms include baroreceptors and chemoreceptors. Hormonal mechanisms include secretion of epinephrine and norepinephrine by the adrenals; secretion of renin by the kidneys, with subsequent formation of angiotensin I and II; secretion of antidiuretic hormone by the hypothalamus; and secretion of prostaglandins by various tissues. Physical mechanisms include vascular stress-relaxation and capillary fluid shift.
• The heart responds to increased filling pressure at diastole by contracting more forcefully at systole, in accordance with Starling's law.
• In heart failure, compensatory mechanisms cannot maintain adequate cardiac output, arterial pressure, or renal perfusion, and the heart undergoes cardiogenic shock, which profoundly affects the kidneys, liver, and lungs. When these organs fail to support each other, death ensues if heart action isn't quickly restored.

2 ASSESSING CARDIOVASCULAR DYNAMICS

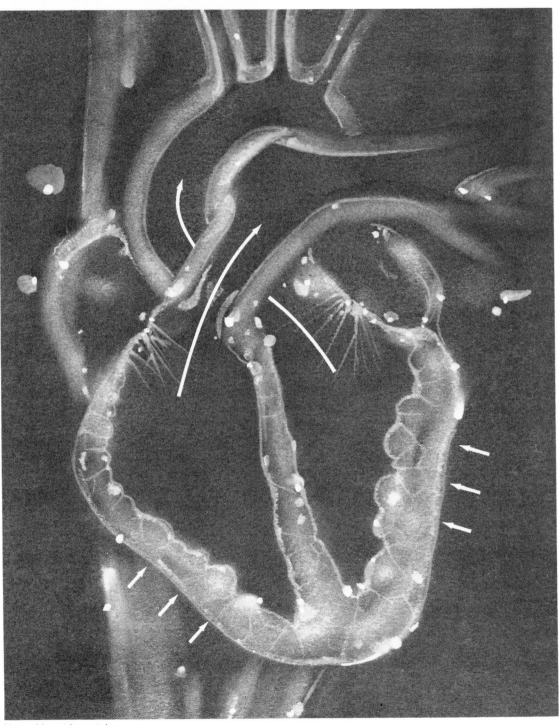

Normal heart in systole

No matter where you practice nursing, the overwhelming prevalence of cardiovascular diseases ensures that some form of cardiovascular assessment is part of your daily responsibility. Complete and accurate assessment of this complex system requires mastery of advanced techniques, including auscultation of heart sounds and murmurs, inspection of neck veins, and palpation of the precordium. If you feel uncertain about these techniques and become uneasy once you're past taking routine vital signs, you're not unusual.

The information in this chapter will help you review or master all the skills necessary for assessing cardiovascular status—beginning with the patient's complaints and symptoms, progressing through all the stages of physical assessment (patient preparation, overall inspection, history taking, and physical examination), and ending with the nursing diagnosis.

This chapter will also help you understand the delicate balance between cardiac and other body functions. Cardiovascular assessment demands a skillful evaluation of the entire circulatory system, including core and peripheral circulation.

Prepare the equipment
Begin by gathering the necessary equipment: stethoscope, blood pressure cuff, and ruler. Then, make sure the height of the bed or examining table allows inspection of the patient in the supine, sitting, and left lateral positions. To enhance your vision, place the light source so light crosses the areas you'll inspect—the extremities, abdomen, neck, and precordium—but doesn't shine directly on them. Also, make sure the room is quiet enough to allow accurate auscultation of heart sounds, which are usually subtle and low-pitched.

Prepare the patient
As you introduce yourself to the patient, form an overall impression of his body type, posture, gait, and movements as well as his overall health and basic hygiene. Also, look for observable cardiac risk factors, such as cigarette smoking, obesity, and xanthomas (fatty cholesterol deposits on the skin). Meanwhile, put the patient at ease and ensure his privacy. Tell him that you'll be conducting the examination, and make sure he's wearing a hospital gown that allows easy access to the neck, chest, arms, and legs. Then, ask him to lie back with his head and thorax comfortably supported at about a 45° angle. During the examination itself, stand at the patient's right side. This allows you to fully inspect the neck area and precordium and to reach comfortably across the precordium for palpation and auscultation.

HISTORY AND OBSERVATION
Now that you've formed a first impression of the patient's physical appearance, assess his mental status, particularly the appropriateness of his responses and the clarity of his speech. Watch his facial expressions for signs of discomfort, withdrawal, fear, or depression.

Look at the patient to gather information about his cardiovascular function: notice the color and condition of his skin—especially on the face, mouth, earlobes, and fingernails—to help evaluate the adequacy of cardiac output. Pallor or cyanosis may indicate poor cardiac output and poor tissue perfusion. Feel the patient's arm to assess its warmth and dryness. If his skin feels cool or clammy, suspect peripheral vasoconstriction. Consider, too, that peripheral vasoconstriction can be an early compensatory response in shock.

Collect subjective data
Begin the patient interview. You'll need the subjective information that only the patient can provide to interpret your examination results. Successful interviewing starts with your attitude toward the patient and toward the interview itself. If you conduct patient interviews as conversations rather than anonymous hospital checklists, the quality of information your patient gives you will improve noticeably. Most importantly, avoid turning the interview into a rapid-fire interrogation, which tends to intimidate the patient and inhibit free discussion. Instead, foster an atmosphere of mutual trust and respect. Show genuine interest and concern by being calm, unhurried, and sympathetic. Address the patient by name. Use eye contact appropriately: look into his eyes from time to time, but don't stare. Allow him to finish his sentences, even if his speech is rambling and slow. Then redirect your questioning as needed.

Help the patient define the problem
Ask the patient what caused him to seek medical help (his chief complaint). You might ask, "Why did you come to the hospital (doctor's office)?" or "What's troubling you?" Pay

attention not only to *what* he says, but to *how* he says it. Does he appear to be upset or in pain? Record the chief complaint in the patient's own words. For example, the patient isn't likely to say he has edema; he'll say his ankles are swollen. Find out when his problem is most likely to occur. If he reports pain, ask him: "What provokes it? Where is it located? Does it radiate? How long does it last? How strong is it? Does it occur with any other symptoms? What are the effects of any treatment or medication?"

The patient with a cardiovascular disorder is apt to complain of chest pain. If he has angina, he may press the midsternal area as he describes the pain. However, if he has early congestive heart failure, he's more likely to complain of fatigue and mildly swollen ankles. Remember that the *timing* of symptoms is often a helpful clue. For example, chest pain after stress or exertion points to angina.

After the patient has described his chief complaint, ask about any other symptoms. In addition to chest pain, be sure to ask specif-

ically about dyspnea, paroxysmal nocturnal dyspnea, orthopnea, unexplained weakness and fatigue, irregular heartbeat, and weight change with edema. Always speak in terms the patient understands. For example, ask him if he has difficulty breathing, not if he experiences dyspnea.

Inquire about previous conditions that predispose to cardiovascular disease, especially hypertension, hyperlipoproteinemia, diabetes mellitus, and rheumatic fever. Note any family history of cardiovascular disease. Look for telltale signs of long-term cardiovascular disease. Find out which drugs he has taken. Also, ask about the patient's life-style—use of alcohol and tobacco; occupation; problems, including any source of unusual stress; physical activity; and dietary habits, including intake of caffeine, starch, fat, and sodium.

Collect objective data
Having completed the interview, you're ready to begin a systematic physical examination. If you're doing a routine cardiovascular as-

Identifying causes of chest pain

Character-istics	Myocardial infarction	Pericarditis	Angina	Pleuropulmonary disorders
Onset	Sudden	Sudden	Buildup of intensity (crescendo) or sudden	Gradual or sudden
Precipitating factors	Not necessarily anything; may occur at rest or follow physical or emotional exertion	Not induced by activity	Physical exertion; emotional stress; eating; cold or hot, humid weather; recumbency; micturition or defecation or no related factors	Pneumonia or other respiratory infection
Location	Substernal, anterior chest, and midline	Substernal, to left of midline or precordial only	Substernal, anterior chest, not sharply localized	Over lung fields to side and back
Radiation	Down one or both arms; to jaw, neck, or back	To back or left supraclavicular area	To back, neck, arms, and jaw; occasionally to upper abdomen or fingers	Anterior chest, shoulder, and neck
Duration	At least 30 min but usually 1 to 2 hr; residual soreness for 1 to 3 days	Continuous; may last for days; residual soreness	Usually less than 15 min but never more than 30 min (average: 3 min)	Continuous for hours
Quality-intensity	Severe, "stabbing," "choking," "squeezing"; intense pressure, deep sensation, vicelike and burning	Moderate to severe or only an "ache"; sharp, "stabbing"; deep or superficial sensation	Mild to moderate; "squeezing"; vague, uniform pattern of attacks; heavy pressure, deep sensation, tightness	Sharp "ache," not severe; "stabbing," "shooting"; deep sensation, crushing
Signs and symptoms	Apprehension, nausea, dyspnea, diaphoresis, dizziness, weakness, pulmonary congestion, tachycardia, decreased blood pressure, gallop heart sound, fatigue	Precordial friction rub; increased pain with muscle movement, inspiration, laughter, coughing, or left lateral positioning; decreased pain with sitting or leaning forward	Dyspnea, diaphoresis, nausea, desire to void; associated with belching, apprehension, or uneasiness	Dyspnea, tachycardia, apprehension, pleural rub, fever; increased pain with coughing, inspiration, or movement; decreased pain with sitting

Recognizing pulse abnormalities

Pulsus alternans

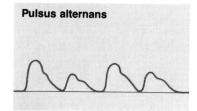

Pulsus paradoxus

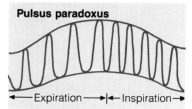

←——Expiration——→|←— Inspiration —→

Pulsus bigeminus

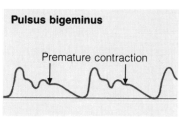

Premature contraction

Pulsus alternans is an alteration in pulse size and intensity occurring with every other beat. The rhythm of pulsus alternans is regular, but its volume varies. If you take the blood pressure of a patient with this abnormality, you'll first hear a loud Korotkoff sound and then a soft sound, continually alternating. Pulsus alternans frequently accompanies left ventricular

failure and states of poor contractility.

Pulsus paradoxus is an exaggerated decrease in blood pressure during inspiration resulting from an increase in negative intrathoracic pressure. A pulsus paradoxus that exceeds 10 mm Hg is considered abnormal and may result from pericardial tamponade, constrictive pericarditis, severe lung disease, or advanced heart failure.

Pulsus bigeminus is a basic heart rhythm irregularity in which premature beats alternate with sinus beats. The premature beat usually has such a poor stroke volume (because of its timing in the cardiac cycle and its inadequate diastolic filling period) that it doesn't perfuse to the periphery. Because only the sinus beat perfuses to the periphery, the pulse may be slower than normal.

---

sessment, examine the patient from the periphery toward the center in the following order: arms and legs, abdomen, neck, and precordium. However, if your overall impression of the patient suggests a potentially life-threatening disorder, examine him from the center toward the periphery to promote more rapid identification of the disorder. If the cardiovascular assessment is part of a multisystem or complete physical assessment, proceed from his head to his feet.

As you know, your examination requires skillful use of inspection, palpation, percussion, and auscultation. Inspection requires keen observation. Palpation provides clinical information through the trained and skillful use of your sense of touch. Percussion involves tapping the body surface lightly—with a sharp, quick motion—to produce sounds that help determine the size, shape, position, and density of underlying organs and tissues. Auscultation detects body sounds, with the unaided ear or a stethoscope. Your level of expertise in these skills determines the quality of your assessment.

PHYSICAL EXAMINATION

As you do in every examination, begin by taking and recording your patient's temperature. (If you suspect dyspnea, take the patient's temperature with an electronic thermometer.)

Then, count respirations for 1 minute, noting chest symmetry; ease of breathing; use of thoracic, abdominal, or accessory muscles; coughing; sternal and intercostal retraction; and nasal flaring. Take the radial pulse for 1 minute to note normal or abnormal rate and rhythm (see *Recognizing pulse abnormalities*). Note pulse quality and take blood pressure readings in both arms (see *Perfecting blood pressure technique,* page 24).

Check peripheral circulation

Continue your examination by inspecting the skin color of your patient's extremities. Don't forget to follow up on suspicions you formed based on the overall inspection and patient history. Describe skin color as *normal, cyanotic, mottled,* or *excessively pale.* (If your patient is black, examine the buccal membranes, lips, tongue, nail beds, and palms for pallor.) Note if the patient has any petechial hemorrhages, Osler nodes (tender, painful raised areas) on the fingers or palms, or Janeway lesions (nontender nodules) on the palms, which often point to bacterial endocarditis.

Test the patient's arms and legs for normal sensations to both light and deep palpation. Note areas of tenderness and increased warmth or coolness. Also, determine if both arms and legs are of equal size.

Examine the patient's fingernails and toe-

Perfecting blood pressure technique

Systolic

phase I

phase II

phase III

1st diastolic

phase IV

2nd diastolic

phase V

190
180
170
160
150
140
130
120
110
100
90
80
70
60
50
40
30
20
10
0

When you take blood pressure, you're measuring the lateral force that blood exerts on arterial walls as the heart contracts (systolic pressure) and relaxes (diastolic pressure). As you know, systolic pressure normally ranges from 110 to 140 mm Hg; diastolic pressure, from 60 to 90 mm Hg. Obtaining an accurate reading depends on how well you prepare the patient, select the equipment, and carry out the procedure, as described below.

• Before taking the patient's blood pressure, encourage him to relax. Don't take blood pressure after meals, during or directly after exercise or an emotional upset or just before or after urination or defecation.

• Choose a cuff of the correct size. The cuff's bladder should be 20% to 25% wider than the patient's arm circumference. Also, be sure to check that the cuff works properly. Don't use a cuff that inflates or deflates erratically or has faulty pressure bulb screw clamps.

• After you prepare the patient and the equipment, support the patient's arm at heart level on a table or bed. Then, center the cuff over the brachial artery, and wrap it smoothly and securely around the patient's upper arm.

• Palpate the brachial pulse and rapidly inflate the cuff until the pulse disappears. Continue inflating the cuff until pressure rises an additional 30 mm Hg.

• Place the bell of the stethoscope lightly over the brachial artery. Then, deflate the cuff at 2 to 3 mm Hg/second. If you deflate the cuff too slowly, venous congestion in the arm can result in a spuriously high reading. However, if you deflate the cuff too quickly, diastolic pressure can't be accurately assessed.

• Listen for the Korotkoff sounds as you deflate the cuff. These sounds occur in five phases: phase I—clear tapping sounds; phase II—tapping sounds along with a blowing murmur or whooshing sound; phase III—louder and higher-pitched tapping sounds; phase IV—muffled sounds; and phase V—silence.

When you hear the first two consecutive tapping sounds of phase I, record the systolic pressure. For an accurate reading, keep the mercury column on a level surface and view the meniscus at eye level.

When you hear the first two consecutive muffled sounds of phase IV, record the diastolic phase IV pressure. With the onset of silence, record the diastolic phase V pressure. For example, 120/90/80 is a reading in which the systolic pressure equals 120; the diastolic phase IV pressure, 90; and the diastolic phase V pressure, 80.

If you fail to hear all five phases of the Korotkoff sounds, you'll have to record blood pressure somewhat differently. This often happens in children and, at times, in adults. For example, the muffled sounds of phase IV may continue, without fading into silence. When this happens, record one diastolic pressure—the first two muffled sounds of phase IV.

Phase IV may occasionally be absent. Silence—not muffled sounds—follows the loud tapping sounds of phase III. If this occurs, record one diastolic pressure—the onset of silence of phase V. An auscultatory gap—an interval of silence lasting 5 to 10 seconds—can also interrupt the sequence of Korotkoff sounds. This gap occurs after the tapping sounds of phase I and may take the place of phase II. If this happens, record the pressures when the silence begins and when the pulse sounds return. To prevent a false reading due to an auscultatory gap, inflate the cuff 30 mm Hg above the point at which the pulse disappears.

In the blood pressure measurement at left, the interval of silence or absence of pulse sounds known as the *auscultatory gap* is nonexistent.

nails for changes in thickness and for such qualitative changes as color, contour, consistency, and adherence to the nail bed. In a patient with chronic heart disease and, consequently, prolonged hypoxemia, check for clubbed fingers—chronic thickening and enlargement of the nails as well as bulbous enlargement of the ends of fingers. In such a patient you may find exaggerated curves in the nails and spongy softening of the end root.

Now, inspect the patient's skin for texture and hair patterns. In a patient with chronically poor circulation, the skin is thin, waxy, fragile, and shiny; normal body hair on the arms and legs is absent. These changes, characteristic of arterial insufficiency, are also typical in chronic diabetes mellitus. Remember to look for areas of unusual pigmentation that may indicate new skin lesions, rashes, scarring from past injury, or ulceration, which may show deficient arterial circulation.

Also inspect the patient's arms, hands, legs, feet, and ankles for edema—the common result of abnormal accumulation of serous fluid in the connective tissues. (If the patient has been confined to bed, remember to check for edema in the buttocks and sacral area because edema occurs in the most dependent body parts.) For reliable assessment, palpate for edema against a bony prominence and describe its characteristics:
• type (pitting or nonpitting)
• extent and location (ankle-foot area, foot-knee area, hands or fingers)
• degree of pitting (described in terms of depth): 0″ to ¼″ is mild (1 +); ¼″ to ½″, moderate (2 +); and ½″ to 1″, severe (3 +)
• symmetry (unilateral or symmetrical).

Evaluate vascular integrity
To assess the adequacy of arterial flow, test vascular filling time. Have the patient lie down and raise his legs or arms 12″ (30 cm) above heart level; then ask him to move his feet or hands up and down for 60 seconds. This maneuver helps drain venous blood from the extremity, thereby revealing the color of arterial blood. Next, tell the patient to sit up and dangle his legs or arms, which should show mild pallor. The original color should return in about 10 seconds; the veins should refill in about 15 seconds. If one or both of the patient's feet or hands persistently show marked pallor, delayed return of color ending with a mottled appearance, or delayed venous filling, suspect arterial insufficiency. If you note marked redness of the arms or legs, again

suspect arterial insufficiency.

To assess the adequacy of venous flow, inspect and palpate the patient's legs for superficial veins. When the legs are in a dependent position, check for signs of normal circulation: venous distention, nodular bulges at venous valves (bifurcations of veins), and collapsing veins on elevation. Also check for signs of venous insufficiency: dilatated, tortuous veins with poorly functioning valves, peripheral cyanosis, peripheral edema that pits with pressure, unusual ankle pigmentation, skin thickening, and ulceration around the ankles.

Inspect and palpate for evidence of deep vein inflammation or clot formation. Ask the patient about pain, tenderness, or a sense of fullness in the calf, which may be aggravated during standing or walking. Next, check the feet for edema and dependent cyanosis. Gently press the calf muscle with your palm; pain indicates possible thrombophlebitis. To test for Homans sign, support the entire leg, which must be extended or slightly bent, and firmly and abruptly dorsiflex the patient's foot. Deep calf pain during this maneuver indicates thrombophlebitis.

Perform the Allen test
This test, which evaluates arterial circulation to the hands, isn't part of a routine assessment but *is necessary* before arterial line insertion. First, tell the patient to rest his right arm on a table, and support the wrist with a rolled washcloth. Then, occlude the radial and ulnar arteries by exerting pressure with your fingers. Ask the patient to repeatedly clench and open his fist to encourage the palm to blanch. (If your patient can't clench his fist, encourage blanching by occluding the ulnar and radial arteries, elevating the hand, and massaging the palm.) Release pressure on the ulnar artery, and ask the patient to open his hand. If it flushes, even though the radial artery remains occluded, the ulnar artery is patent. If it remains blanched, suspect ulnar artery occlusion. (Remember, though, that slow return of blood to the hand may result from poor cardiac output or, in a patient in shock, from poor capillary refill.) Repeat the test, this time releasing just the radial artery. Then, repeat the test on the patient's left arm. Record your findings.

Assess peripheral pulses
Now that you've evaluated the overall competence of the vascular system, you're ready to assess the peripheral pulses—important

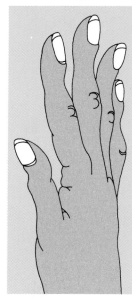

Peripheral pulse points

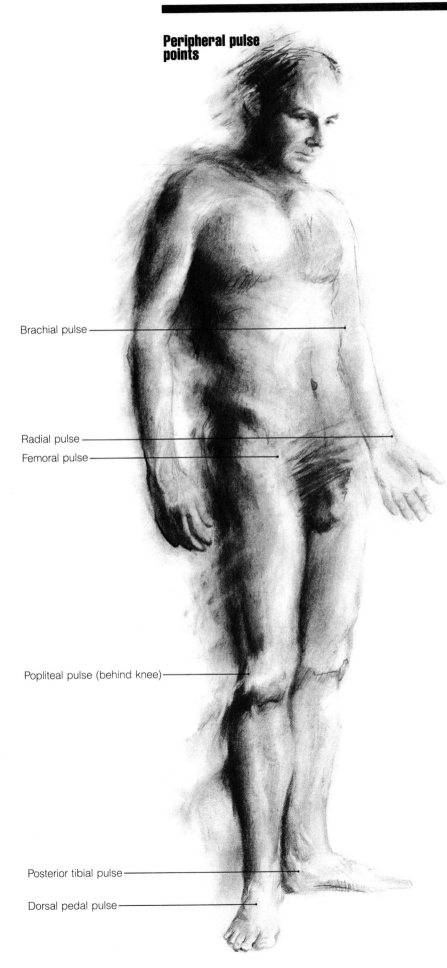

Brachial pulse

Radial pulse

Femoral pulse

Popliteal pulse (behind knee)

Posterior tibial pulse

Dorsal pedal pulse

clues to cardiac function and the quality of peripheral perfusion—for rate, rhythm, amplitude, and symmetry. Using your dominant hand, palpate peripheral pulses lightly with the pads of your index, middle, and, when appropriate, ring fingers. Use three fingers where space permits; use two fingers to palpate a small or angled area (for example, the area of the femoral pulses).

To determine *rate,* count all pulses for at least 30 seconds (60 seconds when recording vital signs). The normal rate is between 60 and 100 beats/minute.

To estimate *amplitude,* or *volume,* palpate the blood vessel during ventricular systole. Pulse amplitude reflects the adequacy of the circulating volume, the vessel tone, the strength of left ventricular contraction, and the elasticity of the arterial walls. Normal arteries are soft and pliable. Sclerotic arteries are more resistant to occlusion by external pressure; when you palpate them, they feel beaded and cordlike. Describe pulse amplitude by using this scale:

3 + : bounding, increased

2 + : normal

1 + : weak, thready, decreased

0:     absent.

To determine *symmetry,* simultaneously palpate pulses (except for the carotid pulse) on both sides of the patient's body; inequality is diagnostically significant. Always assess peripheral pulses methodically, moving from the patient's arms to the legs. Palpate the patient's *brachial pulses* medial to the biceps tendons. Then, palpate the *radial pulses* on the palmar surface of the patient's relaxed, slightly flexed wrists, medial to the radial styloid processes. (Remember, the radial pulse is the most commonly used indicator of pulse rate and rhythm.)

If you detect an irregular radial pulse, ask another nurse to help you take the patient's *apical-radial* pulse. First, locate the apical and radial pulses. Then, palpate the radial pulse while the assisting nurse auscultates the apical pulse with a stethoscope. Determine a time to begin counting. Then, using the same watch, count beats at the same time for 60 seconds. If another nurse isn't available to help, auscultate the apical pulse for 1 minute. Then, immediately palpate the radial pulse for 1 minute. In both methods, a pulse deficit—the difference between the apical and radial pulse rates—greater than 10 beats/minute indicates dysrhythmias that aren't perfused to the periphery.

To assess the patient's *femoral pulses,* use the pads of your fingers to deeply palpate the area below the inguinal ligaments, midway between the anterior superior iliac spine and the symphysis pubis. Then, auscultate each femoral area for blowing sounds called *bruits,* which indicate the presence of arteriosclerotic plaques.

To assess the *popliteal pulses,* which are relatively deep in the soft tissues behind the knees, place the patient in the supine or semi-Fowler position and flex the knees slightly. Use both hands to deeply palpate the pulses. Or you can locate the pulses more easily by placing both thumbs on the patient's knees and palpating behind them with the first two fingers of both hands.

Assess the patient's *pedal pulses* by using the pads of your fingers to palpate the dorsum of the feet. To prevent excessive traction on the arteries, dorsiflex the feet, preferably to 90°, and palpate where the vessels pass over the dorsum. To locate the pulses, place your palms lightly on the dorsum until you feel the dorsalis pedis pulse points. (Remember, the pedal pulses are superficial and can be obscured by heavy palpation.) Maintaining dorsiflexion of the patient's feet, use the pads of your fingers to locate the posterior tibialis pulses on the posterior or inferior medial malleolus of the ankles.

Assess the upper abdomen
Be sure to check the upper abdomen for evidence of cardiovascular disease. Visible or palpable pulsations in the upper central abdomen (epigastric area) may be normal. However, abnormally large aortic pulsations may result from an aneurysm of the abdominal aorta or from aortic valvular regurgitation. Exaggerated epigastric pulsations may also result from right ventricular hypertrophy or an aortic abnormality. To distinguish between them, place your palm on the epigastric area and slide your fingers under the rib cage. You'll feel aortic pulsations with your palm, right ventricular impulses with your fingertips.

Next, use the bell of the stethoscope to auscultate the epigastric area in the abdominal midline to the umbilicus, listening carefully for bruits.

Examine the jugular pulse: Clue to right ventricular failure
Internal and external jugular vein pulsations provide valuable information about the adequacy of circulating volume, right ventricular function, and venous pressure. External jugular veins, which lie superficially, are visible above the clavicle. Internal jugular veins, which are larger than the external veins, lie deeper along the carotid arteries and transmit their pulsations outward to the skin overlying these vessels.

Normally, the jugular veins protrude when the patient lies down and flatten when he stands up. The semi-Fowler position is best for inspecting them, because at a 45° elevation the jugular veins shouldn't be prominent if right ventricular function is normal. Position the patient properly, and turn his head slightly away from you. Use a small pillow to support the head, but don't flex the neck sharply. Remove clothing around the neck and thorax to prevent circulatory constriction. Use tangential lighting—arrange the lighting to cast small shadows along the neck.

You can learn about right heart dynamics by analyzing the venous waveform of the patient's right internal jugular vein. Use the carotid pulse or heart sounds to time the venous pulsations with the cardiac cycle. (See *Relationship of pulses to cardiac cycle,* page 28.)

The jugular venous pulse consists of five waves: three positive, or ascending, waves (*a, c,* and *v*) and two negative waves (*x* and *y*). *Positive,* or ascending, waves produce an undulating pulsation normally seen ⅜″ to ¾″ (1 to 2 cm) above the clavicle, just to the medial side of the sternocleidomastoid muscle, as follows:
• The *a wave* is the initial pulsation of the jugular vein, produced by right atrial contraction and retrograde transmission of the pressure pulse to the jugular veins. It occurs just before the first heart sound.

The *a* wave may be exaggerated in chronic obstructive pulmonary disease, pulmonary embolism, and pulmonic or tricuspid stenosis—conditions causing elevated right atrial pressure. A giant *a* wave, or *cannon wave,* occurs when the atrium contracts against a closed tricuspid valve during ventricular systole. The cannon wave results from ectopic heartbeats, especially premature ventricular contractions, atrioventricular (AV) dissociation, or complete AV block.
• The *c wave* begins shortly after the first heart sound and results from closure of the tricuspid valve at the beginning of ventricular systole.
• The *v wave* peaks just after the second heart sound, when the tricuspid valve opens.

It results from continued passive atrial filling and ventricular contraction.

Negative, or descending, waves complete the jugular venous pulse:
• The *x descent,* the descent of the *a* and *c* waves, results from right atrial diastole, as well as from the tricuspid valve's being pulled down during ventricular systole, reducing right atrial pressure.
• The *y descent* is the fall in right atrial pressure from the peak of the *v* wave after the opening of the tricuspid valve. It occurs during rapid atrial emptying into the ventricle in early diastole.

Estimate venous pressure
You can obtain more information about right ventricular function by estimating venous pressure (see *Estimating venous pressure*). Venous pressure, the force exerted by blood in the venous system, normally ranges from 6 to 8 cmH_2O. It reflects the influence of circulating blood volume, vessel wall tone, vein patency, respiratory function, pulmonary pressures, the force of gravity, and, of course, right ventricular function. After estimating venous pressure, observe the jugular veins for the degree and height of distention. Characterize the degree as flat, mild, moderate, or severe; characterize the height in fingerbreadths. To confirm true venous distention, observe the veins bilaterally. (Unilateral jugular venous distention may result from local obstruction.)

Examine the carotid pulse: Essential clue to heart function
The carotid pulse correlates with central aortic pressure and reflects cardiac function more accurately than peripheral pulses. The carotid pulse should be easy to palpate even during diminished cardiac output.

Examine the carotid pulse for rate, rhythm, equality, contour, and amplitude. Observe the carotid area for exaggerated waves indicating a hypervolemic or hyperkinetic left ventricle, as in aortic regurgitation. With the patient in semi-Fowler position and his head turned toward you, palpate the carotid arteries as follows:
• To prevent possible cerebral ischemia, palpate *only one* carotid artery at a time.
• Feel the trachea and roll your fingers laterally into the groove between it and the sternocleidomastoid muscle.
• To avoid a sharp drop in heart rate, don't massage or exert excessive pressure on the carotid area.
• In a patient with a regular rhythm, palpate the carotid pulse for 30 seconds; if the rhythm is irregular, palpate for 1 to 2 minutes. Remember, you can't determine the exact pattern of irregularity or the presence of an apical-radial pulse deficit until you analyze the precordium and apical pulse.
• Describe the amplitude of the carotid pulse as normal, increased (hyperkinetic), or decreased (hypokinetic). Increased amplitude is characterized by large, bounding pulsations that have a rapid upstroke, a brief peak, and a fast downstroke. It commonly occurs during exercise or with anxiety or fear (because of high levels of circulating catecholamines) and may also accompany hyperthyroidism, anemia, aortic regurgitation, complete heart block, extreme bradycardia, and hypertension. A bounding carotid pulse may indicate that the left ventricle is generating excessive pressure to accomplish adequate cardiac output.

Decreased amplitude is characterized by small, weak pulsations that demonstrate diminished pressure; a slow, gradual velocity of

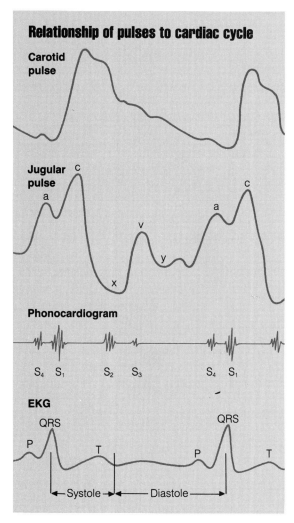

Relationship of pulses to cardiac cycle

Carotid pulse

Jugular pulse
c
a
v
y
x

Phonocardiogram
S₄ S₁   S₂ S₃   S₄ S₁

EKG
QRS   QRS
P   T   P   T
←— Systole —→ ←—— Diastole ——→

Estimating venous pressure

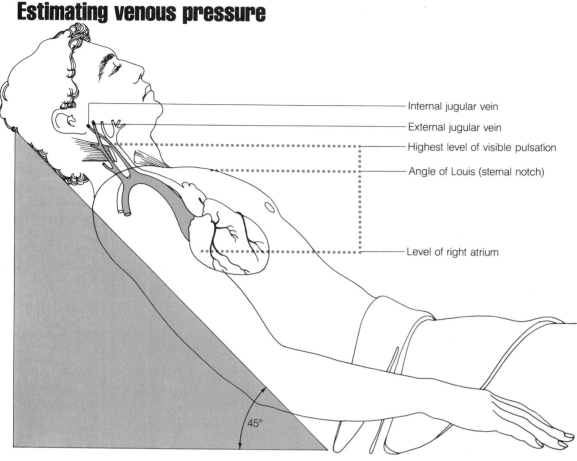

- Internal jugular vein
- External jugular vein
- Highest level of visible pulsation
- Angle of Louis (sternal notch)
- Level of right atrium

45°

This illustration shows how to measure venous pressure indirectly. To begin, place the patient at a 45° angle. Observe the internal jugular vein to determine the highest level of visible pulsation (meniscus). (Although you can use the external or the internal jugular vein, the internal jugular is the more reliable indicator of venous pressure.)

Next, locate the angle of Louis, or sternal notch. To do so, palpate the clavicles where they join the sternum (the suprasternal notch). Place your first two fingers on the suprasternal notch. Then, without lifting them from the skin, slide them down the sternum until you feel a bony protuberance—the angle of Louis.

To estimate venous pressure, measure the vertical distance between the highest level of visible pulsation and the angle of Louis (sternal notch). Normally, this vertical distance is less than 3 cm. Add 5 cm to this figure to estimate the total distance between the highest level of pulsation and the right atrium. If your total exceeds 10 cm, consider venous pressure elevated and suspect right ventricular failure.

upstroke; a delayed systolic peak; and a prolonged downstroke. It results from left ventricular failure, severe shock, constrictive pericarditis, and aortic stenosis.

After palpating both carotid pulses, carefully auscultate one carotid artery at a time. First, turn the patient's head slightly away from you to allow room for the stethoscope. Then, place the bell on the skin overlying the carotid artery. Ask the patient to hold his breath. (Avoid using the Valsalva maneuver—forced exhalation against a closed glottis—which may provoke dysrhythmias in some patients.) Normally, blood flow through the arteries is silent. But you may hear bruits in a patient with occlusive artery disease, arte-

riovenous fistula, or various high cardiac output conditions (such as anemia, hyperthyroidism, or pheochromocytoma). If you do, gently repalpate the artery with the pads of your fingers to detect the thrill (a vibrating sensation similar to the one you feel on a purring cat's throat) that frequently accompanies the bruit. A thrill reflects turbulent blood flow caused by arterial obstruction.

Core assessment: Examine the heart
Now you're ready to inspect *the precordium,* the part of the chest wall that lies over the heart. Begin by identifying the critical anatomic landmarks: the suprasternal notch and the sternal notch, or angle of Louis. Other

Cardiac landmarks

Anterior chest

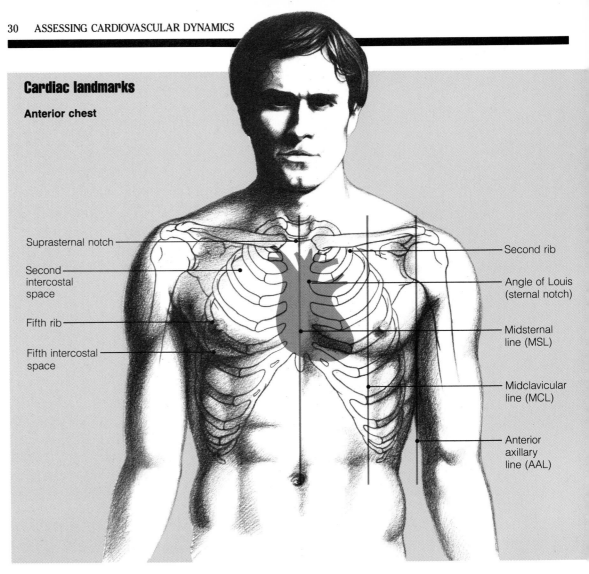

Suprasternal notch

Second intercostal space

Fifth rib

Fifth intercostal space

Second rib

Angle of Louis (sternal notch)

Midsternal line (MSL)

Midclavicular line (MCL)

Anterior axillary line (AAL)

important thoracic landmarks include the midsternal line (MSL), the midclavicular line (MCL), the midaxillary line (MAL), the anterior axillary line (AAL), and the posterior axillary line (PAL).

Place the patient in the supine position, and elevate the upper trunk 30° to 45°. Remember, you can best examine the precordium by standing to the right of the patient and using lighting that casts shadows across the chest area. First, observe the patient's thorax for shape, size (including thickness), symmetry, obvious pulsations, and retractions. (Certain congenital heart diseases can cause left-chest prominence.) Then, inspect the right and left lower sternum for excessive pulsations and any bulging, lifting, heaving, or retraction. A slight retraction of the chest wall just medial to the MCL in the fourth intercostal space (ICS) is a normal finding, but retraction of the rib is abnormal and may result from pericardial disease. When the work and force of the right ventricle increase markedly, a diffuse and lifting pulse can usually be seen or felt along the left sternal border. This impulse,

called a *parasternal lift,* indicates right ventricular hypertrophy (less common than left ventricular hypertrophy).

Next, *observe the apical impulse,* which is normally located in the fifth ICS at about the MCL. You can see this apical impulse as a pulsation produced by the thrust of the contracting left ventricle against the chest wall during systole. The apical impulse, which is evident in about half the normal adult population, occurs almost simultaneously with the carotid pulse. Consequently, simultaneous palpation of a carotid pulse helps identify it.

The apical impulse accurately reflects the size and location of the left ventricle. A sustained, forceful, laterally displaced apical impulse reflects left ventricular dilatation (volume overload) and is commonly associated with hypertrophy (pressure overload).

Palpate the precordium

Palpate the apex to the left sternal border and the base of the heart. (You can also palpate the epigastrium, the right sternal border, and the clavicular and left axillary areas.) Begin

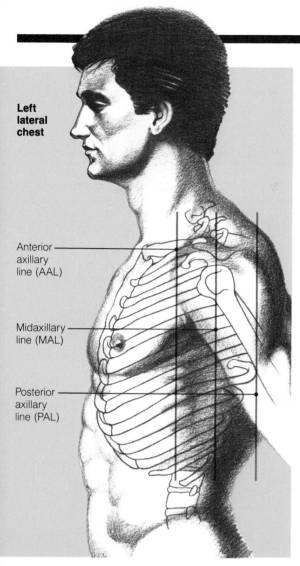

Left lateral chest

Anterior axillary line (AAL)

Midaxillary line (MAL)

Posterior axillary line (PAL)

by placing your right palm over the apex area—the midclavicular line at the fifth ICS—to *locate the point of maximum impulse (PMI)*. Locating the PMI helps you to evaluate heart size and to hear heart sounds for recording apical rates. It also helps you to hear the mitral valve and other heart sounds, such as the gallop rhythms of S_3 and S_4.

Using light palpation, you should feel a tap with each heartbeat over an area the size of a nickel. The PMI correlates with the first heart sound and carotid pulsation. If you have difficulty palpating the PMI, turn the patient to the left lateral position, thereby bringing the heart closer to the left chest wall.

The PMI may be abnormal in size, strength, and location. Usually, a weak PMI indicates poor stroke volume and a weakened contractile state, such as decompensated congestive heart failure from increased lung volume. However, the PMI may normally be imperceptible in an obese or muscular person. (Occasionally, in a patient with left ventricular hypertrophy, you may feel a lifting sensation under your examining hand in the PMI area.)

A PMI that's sustained, forceful, and diffuse over a large area or one that's displaced toward the axillary line usually indicates left ventricular hypertrophy. However, such displacement can also indicate left ventricular dilatation.

Palpate the apex for thrills
After assessing the PMI, *palpate the apex for thrills.* High flow rates (and possibly mitral regurgitation and stenosis) cause turbulent blood flow, which in turn causes thrills at the apex. These thrills can result from turbulent blood flow:
• across a damaged valve
• through a partially obstructed vessel
• through artificial changes between arteries and veins (such as a shunt for dialysis)
• through abnormal openings between heart chambers (such as ventricular or atrial septal defects).

Palpate the left sternal border
Place your right palm on the patient's left sternal border area. Palpate for thrills and for a diffuse, lifting systolic impulse that indicates right ventricular hypertrophy (less common than left ventricular hypertrophy). This impulse may be associated with a systolic retraction at the apex caused by posterior displacement and rotation of the left ventricle by the enlarged right ventricle. This finding may indicate pulmonic valve disease, pulmonary hypertension, or abnormalities associated with chronic lung disease leading to right ventricular failure.

Palpate the base of the heart
Place your hand over the base, located at the second left and right ICS at the sternal borders. (Keep in mind that the sternal notch, or angle of Louis, marks the exact location of the second ICS.) Usually, you won't feel any pulsations or thrills at the base of the heart; however, the presence of such pulsations can indicate excessive systemic or pulmonary pressures, as well as aortic or pulmonic valve disease. When your hand covers the base, the aortic valve lies beneath your palm and the pulmonic valve area beneath your fingertips. Remember that these areas don't correspond to the exact location of the valves but to the sites where their sounds are normally detected.

Palpate for a thrill in the second ICS or the first and third right ICS. A thrill may indicate aortic stenosis. In the patient with systemic

Choosing—and using—a stethoscope

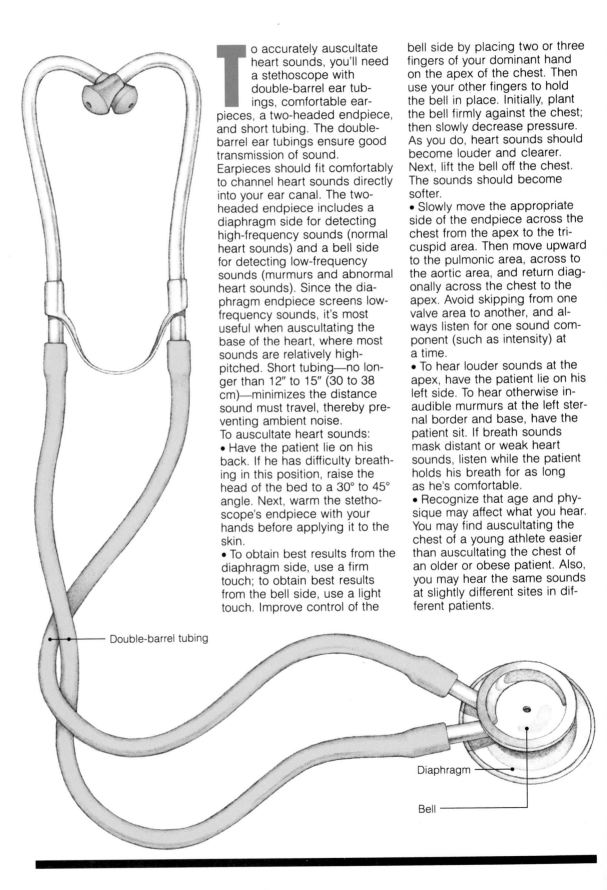

To accurately auscultate heart sounds, you'll need a stethoscope with double-barrel ear tubings, comfortable earpieces, a two-headed endpiece, and short tubing. The double-barrel ear tubings ensure good transmission of sound. Earpieces should fit comfortably to channel heart sounds directly into your ear canal. The two-headed endpiece includes a diaphragm side for detecting high-frequency sounds (normal heart sounds) and a bell side for detecting low-frequency sounds (murmurs and abnormal heart sounds). Since the diaphragm endpiece screens low-frequency sounds, it's most useful when auscultating the base of the heart, where most sounds are relatively high-pitched. Short tubing—no longer than 12″ to 15″ (30 to 38 cm)—minimizes the distance sound must travel, thereby preventing ambient noise.

To auscultate heart sounds:
• Have the patient lie on his back. If he has difficulty breathing in this position, raise the head of the bed to a 30° to 45° angle. Next, warm the stethoscope's endpiece with your hands before applying it to the skin.
• To obtain best results from the diaphragm side, use a firm touch; to obtain best results from the bell side, use a light touch. Improve control of the bell side by placing two or three fingers of your dominant hand on the apex of the chest. Then use your other fingers to hold the bell in place. Initially, plant the bell firmly against the chest; then slowly decrease pressure. As you do, heart sounds should become louder and clearer. Next, lift the bell off the chest. The sounds should become softer.
• Slowly move the appropriate side of the endpiece across the chest from the apex to the tricuspid area. Then move upward to the pulmonic area, across to the aortic area, and return diagonally across the chest to the apex. Avoid skipping from one valve area to another, and always listen for one sound component (such as intensity) at a time.
• To hear louder sounds at the apex, have the patient lie on his left side. To hear otherwise inaudible murmurs at the left sternal border and base, have the patient sit. If breath sounds mask distant or weak heart sounds, listen while the patient holds his breath for as long as he's comfortable.
• Recognize that age and physique may affect what you hear. You may find auscultating the chest of a young athlete easier than auscultating the chest of an older or obese patient. Also, you may hear the same sounds at slightly different sites in different patients.

Double-barrel tubing

Diaphragm

Bell

hypertension, you may palpate an exaggerated vibration, indicating aortic valve closure, during the second heart sound. A thrill in the second and third left ICS may indicate pulmonic valve stenosis. The most common causes of such abnormal pulsations in the area of the pulmonary artery and pulmonic valve are pulmonary hypertension and atrial septal defect.

Learn to identify heart sounds
Auscultation is the only way to identify many valvular abnormalities, but it's an assessment skill that's difficult to master. You need continual practice to achieve accuracy. But don't be discouraged; practice as much as you can. Initially, auscultation can take 10 to 15 minutes to complete. So the patient won't become alarmed, be sure to tell him that this examination requires extensive and careful listening. To make your auscultation as successful as possible, minimize room noise by closing doors and windows.

Listen for first sounds: S_1 and S_2
S_1 is the lub and S_2 the dub of the lub-dub sound made by the normal heart. To identify S_1, produced by the closing of the mitral and tricuspid valves, auscultate the PMI with the diaphragm of the stethoscope while you watch or palpate the carotid pulse. You'll hear S_1 just before or at the same time as carotid pulsation. At the apex, S_1 is louder, longer in duration, and lower in pitch than S_2. At the tricuspid area, splitting—the closure of the mitral valve before the tricuspid valve—is normal but usually inaudible. However, abnormal S_1 splitting (greater than 0.03 seconds) may be audible.

To identify S_2, produced by the closing of the aortic and pulmonic valves, place the diaphragm of the stethoscope over the aortic valve area. Identify the loudest sound and then slowly move the stethoscope diagonally toward the PMI. The loudest sound, S_2, should become softer. Normal S_2 splitting can be heard best in the pulmonic area during inspiration. It appears when decreased intrathoracic pressure draws additional blood into the right ventricle, delaying closure of the pulmonic valve; it disappears when the patient exhales or sits up. Abnormal S_2 splitting—usually due to overfilling of the right ventricle, which isn't affected by breathing or position changes—is sometimes heard in the patient with pulmonic valve stenosis, atrial ventricular defects, or right bundle branch block.

Listen for extra sounds: S_3 and S_4
You may hear a third heart sound, S_3, early in diastole. It usually occurs in a dilatated ventricle and results from the rapid flow of blood into the ventricles. You can hear it best at the apex, through the bell of the stethoscope, with the patient lying on his left side. In bradycardia, S_3 sounds like the "y" in Kentucky; in tachycardia, like a galloping horse—thus the term *gallop rhythm* or ventricular gallop. It can be perfectly normal in a child or adolescent, or even in a young adult with an extremely thin chest wall. In any other adult, it probably indicates left ventricular failure.

You may also hear a fourth heart sound—S_4. Some say it sounds like the "Tenn" in Tennessee. This atrial flow sound occurs late in diastole (atrial kick). It's heard best at the apex under the same conditions as S_3.

These last two sounds are the so-called gallop rhythms: S_3 is a *ventricular gallop*, S_4 an *atrial gallop*. S_3 occurs directly after S_2; S_4, directly before S_1. A *summation gallop*, combining S_3 and S_4, is a loud single sound that occurs in mid-diastole. A ventricular or summation gallop should be reported to a doctor immediately.

Listen for murmurs
Murmurs—sounds produced by abnormal turbulence—result from an increased rate of blood flow, increased or decreased blood vessel diameter, decreased blood viscosity, or a rough inner surface of a blood vessel wall. Murmurs are classified by:
• timing (place in cardiac cycle)
• location (point of maximal intensity; reference points are valve areas and intercostal spaces)
• pitch (low, medium, high)
• intensity (graded on a scale from I, barely audible, to VI, audible without stethoscope)
• duration (short, medium, long)
• quality (recorded in descriptive terms such as blowing, harsh, rumbling).

If you're just starting to learn about murmurs, classify them by timing, location, and intensity. With experience you'll be able to classify the more subtle characteristics and their interactions.

The velocity of blood flow determines pitch and loudness. For example, exercise or increased body temperature increases blood flow and causes a murmur to become louder and higher pitched. The location of a murmur also affects its loudness; murmurs are loudest at their site of origin, and the closer the site

Implications of abnormal heart sounds

Areas of auscultation

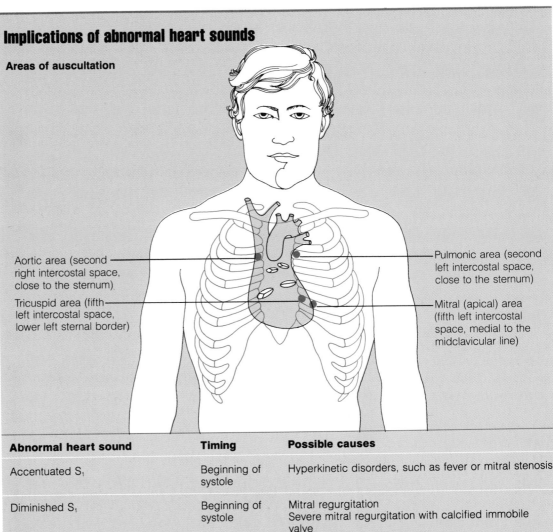

Aortic area (second right intercostal space, close to the sternum)

Tricuspid area (fifth left intercostal space, lower left sternal border)

Pulmonic area (second left intercostal space, close to the sternum)

Mitral (apical) area (fifth left intercostal space, medial to the midclavicular line)

Abnormal heart sound	Timing	Possible causes
Accentuated S_1	Beginning of systole	Hyperkinetic disorders, such as fever or mitral stenosis
Diminished S_1	Beginning of systole	Mitral regurgitation Severe mitral regurgitation with calcified immobile valve Heart block
Accentuated S_2	End of systole	Pulmonary or systemic hypertension
Diminished or inaudible S_2	End of systole	Aortic or pulmonary stenosis
Persistent S_2 split	End of systole	Delayed closure of the pulmonic valve, usually from overfilling of the right ventricle causing prolonged systolic ejection time
Persistent S_2 split that widens during inspiration	End of systole	Pulmonic valve stenosis Atrial ventricular septal defect Right bundle branch block
Reversed or paradoxical S_2 split that appears in expiration and disappears in inspiration	End of systole	Delayed ventricular stimulation: left bundle branch block or prolonged left ventricular ejection time
S_3 (ventricular gallop)	Early diastole	Normal in children and young adults Overdistention of ventricle in rapid-filling segment of diastole: mitral insufficiency or ventricular failure
S_4 (atrial gallop or presystolic extra sound)	Late diastole	Forceful atrial contraction from resistance to ventricular filling late in diastole: left ventricular hypertrophy, pulmonary stenosis, hypertension, coronary artery disease, and aortic stenosis
Pericardial friction rub (grating or leathery sound at left sternal border; usually muffled, high-pitched, and transient)	Throughout systole and diastole	Pericardial inflammation

Identifying heart murmurs

Timing	Quality	Pitch	Location	Radiation	Condition
Midsystolic (systolic ejection)	Harsh, rough	Medium to high	Pulmonic	Toward left shoulder and neck	Pulmonic stenosis
	Harsh, rough	Medium to high	Aortic and suprasternal notch	Toward carotid arteries or apex	Aortic stenosis
Holosystolic (pansystolic)	Harsh	High	Tricuspid	Precordium	Ventricular septal defect
	Blowing	High	Mitral, lower left sternal border	Toward left axilla	Mitral insufficiency
	Blowing	High	Tricuspid	Toward apex	Tricuspid insufficiency
Early diastolic	Blowing	High	Mid-left sternal edge (not aortic area)	Toward sternum	Aortic insufficiency
	Blowing	High	Pulmonic	Toward sternum	Pulmonic insufficiency
Mid- to late diastolic	Rumbling	Low	Apex	Usually none	Mitral stenosis
	Rumbling	Low	Tricuspid, lower sternal border	Usually none	Tricuspid stenosis

of origin to the anterior chest wall, the louder the murmur on auscultation. Loudness varies if the sounds radiate outward. Pitch varies with the quantity of tissue the sounds must pass through before reaching the chest wall and with the direction of blood flow.

When timing a murmur, establish if it occurs during diastole or systole. Remember, if you hear a murmur between S_1 and S_2, it's a systolic murmur; between S_2 and the next S_1, a diastolic murmur. Also establish the point in systole or diastole at which the murmur occurs—for example, mid- diastole or late systole.

The intensity of murmurs varies greatly and is graded from I to VI:
• Grade I, very faint
• Grade II, soft and low
• Grade III, prominent but not palpable
• Grade IV, prominent and palpable (you can feel a thrill)
• Grade V, very loud
• Grade VI, audible with the stethoscope off the chest.

Finally, integrate your data
The subjective and objective data you've gathered throughout your assessment will help you arrive at a nursing diagnosis. A nursing diagnosis describes a combination of signs and symptoms that indicate an actual or potential health problem requiring nursing intervention. This isn't much different from what you've always done. What's changing, though,

is the systematic definition, explanation, and classification of these problems by the National Group for the Classification of Nursing Diagnoses. The group's goal is to standardize diagnostic labels so patients' problems and needs can be clearly communicated from one nurse to another. These labels are being tested by research that will eventually lead to the establishment of specific outcome criteria and nursing interventions for each diagnosis. Until a full set of accepted cardiovascular diagnoses are developed, you can help identify possible diagnoses for future acceptance.

When writing a nursing diagnosis, keep it simple. Establish a baseline assessment using a nursing data base; then write your diagnostic statement—reflecting a problem related to etiology. Remember, your nursing diagnosis should represent a specific problem requiring nursing intervention. If you know the cause of the problem, your nursing diagnosis should clearly describe it.

Throughout the day, keep your diagnoses in mind as you set your goals. Plan, implement, and evaluate your patients' care according to your patient's diagnosis.

Mastering the steps from nursing assessment to nursing diagnosis will help you detect subtle physiologic changes in patients that signal the need for early intervention. Don't be discouraged if you don't master the whole approach at once. You'll need a lot of practice. Careful, competent cardiovascular assessment takes much patience... and many patients!

Points to remember

• The stages of cardiovascular assessment include patient preparation, overall inspection, history taking, physical examination, and formulation of a nursing diagnosis.
• The patient interview provides valuable subjective information to help you interpret your examination results. To make this interview successful, think of it as a conversation rather than an anonymous hospital checklist.
• The physical examination should proceed in a systematic way. Examine the patient from the periphery toward the center in the following order: arms and legs, abdomen, neck, and precordium. However, if your overall impression of the patient suggests a potentially life-threatening disorder, reverse the order of the examination, moving from the center toward the periphery.
• Mastery of advanced techniques—auscultation of heart sounds and murmurs, inspection of neck veins, and palpation of the precordium—is necessary for complete cardiovascular assessment.
• The results of the patient interview and the physical examination allow you to form a nursing diagnosis—a combination of signs and symptoms that indicate an actual or potential health problem requiring nursing intervention.

3 UPDATING DIAGNOSTIC CONCEPTS

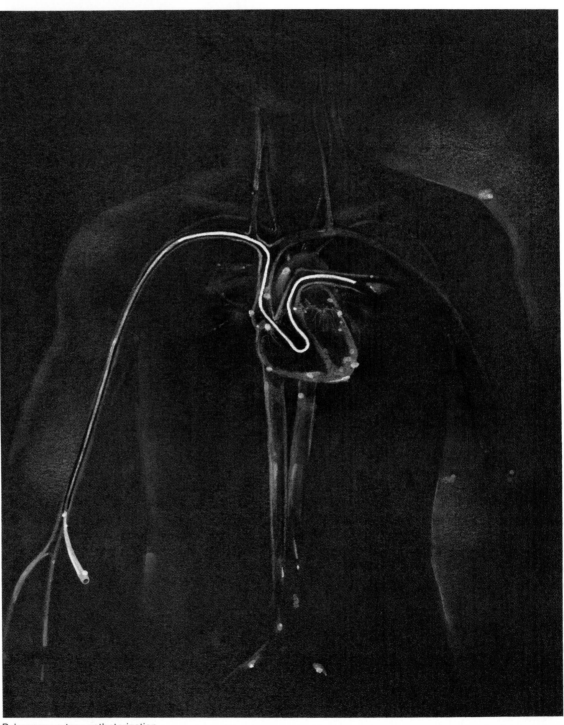

Pulmonary artery catheterization

Today, safe and effective nursing care means, in part, keeping up with rapid advances in cardiovascular testing. These advances have allowed earlier diagnosis and treatment of cardiovascular disorders, leading to the recent decline in the death rate from these disorders. For example, in certain patients, echocardiography—a noninvasive, risk-free test—can provide as much diagnostic information on valvular heart disease as cardiac catheterization—an invasive, high-risk test. And the risk of mortality associated with cardiac catheterization is now lower due to improved equipment and monitoring capabilities.

Technological advances have also improved the precision of diagnostic tests. Previously, diagnosis of acute myocardial infarction (MI) depended solely on serial 12-lead electrocardiograms and cardiac enzyme studies. Today, electrophysiologic and nuclear imaging tests can pinpoint the exact location and extent of cardiac damage within hours of an acute MI, allowing more effective treatment. Understanding these new diagnostic tests as well as reviewing the familiar ones will help you improve your nursing care.

ELECTROCARDIOGRAPHY

Electrocardiography, a routine part of every cardiovascular evaluation, is one of the most valuable diagnostic tests. Research and technological advances have led to the development of several forms of this test (see *Electrocardiography: Its forms and objectives*). Besides becoming familiar with these EKG forms, you'll also need to acquire the skills to interpret their resulting tracings. Not too long ago, only critical-care nurses needed proficiency in interpreting EKG tracings. But today some hospitals require these skills in nurses who work in emergency departments, operating rooms, and labor and delivery rooms. To achieve this proficiency, you'll need to review the EKG and its fundamental mechanisms in order to recognize standard tracings and detect electrical or mechanical problems that can cause spurious test results.

Review EKG basics

Electrocardiography graphically records electrical current (electrical potential) generated by the heart. Current radiates from the heart in all directions and, on reaching the skin, is measured by electrodes connected to an amplifier and strip chart recorder. In standard electrocardiography, five electrodes attached to the arms, legs, and chest measure current from 12 different views, or leads: three standard bipolar limb leads (I, II, and III), three unipolar augmented limb leads (aVR, aVL, and aVF), and six unipolar chest leads (V_1 to V_6).

The *standard limb leads* are called bipolar leads because each has two electrodes that simultaneously record the heart's electrical current flowing toward two extremities. That is, lead I records electrical current between the right and left arms; lead II, between the right arm and left leg; and lead III, between the left arm and left leg. The right arm is always the negative pole, while the left leg is always the positive pole. The left arm can be either positive or negative, depending on the lead—in lead I, it's positive; in lead III, it's negative. When current flows toward the positive pole, the EKG waveform deflects upward (positive). When current flows toward the negative pole, the waveform inverts (negative). For example, in lead II the flow of current is from the negative to the positive pole, so the EKG deflects upward.

The *augmented limb leads,* which use the same electrode placement as the standard limb leads, measure electrical current between one augmented limb electrode and the electrical midpoint of the remaining two electrodes, which is determined electronically by the EKG machine. Like the standard leads, the augmented leads measure electrical current from a vertical plane.

The six unipolar *chest leads,* which measure electrical current from a horizontal plane, are designated by the letter "V" and a number representing the electrode's position on the chest wall, or precordium. These positions are: V_1—fourth intercostal space, right sternal border; V_2—fourth intercostal space, left sternal border; V_3—midway between V_2 and V_4, on a line joining these positions; V_4—fifth intercostal space at midclavicular line; V_5—midway between V_4 and V_6, on the anterior axillary line horizontal to V_4; and V_6—left midaxillary line horizontal to V_4 and V_5.

Lead V_1 best represents the right and left atria and the right ventricle, while leads V_2 through V_6 represent the left ventricle. Leads II, III, and aVF represent the inferior or diaphragmatic part of the heart. Leads I and aVL show reciprocal changes from the left ventricle. If you keep in mind that each lead pictures a different anatomical area, you'll be able to pinpoint areas of cardiac damage when you find abnormal tracings.

The EKG machine averages the electrical

Electrocardiography: Its forms and objectives

Various forms of electrocardiography—resting, exercise, and continuous ambulatory—provide important information for diagnosis of cardiovascular disorders.

Resting EKG:
• helps identify primary conduction abnormalities, cardiac dysrhythmias, cardiac hypertrophy, pericarditis, electrolyte imbalance, myocardial ischemia, and the site and extent of MI
• helps monitor recovery from MI
• evaluates pacemaker performance and the effectiveness of cardiotonic glycosides and antiarrhythmics.

Exercise EKG:
• helps determine the heart's functional capacity and the origin of chest pain
• screens for asymptomatic coronary artery disease (particularly in men over age 35)
• helps define limits for an exercise program and identifies dysrhythmias that develop during exercise
• evaluates the effectiveness of antiarrhythmic and antianginal drugs.

Continuous ambulatory EKG:
• detects cardiac dysrhythmias and evaluates the effectiveness of antiarrhythmic drugs
• evaluates chest pain
• evaluates cardiac status after acute MI or pacemaker implantation
• allows assessment and correlation of dyspnea, central nervous system symptoms (such as syncope and lightheadedness), and palpitations to actual cardiac events and patient activities.

Standard 12-lead EKG

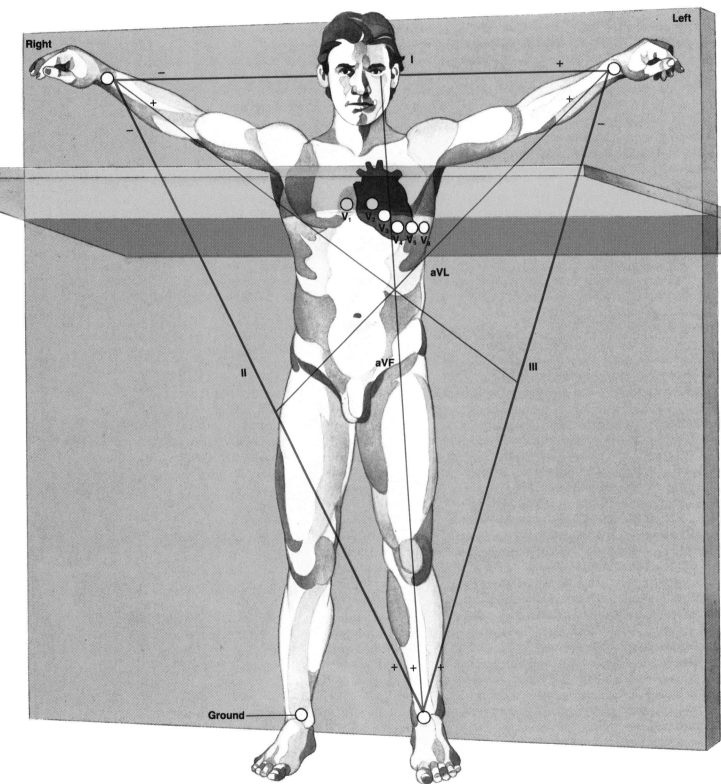

Normally, five electrodes (four limb, one chest) record the heart's electrical potential from 12 different views (leads). One electrode serves as a ground. Standard bipolar limb leads (I, II, III) detect variations in electrical potential at two points (the negative pole and the positive pole) and record the difference. The unipolar aug- mented limb leads (aVR, aVL, and aVF) measure electrical potential between one augmented limb lead and the electrical midpoint of the remaining two leads. Six unipolar chest leads (V₁ through V₆) view electrical potential from a horizontal plane that helps locate pathology in the lateral and posterior walls of the heart.

Normal EKG waveforms

Lead I

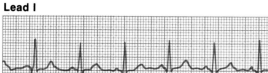

Lead II

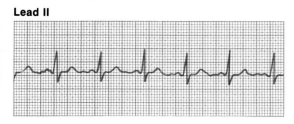

Lead III

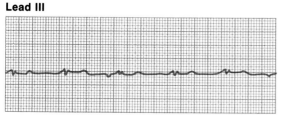

Lead aVR

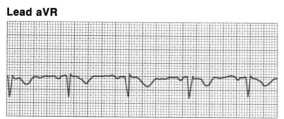

Lead aVL

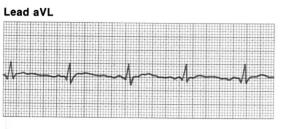

Lead aVF

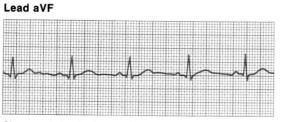

Lead V₁

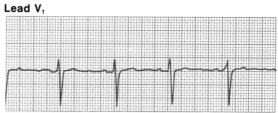

Lead V₂

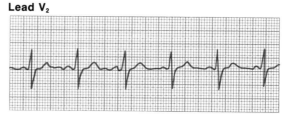

Lead V₃

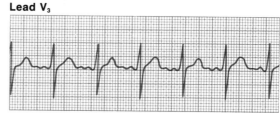

Lead V₄

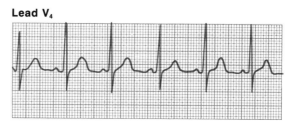

Lead V₅

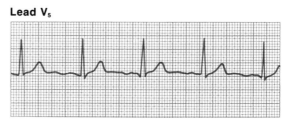

Lead V₆

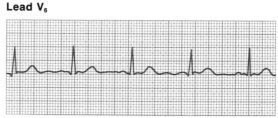

Since each lead takes a different view of heart activity, it generates its own characteristic tracing. The tracings shown here are representative of those produced by each of the 12 leads. A positive (upward) deflection indicates that current is flowing toward the positive electrode placed on the side facing the advancing wave of depolarization. Conversely, a negative (downward) deflection indicates that the wave of depolarization is flowing away from the positive electrode. A biphasic deflection (equally positive and negative) indicates that the wave of depolarization is flowing perpendicularly to the positive electrode.

current under the three limb electrodes and compares this with the electrical current under the positive chest electrode. Recordings made with the V connection show variations in electrical current that occur under the chest electrode as its position is changed. After electrical currents are transmitted to the EKG machine, these forces are amplified and graphically displayed on a strip chart recorder. The graphic display, or tracing, usually consists of the P wave, the QRS complex, and the T wave. The P wave shows atrial depolarization; the QRS complex, ventricular depolarization; and the T wave, ventricular repolarization. The illustration on page 39 shows the normal waveforms for each of the standard 12 leads. Occasionally, artifacts and other types of electrical interference produce distortions in the EKG waveform, resulting in spurious tracings. Such distortions include waveforms with a low amplitude and a wandering or fuzzy baseline. These can result from patient movement, muscle tremors (especially common in the elderly and in those with Parkinson's disease), inadequate skin preparation, loose or overly dry electrodes, poor electrical connections or grounding, broken lead wires, malfunctioning equipment, and static electricity.

Exercise electrocardiography
Commonly known as the stress test, exercise electrocardiography provides diagnostic information that can't be obtained from resting electrocardiography alone. In fact, it's one of the best noninvasive tests for assessing cardiovascular response to an increased work load. In this test, the patient pedals a stationary bicycle or walks on a treadmill as EKG and blood pressure readings are taken to evaluate heart action during physical stress. The body responds to this stress by increasing its demand for oxygen, which increases respiratory rate, cardiac output, and extraction of oxygen by the tissues. The test continues until the patient reaches a predetermined target heart rate or experiences chest pain, fatigue, or other signs and symptoms that reflect exercise intolerance. These may include severe dyspnea, claudication, weakness or dizziness, hypotension, pallor or vasoconstriction, disorientation, ataxia, ischemic EKG changes with or without pain, rhythm disturbances or heart block, and ventricular conduction abnormalities.

Serial stress testing at 3- to 6-month intervals evaluates long-term exercise training programs by verifying the presence or absence of increased exercise tolerance. Increased exercise results in more efficient oxygen extraction at the peripheral or cellular level, which decreases myocardial oxygen demand. This results in increased exercise tolerance. In a patient with increased exercise tolerance, the EKG shows a decrease in heart rate and systolic blood pressure at any given level of activity.

Continuous ambulatory electrocardiography
Like exercise electrocardiography, continuous ambulatory electrocardiography can provide considerably more diagnostic information than standard resting electrocardiography. For instance, the standard EKG records only 45 seconds of heart activity and, as a result, doesn't capture the effects of physical and psychological stresses during normal daily activities. Consequently, it can fail to detect intermittent but potentially lethal dysrhythmias. In contrast, continuous ambulatory electrocardiography (also called Holter monitoring after the scientist who developed this test) allows continuous recording of heart activity as the patient follows his normal routine. In this test, which is usually performed for 24 hours or about 100,000 cardiac cycles, the patient wears a small reel-to-reel or cassette tape recorder connected to bipolar electrodes placed on his chest, and he also keeps a diary of his activities and any associated symptoms. After the monitoring period, the tape is analyzed by a microcomputer to allow correlation of cardiac irregularities, such as dysrhythmias and ST segment changes, with activities noted in the patient's diary.

Continuous ambulatory electrocardiography can also employ patient-activated monitors, which can be worn for 5 to 7 days. The patient manually initiates recording of heart activity when he experiences symptoms.

CARDIAC ENZYMES: CLUES TO MYOCARDIAL INFARCTION
Like the analysis of EKG tracings, analysis of cardiac enzyme levels aids diagnosis of acute MI. After infarction, damaged cardiac tissue releases significant amounts of enzymes into the blood, allowing serial measurement of their levels to reveal the extent of damage or to monitor the progress of healing.

The cardiac enzymes include creatine phosphokinase (CPK), lactic dehydrogenase (LDH), and serum glutamic-oxaloacetic transaminase

Cardiac monitoring facts

Like other forms of electrocardiography, cardiac monitoring uses electrodes applied to the patient's chest to pick up patterns of cardiac impulses for display and analysis on a monitor screen. The monitor displays the patient's heart rate and rhythm, sounds an alarm if the heart rate rises above or falls below the allowable per minute setting, and provides printouts of cardiac rhythms. Cardiac monitoring allows continuous observation of the heart's electrical activity in patients with a symptomatic dysrhythmia or any cardiac pathology that might lead to life-threatening dysrhythmias. It's also used to evaluate effects of therapy.

Two types: Hardwire and telemetry monitoring

Hardwire monitoring permits continuous observation of a patient directly connected to the monitor console. In contrast, telemetry monitoring permits continuous monitoring of an ambulatory patient who isn't connected to a monitor. In telemetry monitoring, cardiac impulses travel from a small transmitter worn by the patient to antenna wires in the ceiling that relay patterns to the monitor screen. Telemetry monitoring permits greater patient mobility than hardwire monitoring, and avoids electrical hazards by isolating the monitor system from leakage and accidental shock. But telemetry monitoring is limited; its relay wires pick up the heartbeat only within 50′ to 2,000′ (15 to 610 m) of the central console, depending on the equipment and the unit's floor plan.

Three-electrode monitor

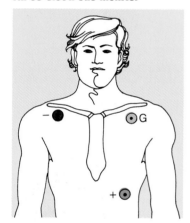

Lead II
Positive (+): left side of chest, lowest palpable rib, midclavicular line
Negative (−): right shoulder, below clavicular hollow
Ground (G): left shoulder, below clavicular hollow

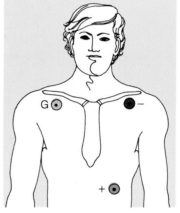

MCL₁
Positive (+): right sternal border, lowest palpable rib
Negative (−): left shoulder, below clavicular hollow
Ground (G): right shoulder, below clavicular hollow

MCL₆
Positive (+): left side of chest, lowest palpable rib, midclavicular line
Negative (−): left shoulder, below clavicular hollow
Ground (G): right shoulder, below clavicular hollow

(SGOT). Two of these enzymes, CPK and LDH, occur in multiple forms, or isoenzymes, that differ in molecular details but retain their fundamental identity. For example, CPK is present in heart muscle, skeletal muscle, and brain tissue. Its isoenzymes are combinations of the subunits M (muscle) and B (brain); CPK-BB is found primarily in brain and nerve tissue; CPK-MM, in skeletal muscle; and CPK-MB, in heart muscle. Elevated levels of CPK-MB reliably indicate acute MI, since this isoenzyme isn't prevalent in other tissues. Typically, CPK-MB levels rise 4 to 8 hours after the onset of acute MI, peak after 20 hours, and may remain elevated up to 72 hours.

Lactic dehydrogenase is present in almost all body tissues, but its five isoenzymes are organ-specific. The isoenzymes LDH_1 and LDH_2 appear primarily in the heart, red blood cells, and kidneys; LDH_3, primarily in the lungs; and LDH_4 and LDH_5, in the liver and skeletal muscle. Typically, LDH_1 and LDH_2 levels rise 8 to 12 hours after acute MI, peak in 24 to 48 hours, and return to normal in 10 to 14 days if tissue necrosis doesn't persist. A flipped LDH, in which LDH_1 levels exceed LDH_2 levels (the reversal of their normal pat-

Serum enzyme and isoenzyme levels after myocardial infarction

Normal range

CPK-MB: 0 to 7 IU/liter
Total LDH: 48 to 115 IU/liter
LDH$_1$: 18.1% to 29%
SGOT: 8 to 20 units/liter

Key

——————— CPK-MB
——————— LDH$_1$
- - - - - - - SGOT

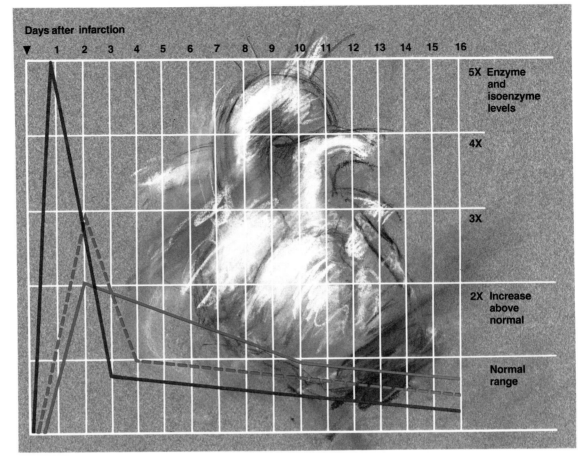

tern), reliably indicates acute MI. As a result, LDH isoenzyme analysis is especially useful when CPK hasn't been measured within 24 hours of an acute MI.

Serum glutamic-oxaloacetic transaminase is present in the heart, liver, skeletal muscles, kidneys, pancreas and, to a lesser extent, in red blood cells. Although a high correlation exists between MI and elevated SGOT, testing for the presence of SGOT is sometimes considered superfluous in diagnosing MI because of this enzyme's low organ specificity. For example, the test doesn't allow for differentiation between acute MI and the effects of hepatic congestion because of heart failure.

CARDIAC RADIOGRAPHY
Cardiac radiography is one of the most frequently used tests for evaluating cardiac disease and its effect on the pulmonary vasculature. Routinely, posteroanterior and left lateral views are taken, allowing visualization of cardiac enlargement, pulmonary congestion and, at times, cardiac calcifications.

Although a radiologist interprets X-rays, it's important for you to be able to distinguish between normal X-ray findings and findings associated with common cardiac abnormali-

ties. The X-rays on page 43 show a normal and an enlarged heart. In an X-ray of the normal heart, you'll be able to see the cardiac silhouette and the pulmonary artery. On the right side of the cardiac silhouette, you'll see the superior vena cava and the right atrium; on the left side, the aortic "knob," the main pulmonary artery and left branch, the left atrial appendage, and the left ventricle.

Recognize cardiac enlargement
On the right side of the cardiac silhouette, prominence of the superior vena cava or right atrium indicates right heart enlargement. Prominence of the superior vena cava can result from long-term congestive heart failure, chronic obstructive pulmonary disease, atrial septal defect, or abnormal pulmonary veins that enter the cava. Prominence of the right atrium can result from atrial septal defect, tricuspid valve disease, and Ebstein's anomaly.

On the left side of the cardiac silhouette, prominence of the aorta, left atrium, pulmonary artery, or left ventricle also indicates cardiac enlargement. Prominence of the aorta—or of both the aorta and its knob—can stem from hypertension, aortic valve disease, aortic dysplasia or aortic aneurysm.

Prominence of the left atrium can stem from mitral valve disease, ventricular septal defect, and patent ductus arteriosus. Similarly, prominence of the pulmonary artery, indicating pulmonary hypertension, can result from ventricular septal defect, patent ductus arteriosus, pulmonary valve disease, and atrial septal defect. Prominence of the left ventricle can result from hypertension, aortic valve disease, subvalvular aortic stenosis, ventricular septal defect, patent ductus arteriosus, coronary artery disease, and cardiomyopathy.

Recognize pulmonary congestion

When the heart fails to eject blood efficiently, the blood remaining in it after systole pools in the pulmonary system, causing pulmonary vascular congestion. On a chest X-ray, this congestion may appear initially as dilatation of pulmonary venous shadows in the superior lateral aspect of the hilus, and as vascular shadows horizontally and inferiorly along the right margin of the heart. Chronic pulmonary venous hypertension produces an "antler" pattern, caused by dilated superior pulmonary veins and normal or constricted inferior pulmonary veins. Acute alveolar edema results in increased densities in central lung fields, producing a butterfly shape; interstitial pulmonary edema produces a cloudy, cottony appearance.

PULMONARY ARTERY CATHETERIZATION

Because of technologic advances, it's becoming more common to depend on invasive procedures that allow continuous hemodynamic monitoring to help determine treament goals. One of these procedures, pulmonary artery (Swan-Ganz) catheterization, provides instantaneous cardiopulmonary pressure measurements. At one time limited to the cardiac catheterization laboratory, this procedure is now performed at bedside in an intensive care unit. In fact, pulmonary artery catheterization is the best bedside procedure for evaluating left ventricular function and the response of the left ventricle to therapy, particularly administration of fluids, inotropic agents, and vasodilators. It uses a balloon-tipped, flow-directed catheter, connected to a transducer and a monitor, and allows measurement of pulmonary artery pressure (PAP), pulmonary capillary wedge pressure (PCWP), cardiac output, and mixed venous oxygen saturation, which evaluates pulmonary vascular resistance and tissue oxygenation.

Normal and abnormal cardiac outlines

Normal

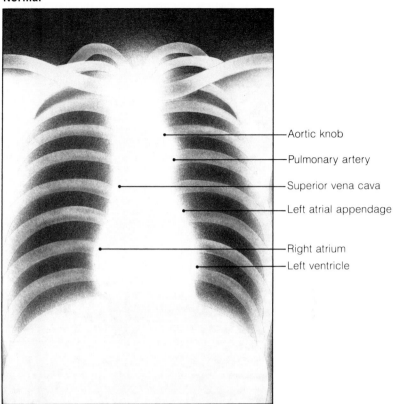

— Aortic knob

— Pulmonary artery

— Superior vena cava

— Left atrial appendage

— Right atrium
— Left ventricle

Abnormal

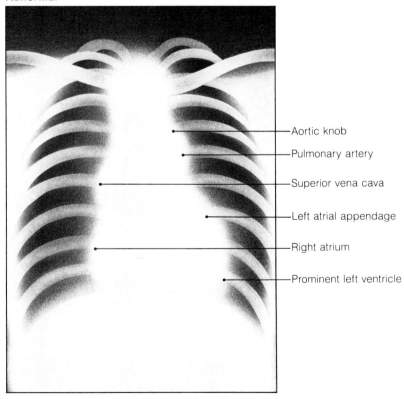

— Aortic knob

— Pulmonary artery

— Superior vena cava

— Left atrial appendage

— Right atrium

— Prominent left ventricle

The posteroanterior chest X-ray permits visualization of the position, size, and contour of the heart and great vessels. Note the prominent left ventricle in the enlarged silhouette.

Pulmonary artery catheterization, performed by a doctor with a nurse assisting, involves the insertion of a multilumen catheter into the internal jugular or subclavian vein, or occasionally into the basilic vein of the antecubital fossa. The catheter enters the right atrium through the superior vena cava. When it's in the right atrium, the doctor inflates the balloon to assist in propelling the catheter through the tricuspid valve and into the right ventricle. The catheter then travels through the pulmonary semilunar valve into the pulmonary artery and eventually into a branch of the pulmonary artery with a smaller diameter than that of the balloon, which becomes wedged in the vessel. Here, it allows measurement of PCWP. As the catheter passes through the right atrium, right ventricle, and pulmonary artery, the pressures and corresponding waveforms are monitored. (For characteristic waveforms, see the chart *Interpreting hemodynamic waveforms* on page 46.) Meanwhile, samples of blood from any of these areas can be withdrawn and sent to the laboratory for analysis of oxygen content.

After catheter insertion, the pressure readings obtained during the procedure are evaluated to help diagnose cardiac dysfunction. Comparison of right atrial pressure and pulmonary artery end-diastolic pressure (PAEDP) or PCWP provides valuable information about several disorders:
• Acute left ventricular dysfunction elevates left ventricular filling pressure, but causes only a slight change in right atrial pressure.
• Hypovolemia produces a low right atrial pressure and a low left ventricular filling pressure.
• Cardiac tamponade, pericardial constriction, right ventricular infarction, septal defects, restrictive cardiomyopathy, or severe biventricular congestive failure are possible when the right-sided filling pressure approximately equals the left-sided filling pressure.

Continuous hemodynamic monitoring
After insertion, the balloon can be deflated so that the catheter floats back into the pulmonary artery. Using a constant infusion valve, PAEDP can then be continuously monitored by a computer to detect a change in the patient's hemodynamic status or to detect monitoring problems, such as wedging of the catheter tip and recoil of the catheter into the right ventricle. However, the catheter-fling artifact—the rapid movement of the tip of the pulmonary artery catheter—can pose a problem when monitoring PAEDP. The standard bedside diastolic pressure readout shows the minimum (valley) of the fling artifact, thus underestimating the true PAEDP. As a result, PAEDP should be measured at the midpoint of the oscillations just before systole, using a calibrated strip chart recorder.

Pulmonary capillary wedge pressure can be recorded by inflating the balloon and allowing the catheter to advance until it obstructs a branch of the pulmonary artery. Then the catheter's distal port records pressure that is transmitted backward through the capillary bed from the left atrium, yielding a measure of left ventricular filling pressure.

During PCWP monitoring, be alert for these complications:
• Prolonged overinflation of the balloon can obstruct blood flow to a portion of the lung, causing pulmonary infarction.
• Balloon rupture may cause a life-threatening air embolism.
• Inflation of the balloon when the catheter tip is positioned in a small arterial branch may rupture the vessel wall, resulting in pulmonary hemorrhage.
• With repeated balloon inflations, the catheter tip usually becomes wedged in a distal branch of the pulmonary artery. If the catheter remains in a wedged position, pulmonary infarction will occur. When the catheter tip is withdrawn from the wedged position, however, it occasionally recoils into the right ventricle or atrium.

Cardiac output
Measured to help evaluate cardiac function, cardiac output is the amount of blood ejected from the ventricles, expressed in liters per minute. It's usually measured at bedside using a four- or five-lumen pulmonary artery catheter with a thermodilution tip. A predetermined amount of chilled or room temperature solution is injected into the right atrium through the proximal lumen of the catheter, which empties into the right atrium or superior vena cava. A minicomputer then calculates cardiac output from temperature changes of the blood detected by a thermistor in the catheter tip, and the cardiac output is displayed on a digital readout.

Periodic measurement of cardiac output helps determine a patient's response to drug therapy or the need for alternate treatments. Low cardiac output results from decreased myocardial contractility because of myocardial infarction, drugs, acidosis, or hypoxia;

Pulmonary artery catheters

Four types of pulmonary artery catheters are available to help evaluate cardiovascular and pulmonary functions. The *double-lumen catheter* monitors pulmonary artery and pulmonary capillary wedge pressures. It's also used for obtaining samples of mixed venous blood, and for infusion of solutions. The *triple-lumen catheter* has the same capabilities as the double-lumen catheter, but also allows monitoring of right atrial (central venous) pressure. The *four-lumen, flow-directed thermodilution catheter* has the same capabilities as double- and triple-lumen catheters but also allows evaluation of cardiac output.

The *five-lumen pulmonary catheter* (shown here) has the same capabilities as the other catheters but also allows atrial, ventricular, and atrioventricular sequential pacing. By performing the same functions that previously required two or more catheters, it helps reduce patient trauma and discomfort. The five-lumen pulmonary catheter is particularly effective in patients who require hemodynamic monitoring and temporary pacing, suffer acute MI with conduction defects, require cardiac surgery or override of atrial or ventricular dysrhythmias, or require diagnosis of complex dysrhythmias.

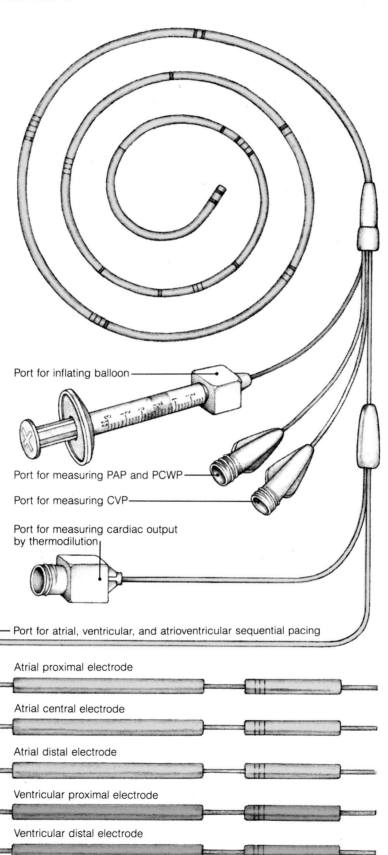

Port for inflating balloon

Port for measuring PAP and PCWP

Port for measuring CVP

Port for measuring cardiac output by thermodilution

Port for atrial, ventricular, and atrioventricular sequential pacing

Atrial proximal electrode

Atrial central electrode

Atrial distal electrode

Ventricular proximal electrode

Ventricular distal electrode

Interpreting hemodynamic waveforms

Right atrium

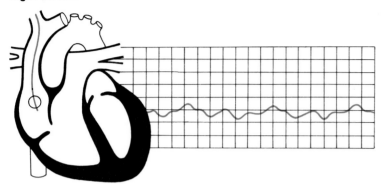

Normal Pressure
Mean: 1 to 6 mm Hg

Physiologic Significance
Right atrial (RA) pressures reflect mean RA diastolic (filling) pressure (equivalent to central venous pressure) and right ventricular (RV) end-diastolic pressure.

Clinical Implications
Increased RA pressure may signal RV failure, volume overload, tricuspid valve stenosis or regurgitation, constrictive pericarditis, or pulmonary hypertension.

Right ventricle

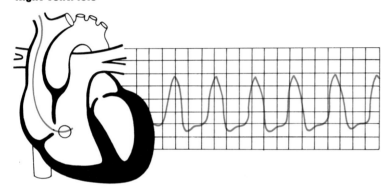

Normal Pressures
Systolic: 15 to 25 mm Hg
Diastolic: 0 to 8 mm Hg

Physiologic Significance
RV systolic pressure equals pulmonary artery systolic pressure; RV end-diastolic pressure reflects RV function and equals RA pressure.

Clinical Implications
RV pressures rise in mitral stenosis or insufficiency, pulmonary disease, hypoxemia, constrictive pericarditis, chronic congestive heart failure, atrial and ventricular septal defects, and patent ductus arteriosus.

Pulmonary artery

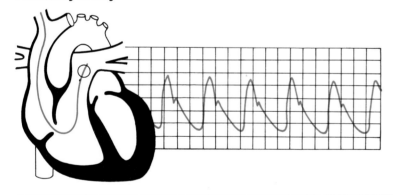

Normal Pressures
Systolic: 15 to 25 mm Hg
Diastolic: 8 to 15 mm Hg
Mean: 10 to 20 mm Hg

Physiologic Significance
Pulmonary artery pressure (PAP) reflects venous pressure in the lungs and mean filling pressure in the left atrium and left ventricle (if the mitral valve is normal), allowing detection of pulmonary congestion. PAP also reflects RV function since, in the absence of pulmonary stenosis, systolic PAP usually equals RV systolic pressure.

Clinical Implications
PAP rises in left ventricular (LV) failure, increased pulmonary blood flow (left or right shunting as in atrial or ventricular septal defects), and in any increase in pulmonary arteriolar resistance (as in pulmonary hypertension or mitral stenosis).

Pulmonary capillary wedge

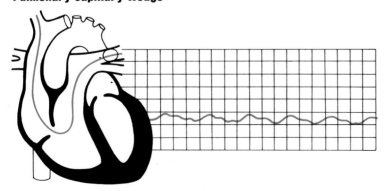

Normal Pressure
Mean: 5 to 12 mm Hg

Physiologic Significance
Pulmonary capillary wedge pressure (PCWP) accurately reflects both left atrial (LA) and LV pressures (if mitral stenosis is not present), because the heart momentarily relaxes during diastole as it fills with blood from pulmonary veins. At this instant, the pulmonary vasculature, left atrium, and left ventricle act as a single chamber with identical pressures. Thus, changes in PAP and PCWP reflect changes in LV filling pressure.

Clinical Implications
PCWP rises in LV failure, mitral stenosis or insufficiency, and pericardial tamponade. It decreases in hypovolemia.

decreased left ventricular filling pressure because of fluid depletion; increased systemic vascular resistance because of arteriosclerosis or hypertension; and impaired ejection of blood because of valvular heart disease. High cardiac output results from septic shock, some arteriovenous shunts, and anxiety. It may be normal in athletes.

Cardiac output relates to body surface area, which is determined from the patient's weight and height, using a nomogram. Dividing cardiac output by the figure obtained from the nomogram reveals the *cardiac index*. This index is useful because a small person requires less circulating blood and, thus, has a lower cardiac output than a large person.

CARDIAC CATHETERIZATION
In the past two decades, cardiac catheterization has become an important diagnostic tool in evaluating cardiac disease. Although you may be unfamiliar with this invasive test since it's performed in a cardiac catheterization laboratory, you're probably aware that post-test patient care requires prompt recognition of possible life-threatening complications (see *Complications of cardiac catheterization* on pages 48 and 49). Such complications occur more often in cardiac catheterization than in most other diagnostic tests. Nevertheless, technologic advances have lowered mortality associated with this test from 0.45% to 0.07% during the last 10 years in patients from 1 to 60 years old. High mortality persists in patients with pulmonary hypertension, dysrhythmias, hypoxia, severe coronary arteriosclerosis, and severe tetralogy of Fallot.

Cardiac catheterization of the right and left heart can detect and locate intracardiac problems (primarily heart valve and muscle insufficiency), provide intracardiac pressure measurements, and allow visualization of cardiac chambers. It's indicated for valvular and congenital heart disease, pulmonary hypertension, and ventricular aneurysm.

In right-heart catheterization, the catheter is inserted into an antecubital vein and, guided by fluoroscopy, advanced through the superior vena cava, right atrium, right ventricle, and, at times, into the pulmonary artery. Or it may be inserted into a femoral vein and advanced through the inferior vena cava.

In left-heart catheterization, the catheter is typically inserted into an antecubital artery or the femoral artery and advanced retrograde, through the aortic valve into the left ventricle. While the catheter is in the left ventricle, injection of a contrast medium permits radiographic visualization of the ventricle and filming (cineangiography) of heart activity. This test helps evaluate wall motion, valve function, and myocardial integrity.

Other procedures performed during cardiac catheterization include His bundle electrography, insertion of transvenous intracardiac pacing wires, and administration of drugs.

Coronary angiography
This test uses the same technique as left heart catheterization, but the catheter is advanced only as far as the coronary ostia (immediately superior to the aortic valve). Injection of a contrast medium through the catheter permits visualization of the coronary arteries. Coronary angiography is indicated for angina, acute myocardial infarction with recurrent chest pain, follow-up evaluation of coronary artery bypass graft surgery, and suspicious EKG findings in a patient responsible for others' lives, such as an aircraft pilot.

ECHOCARDIOGRAPHY
Unlike cardiac catheterization, echocardiography is a noninvasive, risk-free test, easily performed at a patient's bedside or on an outpatient basis. Increasingly, echocardiography is replacing cardiac catheterization in the diagnosis of valvular heart disease and evaluation of its severity. This test allows visualization and recording of size, shape, and behavior of the heart's internal structures, particularly the valves.

Echocardiography relies on the physical principles of pulsed reflected ultrasound. A special transducer placed at an acoustic window (an area where bone and lung tissue are absent) on the patient's chest directs ultrahigh-frequency sound waves toward cardiac structures, which reflect these waves. During the test, the patient may be asked to change positions and perform special breathing techniques to help direct the sound beams through the acoustic window. The same transducer receives the reflected waves and converts them into electrical signals that are displayed as bright dots on the oscilloscope and recorded on a strip chart or videotape.

The two most commonly used techniques are M-mode (motion-mode) and two-dimensional (cross-sectional) echocardiography. In M-mode echocardiography, a single, pencil-like ultrasound beam strikes the heart, producing an "ice-pick" view of cardiac structures. This technique records the motion of

Complications of cardiac catheterization

Left heart

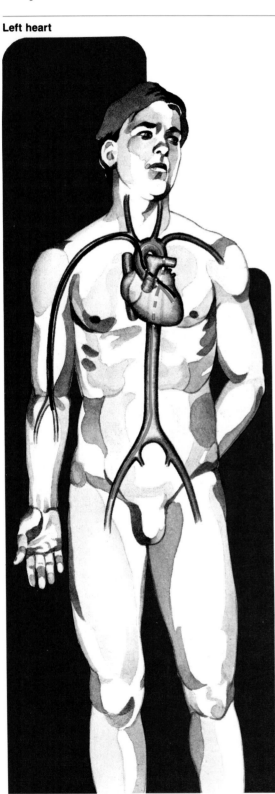

In left heart catheterization, the catheter is inserted into an antecubital artery, or it may be inserted into the femoral artery. Then the catheter is advanced retrograde through the ascending aorta, through the aortic valve, and into the left ventricle.

Cardiac catheterization imposes more patient risk than most other diagnostic tests. Although the incidence of such complications is low, they are potentially life-threatening. Cardiac catheterization requires careful observation during the procedure.

Keep in mind that some complications are common to *both* left heart and right heart catheterization; others result only from catheterization of one side. In either case, notify the doctor promptly and carefully document the complications and their treatment.

Left- or right-side catheterization

Complication	Signs and symptoms	Nursing considerations
Myocardial Infarction *Possible causes:* • Emotional stress induced by procedure • Plaque dislodged by catheter tip that travels to a coronary artery (left-side catheterization only)	• Chest pain, possibly radiating to left arm, back, and/or jaw • Cardiac dysrhythmias • Diaphoresis, restlessness, and/or anxiety • Thready pulse • Nausea and vomiting • Peripheral cyanosis, with cool, clammy skin	• Keep resuscitation equipment available. • Give oxygen or other drugs, as ordered. • Monitor patient continuously, as ordered.
Dysrhythmias *Possible cause:* • Cardiac tissue irritated by catheter	• Irregular heartbeat • Palpitations • Ventricular tachycardia	• Monitor patient continuously, as ordered. • Administer antiarrhythmic drugs, if ordered.
Cardiac tamponade *Possible cause:* • Perforation of heart wall by catheter	• Dysrhythmias • Tachycardia • Decreased blood pressure • Chest pain • Diaphoresis • Cyanosis • Distant heart sounds	• Give oxygen, if ordered. • Prepare patient for emergency surgery, if ordered. • Monitor patient continuously, as ordered.
Infection (systemic) *Possible causes:* • Poor aseptic technique • Catheter contaminated during manufacture, storage, or use	• Fever • Tachycardia • Chills and tremors • Unstable blood pressure	• Collect urine, sputum, and blood samples for culture, as ordered. • Monitor vital signs.
Hypovolemia *Possible cause:* • Diuresis from angiography contrast medium	• Hypotension • Tachycardia • Pallor • Diaphoresis	• Replace fluids by giving patient 1 or 2 glasses of water every hour, or maintain I.V. at a rate of 150 to 200 ml/hr, as ordered. • Monitor fluid intake and output closely. • Monitor vital signs.
Pulmonary edema *Possible cause:* • Excessive fluid administration	• Early stage: tachycardia, tachypnea, dependent rales, diastolic (S_3) gallop • Acute stage: dyspnea; rapid, noisy respirations; cough with frothy, blood-tinged sputum; cyanosis with cold, clammy skin; tachycardia; hypertension	• Administer oxygen and drugs (digitalis, diuretics, morphine), as ordered. • Restrict fluids and insert indwelling catheter. • Monitor the patient continuously, as ordered. • Maintain the patient's airway, and keep him in semi-Fowler position. • Keep resuscitation equipment available. • Apply rotating tourniquets, as ordered.

Complications of cardiac catheterization (continued)

Left- or right-side catheterization

Complication	Signs and symptoms	Nursing considerations
Hematoma or blood loss at insertion site *Possible cause:* • Bleeding at insertion site from vein or artery damage	• Bloody dressing • Limb swelling • Decreased blood pressure • Tachycardia	• Elevate limb, and apply direct manual pressure. • When bleeding stops, apply pressure bandage. If it continues, or if vital signs are unstable, notify doctor.
Reaction to contrast medium *Possible cause:* • Allergy to iodine	• Fever • Agitation • Hives, itching • Decreased urinary output	• Administer antihistamines to relieve itching, and diuretics to treat renal failure, as ordered. • Monitor fluid intake and output closely.
Infection at insertion site *Possible cause:* • Poor aseptic technique	• Swelling, warmth, redness, and soreness at site • Purulent discharge at site	• Obtain drainage sample for culture. Clean site; apply antimicrobial ointment, if ordered; cover the site with a sterile gauze pad. • Review and improve aseptic technique.

Left-side catheterization

Arterial embolus or thrombus in limb *Possible causes:* • Injury to artery during catheter insertion, causing blood clot • Plaque dislodged from artery wall by catheter	• Slow or faint pulse distal to insertion site • Loss of warmth, sensation, and color in arm or leg distal to insertion side • Sudden pain in extremity	• Notify doctor. He may perform an arteriotomy and Fogarty catheterization to remove embolus or thrombus. • Protect affected arm or leg from pressure. Keep it at room temperature, and at a level or slightly dependent position. • Administer a vasodilator to relieve painful vasospasm, if ordered.
Cerebrovascular accident (CVA) *Possible cause:* • Blood clot or plaque dislodged by catheter tip that travels to brain	• Hemiplegia • Aphasia • Lethargy • Confusion, or decreased level of consciousness	• Monitor vital signs closely. • Keep suctioning equipment nearby. • Administer oxygen, as ordered.

Right-side catheterization

Thrombophlebitis *Possible cause:* • Vein damaged during catheter insertion	• Vein is hard, sore, cord-like, and warm. Vein may look like a red line above catheter insertion site. • Swelling at site	• Elevate arm or leg; apply warm, wet compresses. • Administer anticoagulant or fibrinolytic drugs, if ordered.
Pulmonary embolism *Possible cause:* • Dislodged blood clot that travels to lungs	• Shortness of breath • Tachypnea • Tachycardia • Chest pain	• Place patient in high Fowler position. • Give oxygen and anticoagulants, if ordered. • Monitor vital signs.
Vagal response *Possible cause:* • Vagus nerve endings irritated in sinoatrial node, atrial muscle tissue, or atrioventricular junction	• Hypotension • Bradycardia • Nausea	• Monitor heart rate closely. • Administer atropine, if ordered. • Keep patient supine and quiet.

Right heart

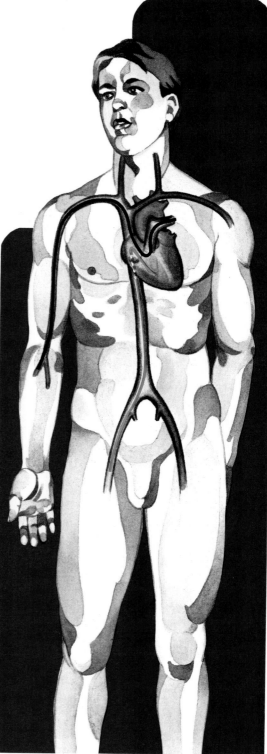

In right heart catheterization, the catheter is inserted into an antecubital vein and advanced through the superior vena cava (or if inserted into a femoral vein, through the inferior vena cava), right atrium, right ventricle, and into the pulmonary artery.

intracardiac structures. In two-dimensional echocardiography, an ultrasound beam rapidly sweeps through an arc, producing a cross-sectional or fan-shaped view of cardiac structures. This technique records lateral motion and shows correct spatial relationships among cardiac structures.

Interpreting the echocardiogram

Myocardial motion is influenced by contractility and other factors such as electrical conduction, relative diastolic volumes of the right and left ventricles, unloading during systole, and motion of adjacent segments.

Normally, the ventricular walls move closer together and thicken during systole. However, absent, reduced, or paradoxical wall motion may result from myocardial ischemia or infarction in the affected area. Thinning of the myocardial wall may indicate acute transmural ischemia that usually results from infarction, although absence of thinning doesn't rule out transmural infarction. Disproportionate thickening of the septum, compared to the posterior wall, indicates asymmetrical septal hypertrophy. Contraction of one ventricle before the other indicates ventricular conduction defects.

Scarred myocardium appears as thin, dense segments, with multiple, linear echoes replacing the speckled appearance of normal myocardium. Because scar tissue is an excellent sound reflector, its echoes are more intense (bright), resulting in a dense appearance. Multiple interfaces between scar and normal tissue cause the echoes to appear as bright dots within the myocardium (reflecting intermittent areas of intact myocardium).

NUCLEAR IMAGING STUDIES

Scientific advances in nuclear engineering, computers, and radiopharmaceuticals have widened the use of nuclear imaging tests. These tests provide information on myocardial metabolism, perfusion, viability, and function that may be otherwise unavailable—even by invasive techniques, which may be less safe, more costly, and less feasible for repeated use. Nuclear imaging tests involve intravenous injection of small amounts of a radioisotope, with minimal radiation exposure. Thus, these tests can be repeated, without harmful side effects, to follow the course of a disorder. The most commonly used nuclear imaging tests include thallium imaging (stress and nonstress), technetium pyrophosphate scanning, and cardiac blood pool imaging.

Thallium imaging

This test evaluates myocardial blood flow and the status of myocardial cells after the I.V. injection of the radioisotope thallium-201. Thallium concentrates in healthy myocardial tissue. Hence, areas with normal blood supply and intact cells rapidly take up the isotope, while necrotic or ischemic tissue doesn't and appears as cold spots on a scan. Cold spots may also result from sarcoidosis, myocardial fibrosis, cardiac contusion, apical clefts, coronary spasm, and artifacts (for example, from breast implants and electrodes). In certain patients with coronary artery disease, this test may fail to show cold spots because the obstruction is very small or because of inadequate stress (in stress imaging), delayed imaging, single-vessel disease (particularly the right or left circumflex coronary arteries), or extensive collateral circulation.

Thallium imaging is performed at rest or after treadmill exercise. The latter form helps evaluate chest pain or questionable cardiac symptoms in a patient who is otherwise difficult to evaluate. For example, stress thallium imaging may show a poor myocardial uptake even though resting imaging demonstrates adequate perfusion. Both tests are used to assess myocardial scarring and perfusion; to detect the location and extent of acute or chronic MI (they do not distinguish an old from a new infarction); to diagnose coronary artery disease; to evaluate the patency of grafts after coronary artery bypass surgery; and to evaluate antianginal therapy or balloon angioplasty.

Technetium pyrophosphate scanning

In contrast to thallium imaging, this test reveals damaged myocardial tissue as hot spots—areas where the radioisotope technetium-99m pyrophosphate accumulates after I.V. injection. In this test, the radioisotope accumulates in damaged myocardial tissue (possibly by combining with calcium in the damaged myocardial cells), where it forms a hot spot on a scan made with a scintillation camera. The test helps detect acute MI and define its location and size, but does not show an old infarction. It allows diagnosis of acute MI when EKG changes or cardiac enzyme tests are inconclusive, or when the location or size of an infarct is questionable.

Cardiac blood pool imaging

This test evaluates regional and global ventricular performance after I.V. injection of red

Additional diagnostic tests

Test	Definition	Diagnostic objectives
Cardiac series	Fluoroscopic visualization of the motion and pulsations of the heart and great vessels during systole and diastole; largely superseded by echocardiography for most diagnostic purposes	To assess structural abnormalities of the heart chambers To detect aortic and mitral valve calcification To evaluate prosthetic valve function To detect abnormalities of the aortic arch and esophageal contours
Lower limb venography (ascending contrast phlebography)	Fluoroscopic visualization of the veins after injection of a contrast medium	To confirm deep vein thrombosis (DVT) To identify the cause of dependent edema To assess vascular status before surgery
Doppler ultrasonography	Transmission of ultrahigh-frequency sound waves through the skin to an artery or vein, which reflects these waves at frequencies that correspond with the velocity of blood flow through the vessel; developed as an alternative to arteriography and venography	To help detect DVT, peripheral arterial aneurysms, and carotid arterial occlusive disease To monitor the patient with arterial reconstruction or bypass graft
Phonocardiography	Graphic recording of the normal and abnormal sounds of the cardiac cycle—gallops, murmurs, and other heart sounds—and the vibrations of the great vessels	To help identify structural valve defects To aid the precise timing of cardiac events To evaluate ventricular function by demonstrating systolic time intervals
Apexcardiography	Graphic recording of chest wall movement caused by low-frequency precordial cardiac pulsations	To help evaluate left ventricular function To help identify heart sounds
Vectorcardiography	Graphic recording of variations in electrical potential during the cardiac cycle, using two simultaneously recorded lead axes to construct a three-dimensional view of the heart; more commonly used in research than in a clinical setting	To detect ventricular hypertrophy, interventricular conduction disturbances, and MI To clarify doubtful EKG results
Carotid pulse tracing	Graphic recording of low-frequency carotid artery vibrations, which reflect pressure changes on the heart's left side during systole and diastole	To help identify aortic valve disease, idiopathic hypertrophic subaortic stenosis, left ventricular failure, and hypertension
Jugular pulse tracing	Graphic recording of low-frequency jugular vein vibrations, which reflect pressure changes on the heart's right side during systole and diastole	To aid diagnosis of right heart failure
Impedance plethysmography (occlusive impedance phlebography)	Graphic recording of changes in electrical resistance (impedance) caused by variations in circulating blood volume—the result of respiration or venous occlusion	To help detect DVT, especially in the popliteal and iliofemoral veins
Cold stimulation test	Recording of color changes in the patient's fingers before and after their submersion in ice water	To help detect Raynaud's syndrome

NMR and DSA: Two promising tests

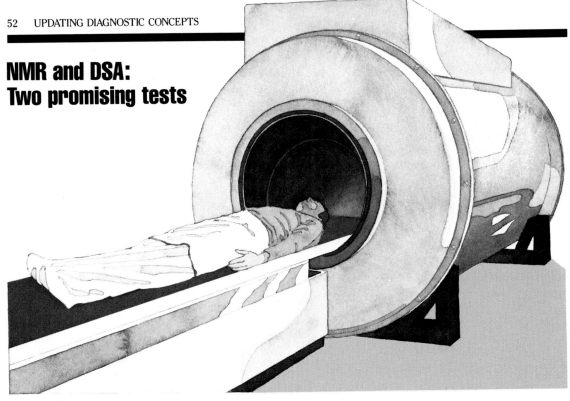

Nuclear magnetic resonance (NMR) and digital subtraction angiography (DSA) may represent major technologic advances in diagnostic testing. Both tests use the computer to produce detailed images of body tissues for evaluating various disorders.

Nuclear magnetic resonance

NMR is a noninvasive imaging technique that detects structural and biochemical abnormalities by directing magnetic and radio waves at body tissues to determine the nuclear response of a test element—chiefly, hydrogen or phosphorus. The technique relies on the natural magnetic properties of certain atoms in the body. Of course, particles that form any atom spin with an electrical charge, and this moving charge creates a magnetic field. Hence, the particles act as tiny magnets. Some NMR studies, called proton NMR, focus on hydrogen protons because of their abundance in the body. These hydrogen protons align themselves within the external magnetic field created by the NMR magnet. Then, for a brief period, the protons are bombarded with radio-frequency signals that deflect them from their induced alignment. When the radio signals stop, the energized protons emit a return signal. The NMR computer analyzes this signal, which varies according to the tissue concentrations of the test element, and the time it takes the protons to return to their original alignment. These "relaxation" times differ for each type of body tissue, but are sometimes prolonged for malignant tissue.

NMR provides greater tissue discrimination than computerized tomography scanning without the risk of ionizing radiation, and may permit safe serial studies of children and pregnant women. However, the NMR magnet affects pacemaker function.

Although use of NMR in cardiovascular testing is still evolving, the procedure may allow visualization of blood flow, cardiac chambers, the interventricular septum, and valvular areas; and detection of vascular lesions, plaque formations, infarctions, tumors, and blood clots. In addition, phosphorus NMR may aid diagnosis of peripheral vascular disease. Soon, in fact, NMR may be able to provide *in vivo* information about cellular processes.

Digital subtraction angiography

DSA is a type of intravenous arteriography. It combines X-ray detection methods and a computerized subtraction technique with fluoroscopy for real-time visualization of the cardiovascular system without interference from adjacent structures, such as bone or soft tissue.

A radiologist injects contrast medium through a catheter threaded into the superior vena cava. As the contrast medium circulates through the arteries, serial X-rays are taken. A computer then "subtracts" structures that block a clear view of the arteries, and projects the enhanced image onto a screen.

DSA is currently used to visualize cerebral blood flow and to detect vascular abnormalities (plaques, tumors, aneurysms), pulmonary embolism, and renal arterial stenosis. The test also permits visualization of arterial bypass grafts and detection of peripheral artery disease. Dynamic studies of heart function are underway, but so far DSA's effectiveness in the study of coronary arteries has been limited by heart-wall motion.

Although DSA doesn't give as sharp an image as coronary arteriography or permit contrast filling of a single artery, the test is considered safer than arteriography. It uses less contrast medium for large vessels, and this medium is injected into a vein, thereby eliminating the risks of arterial puncture. Also, DSA can be performed quickly—on an outpatient basis.

blood cells tagged with the isotope technetium-99m (^{99m}Tc) pertechnetate. In first-pass imaging, a scintillation camera records the radioactivity emitted by the isotope in its initial pass through the left ventricle. Higher counts of radioactivity occur during diastole when there is more blood in the ventricle; lower counts occur during systole as the blood is ejected. The portion of isotope ejected during each heartbeat can then be calculated to determine the ejection fraction. The presence and size of intracardiac shunts can also be determined.

Gated cardiac blood pool imaging, performed after first-pass imaging or as a separate test, has several forms; most use EKG signals to trigger the scintillation camera. In multiple-gated acquisition (MUGA) scanning, the camera records 14 to 64 points of a single cardiac cycle, yielding sequential images that can be studied like motion picture films to evaluate regional wall motion and determine the ejection fraction and other indices of cardiac function. Two representative frames can be selected to allow assessment of left ventricular contraction for areas of dyskinesia or akinesia. In the stress MUGA test, the same test is performed at rest and after exercise to detect changes in ejection fraction and cardiac output. In the nitro MUGA test, the scintillation camera records points in the cardiac cycle after the sublingual administration of nitroglycerin, to assess its effect on ventricular function.

ELECTROPHYSIOLOGIC STUDIES

In electrophysiologic studies (EPS), programmed electrical stimulation (PES) of the heart allows immediate evaluation of conduction abnormalities, and supraventricular and ventricular dysrhythmias by inducing dysrhythmias in a patient with an incapacitating or potentially life-threatening dysrhythmia. Consequently, EPS permits prompt, accurate decisions about therapy for intermittent dysrhythmias without delay for Holter monitor reports or long-term patient follow-up.

Since EPS is invasive and can stimulate possibly lethal dysrhythmias, its use is controversial. However, its proponents argue that its risk is no greater than that of cardiac catheterization, since the test is performed under strictly controlled conditions and immediate treatment is available for any adverse effect. Later complications of EPS may include thromboembolism and infection. A rare but potentially fatal complication is perforation of the heart by the pacing electrode, which may cause pericardial effusion and tamponade.

EPS involves insertion of a multipolar electrode catheter into the femoral vein. The catheter is advanced until one electrode rests in the high right atrium, one adjacent to the bundle of His, and one in the right ventricle. An additional electrode may be placed in the coronary sinus if preexcitation syndromes (such as Wolff-Parkinson-White or Lown-Ganong-Levine) are to be evaluated.

During EPS, the conduction time can be measured from the low right atrium through the node to the His bundle (AH interval) and from the proximal His bundle to the ventricular myocardium (HV interval). Dysrhythmias can be evaluated by pacing the heart and measuring conduction times and refractory periods (the response of cardiac tissue to premature stimulus).

Myocardial mapping, a refinement of EPS, helps determine the site of tachycardia. For the patient with refractory ventricular tachycardia, endocardial, intramural, and epicardial mapping allow consideration of surgical excision of the irritable focus. A His bundle electrogram can help evaluate disturbances in the atrioventricular conduction system. Important for both supraventricular and ventricular tachycardias, this evaluation determines if the dysrhythmia is related to an automaticity mechanism (spontaneous diastolic depolarization of cells) or a reentry mechanism involving the combination of dual pathways, unidirectional block, and slowed conduction.

A final word

Diagnosis of many cardiovascular disorders can be accomplished by thorough analysis of the patient history, and results of the physical exam, and through interpretation of the EKG and chest X-ray findings. However, diagnosis and monitoring of the patient with an unstable, complex cardiac disorder can require the use of additional, specialized techniques, such as cardiac catheterization, hemodynamic monitoring, and echocardiography, to supplement routine assessment. Two new specialized tests—nuclear magnetic resonance (NMR) and digital subtraction angiography (DSA)—show promise and may soon become better known as part of cardiovascular evaluation.

Reviewing the whole range of diagnostic tests can help improve your nursing management skills by deepening your understanding of cardiovascular disorders and their characteristic effects.

Points to remember

• Technologic development and medical research in cardiovascular diagnostic testing has resulted in better equipment and techniques for safer invasive procedures, such as hemodynamic monitoring, cardiac catheterization, and electrophysiologic studies.
• Alternatives to invasive procedures are also available. These include such tests as echocardiography and, soon, nuclear magnetic resonance scanning.
• Improved computer capabilities provide more effective monitoring and imaging techniques in tests such as continuous ambulatory electrocardiography, cardiac monitoring, hemodynamic monitoring, nuclear imaging studies, and digital subtraction angiograpy.
• With these advances, more reliable and precise diagnosis and treatment of cardiovascular disorders are possible.

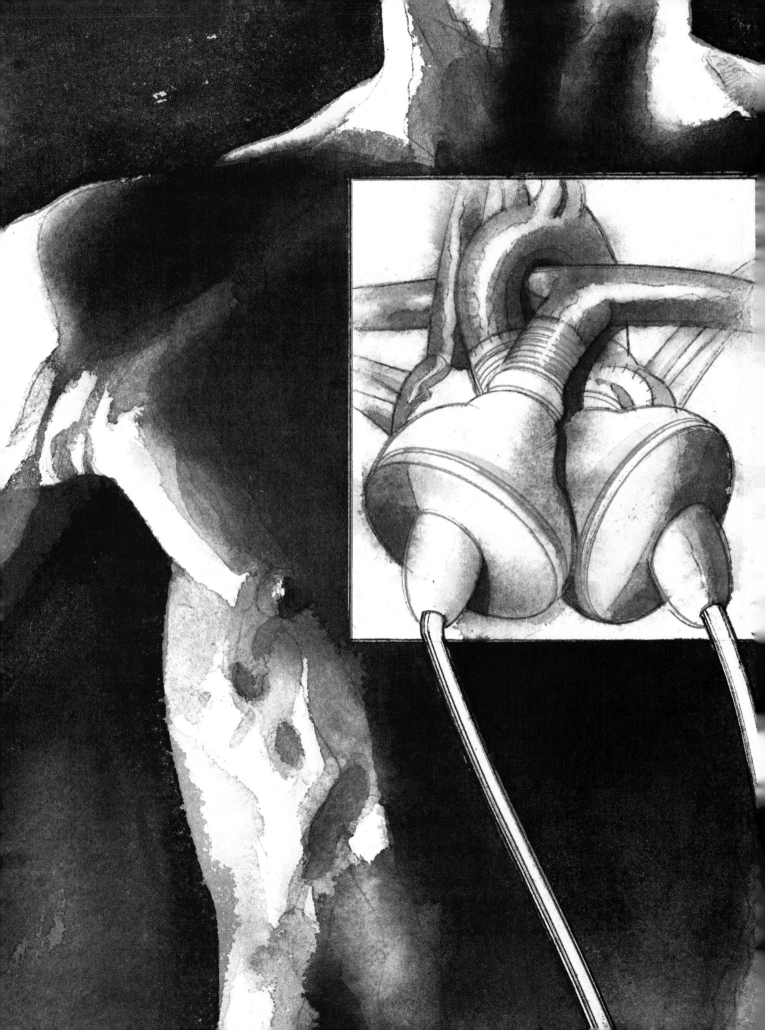

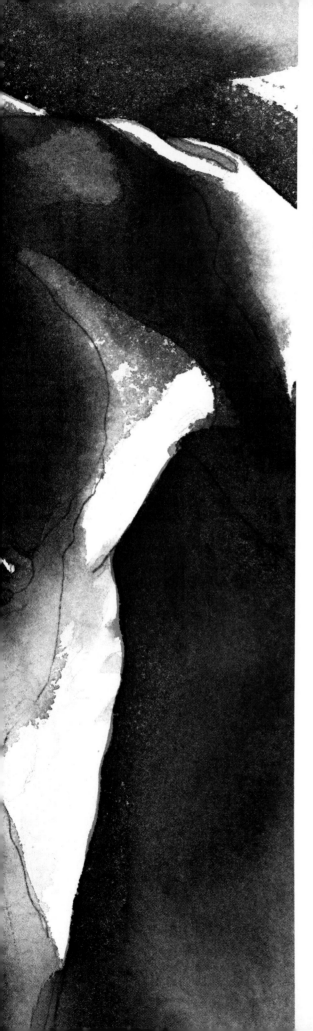

DISORDERS OF CIRCULATION AND PUMP FAILURE

4 CONTROLLING HYPERTENSION

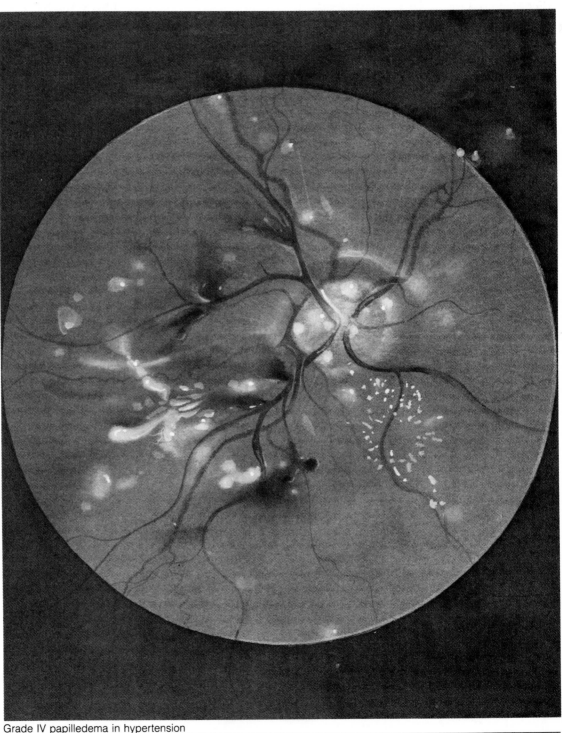

Grade IV papilledema in hypertension

f you're familiar with the latest epidemiologic studies, you know there's a lot of good news about hypertension. The good news is that more people are aware of hypertension, more people know what to do about it, and more people are sticking with the appropriate treatment. Many are benefiting from the stepped-care treatment regimen and from new drugs, including beta blockers. More importantly, continued effective treatment has contributed to a rapidly declining rate of cardiovascular deaths related to hypertension. In addition, the percentage of persons with uncontrolled hypertension is decreasing. Recent decreases in morbidity and mortality are largely the direct results of a massive educational campaign launched in 1972 by the National High Blood Pressure Education Program, the American Heart Association, and other health agencies to enlighten the public and health professionals about hypertension.

The bad news

The bad news is that hypertension is still a massive community health problem. This has become apparent as we have come to know the damaging effects of blood pressures previously considered harmless. Long-term epidemiologic studies now disclose higher-than-normal death rates among people with only slightly elevated blood pressures. In fact, a diastolic reading of 80 to 89 mm Hg *doubles* the normal risk of death from cardiovascular disease. Because some individuals with diastolic blood pressures in this intermediate range go on to develop hypertension, the National Institutes of Health (NIH) is considering recommending frequent blood pressure checks for those with diastolic pressures between 80 and 90 mm Hg.

The 1980 Report of the Joint National Committee on Detection, Evaluation, and Treatment of High Blood Pressure defines hypertension as a diastolic pressure of > 90 mm Hg, measured on at least two occasions—in other words, a *sustained* elevation of diastolic pressure. Several large national surveys indicate that high blood pressure is extremely common. According to the current estimates, 60 million people need clinical support and direction in an active antihypertensive program.

It also means you'll be more involved in patient education and will care for more patients receiving nonpharmacologic and pharmacologic therapy for mild hypertension. More than ever, you need to understand hypertension and how to deal with its variant forms and stages.

Varying stages of hypertension

Hypertension can be classified as primary or secondary. Primary hypertension (also called idiopathic or essential) exists in roughly 90% to 95% of patients, in whom no cause is discernible. Secondary hypertension affects the remaining 5% to 10% of those with the disease. Hypertension, whether primary or secondary, is classified as to severity based on the average of three or more diastolic blood pressure readings taken at rest, several days apart. The degrees of severity are:
Class I (mild) 90 to 104 mm Hg
Class II (moderate) 105 to 114 mm Hg
Class III (severe) 115 mm Hg.
Common usage calls the hypertension in the first category mild. However, even at this lowest level, the risk of cardiovascular sequelae is at least twice that of normotensive persons.

Severe hypertension is further classified as either accelerated or malignant. Accelerated hypertension means the patient's blood pressure has risen to severely elevated levels in a short time. The patient with accelerated hypertension may have Grade III retinopathy (retinal exudates and hemorrhages) and a high diastolic pressure—usually above 120 mm Hg. Malignant hypertension means the patient has Grade IV retinopathy (papilledema, or swelling around the optic disk) and an even higher diastolic pressure—usually above 140 mm Hg.

The severest form of hypertension—hypertensive crisis—occurs when elevated blood pressure causes an immediate threat to the patient's life by compromising cerebral, cardiovascular, or renal function. Hypertensive crisis is not tied to a particular blood pressure level but is based on the patient's total clinical status.

You may also hear hypertension described as labile and resistant. Hypertension is termed *labile* when blood pressure elevations occur intermittently; it's termed *resistant* when it's unresponsive to usual treatment.

What causes hypertension

No single cause of primary hypertension is identifiable, although researchers continue to study various possible causes. Primary hypertension probably reflects an interaction of multiple homeostatic forces, including changes in renal regulation of sodium and extracellu-

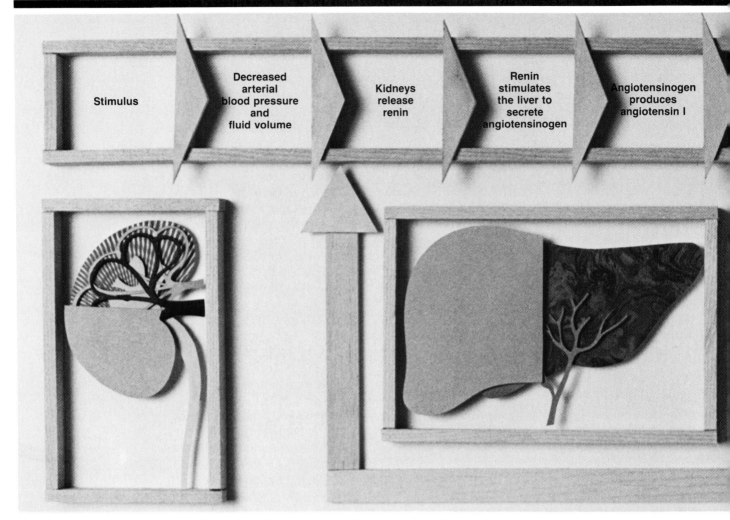

Stimulus

Decreased arterial blood pressure and fluid volume

Kidneys release renin

Renin stimulates the liver to secrete angiotensinogen

Angiotensinogen produces angiotensin I

Renin-angiotensin-aldosterone system

This feedback system aims to correct decreased arterial blood pressure and fluid volume. If this system fails to function properly, hypertension may result.

lar fluids, in aldosterone secretion and metabolism, and in norepinephrine secretion and metabolism.

In people with secondary hypertension, elevated blood pressure results from other abnormalities, notably those of renal function (the most common cause) or cardiovascular, endocrine, or neurologic function. Renovascular hypertension results from decreased renal perfusion, which, in turn, probably results from congenital abnormality, atherosclerosis, or fibroplasia of the renal artery. The resulting renal ischemia stimulates the renin-angiotensin-aldosterone mechanism—surely an integral part of renovascular hypertension. However, because some patients with renal hypertension don't show elevated renin levels, other mechanisms must also act to produce secondary hypertension.

Why blood pressure varies
Blood pressure is the relationship between the volume and flow of circulating fluid (the blood) and its container (the blood vessels). Systolic blood pressure is the pressure exerted within the blood vessels during ventricular

systole (contraction); diastolic blood pressure is the pressure exerted within the vessels during ventricular diastole (at rest).

The variables regulating blood pressure include interactions among several mechanisms: neural (baroreceptors and chemoreceptor); hormonal (norepinephrine, epinephrine, and their effects on alpha and beta receptors; renin-angiotensin-aldosterone activation; hypothalamic secretion of antidiuretic hormone and its release by the posterior pituitary; and secretion of prostaglandins); and physical effects of capillary fluid shift at the cellular level.

PATHOPHYSIOLOGY
In its early stages—often marked by intermittent (labile) elevations of blood pressure—primary hypertension generally causes no changes in vital organs and no symptoms. However, after prolonged elevation of blood pressure, pathologic changes begin in the entire vascular system and in the vital organs it serves—specifically the heart, kidneys, and brain. As hypertension becomes chronic, the large vessels (such as the aorta, coronary

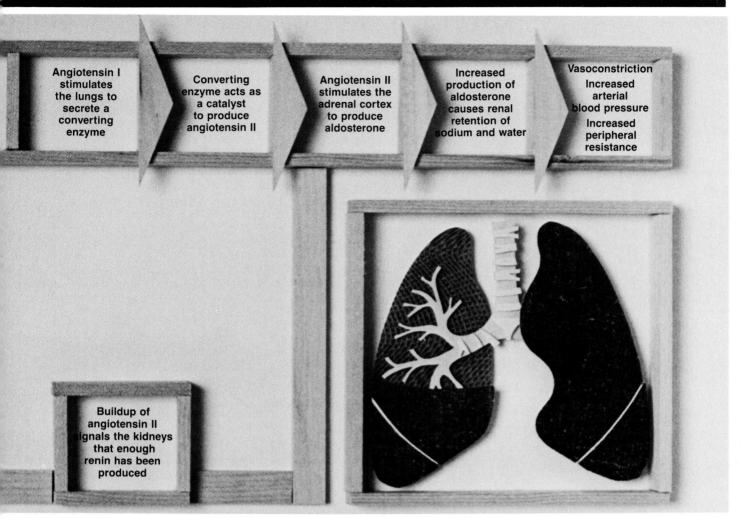

Angiotensin I stimulates the lungs to secrete a converting enzyme

Converting enzyme acts as a catalyst to produce angiotensin II

Angiotensin II stimulates the adrenal cortex to produce aldosterone

Increased production of aldosterone causes renal retention of sodium and water

Vasoconstriction
Increased arterial blood pressure
Increased peripheral resistance

Buildup of angiotensin II signals the kidneys that enough renin has been produced

arteries, basilar artery to the brain, and peripheral vessels) become sclerosed and tortuous; their constricted lumens deliver decreasing amounts of blood to the heart, brain, and legs. Continuing vascular damage may eventually lead to complete occlusion or rupture of large vessels.

The effects of persistent hypertension are no less devastating in the small vessels, causing additional structural abnormalities within the vital organs. Specifically, severely elevated diastolic pressure damages the intimal layer of the small vessels (see page 61), causing accumulation of fibrin, local edema, and, possibly, intravascular clotting. Eventually, these damaging changes diminish cardiac, cerebral, and renal perfusion, causing progressive dysfunction of these most vulnerable vital organs.

Effects on target organs
As diminishing renal perfusion decreases blood supply to the nephrons, the kidney loses some ability to concentrate and form normal urine. This may show in rising levels of blood urea nitrogen (BUN) and serum creatinine and in nocturia. As renal vessels develop

structural abnormalities, they become more permeable and allow leakage of protein into the renal tubules, causing proteinuria in some patients. Renal function can deteriorate to the point of frank renal insufficiency and uremia. The latter is an ominous sign and a hallmark of malignant hypertension.

In the brain, sustained hypertension causes progressive cerebral arteriosclerosis and ischemia, often resulting in small strokes or transient ischemic attacks (TIAs).

The progressive vascular damage resulting from hypertension has devastating effects on the heart. It causes people with hypertension to develop coronary artery disease at two to three times the rate of those with normal blood pressure. As hypertension causes medial hypertrophy, edema, and accelerated arteriosclerosis, coronary perfusion diminishes. These changes may lead to angina, myocardial infarction, or more often, congestive heart failure. This is so because increased aortic pressure causes the left ventricle to increase the force of contractions and thus to increase stroke volume. Sustaining this extra effort over a long time, the left ventricle eventually

Characteristics of secondary hypertension

Cause	Mechanism of hypertension	Symptoms
Renovascular hypertension	Narrowing of renal artery due to atherosclerosis, fibrosis of wall of renal artery, or trauma to renal area	Hypertension; fluid retention with edema
Renal parenchymatous disease (acute and chronic glomerulonephritis)	Immune response to infection in body (usually streptococcal), causing inflammatory changes in glomeruli	Hypertension; sodium and water retention; proteinuria edema; oliguria; orthopnea; dyspnea; pulmonary edema; uremic odor
Coarctation of aorta	Constriction of portion of aorta causes elevated blood pressure proximal to obstruction	Absent or diminished femoral pulses; decreased blood pressure in legs as compared to arms; weight loss
Pheochromocytoma	Adrenal medullary tumor causes excessive secretion of catecholamines	Persistent or intermittent hypertension; sudden attacks of severe headache with palpitation (in 50% of patients); hypermetabolic state; excessive sweating; heat intolerance; flushed, anxious appearance
Primary aldosteronism	Functioning adrenocortical adenoma	Moderate elevation of blood pressure; muscular weakness; polyuria; nocturia; polydipsia; tetany; paresthesia; headache
Cushing syndrome	Excess glycocorticosteroids excreted from adrenal cortex; cause may be adrenocortical adenoma (or carcinoma) or adrenocortical hyperplasia	Mild hypertension; moon facies; "buffalo" hump on back; edema; hirsutism

hypertrophies—leading to congestive heart failure. Of course, certain risk factors (such as smoking and hyperlipidemia) also influence the risk of cardiovascular disease and the cardiac outcome.

Retina: Index of severity
Because the retina is the only site where arteries are visible without invasive examination techniques, its condition reliably indicates the severity of hypertension. Evidence of blood vessel damage in the retina indicates similar damage elsewhere in the vascular system.

MEDICAL MANAGEMENT
Because mild or moderately severe hypertension usually causes no symptoms, measuring the blood pressure is the only way to detect it. But the blood pressure alone doesn't tell the whole story. The normal circadian fluctuations in blood pressure do not allow an accurate diagnosis of hypertension from a single reading. The range of normal fluctuation is such that the highest daytime diastolic pressure can exceed the nighttime systolic pressure. And, as you know, apprehension, pain, or preexisting illness can significantly raise

blood pressure. For these reasons, therapy for Class I or Class II hypertension should begin only after *sustained* elevation is confirmed by at least three readings (on different occasions).

Besides verifying persistent elevation of blood pressure, evaluation for hypertension must determine whether the cause is curable and assess damage, if any.

Because fewer than 10% of all adult cases of hypertension are related to a secondary cause, an exhaustive search is usually unwarranted—except in patients who:
• are under age 35 and have moderate or severe hypertension
• fail to respond to antihypertensive drug therapy
• have a history, physical examination, or initial laboratory findings that suggest secondary causes
• show acceleration of previously well-controlled hypertension
• have accelerated or malignant hypertension.

For most hypertensive patients, medical evaluation should include careful history and analysis of other risk factors; urinalysis and evaluation of urine protein levels to rule out

Vascular damage in hypertension

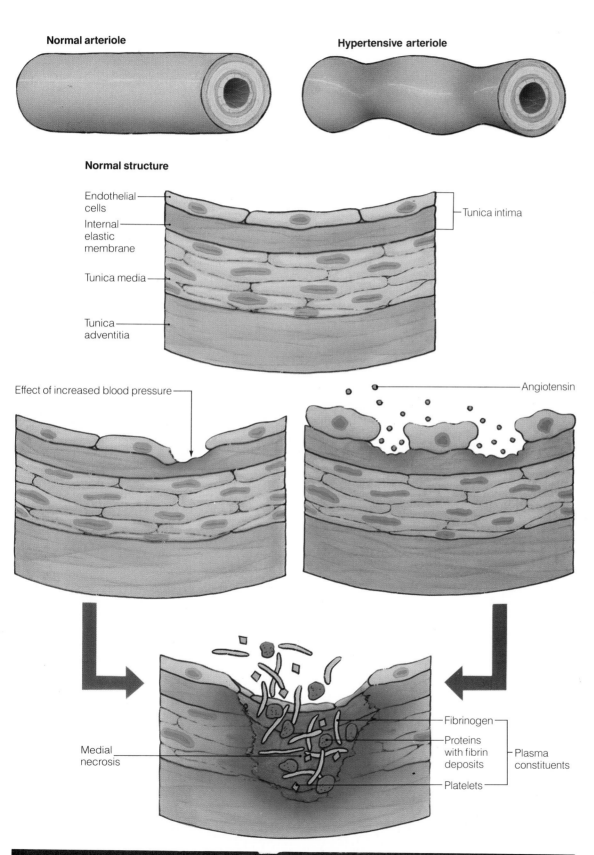

Normal arteriole

Hypertensive arteriole

Normal structure

Endothelial cells

Internal elastic membrane

Tunica media

Tunica adventitia

Tunica intima

Effect of increased blood pressure

Angiotensin

Medial necrosis

Fibrinogen

Proteins with fibrin deposits

Platelets

Plasma constituents

Sustained elevation of blood pressure causes pathologic changes in the entire vascular system. Vascular injury begins with alternating areas of dilation and constriction in the arterioles. Increased intraarterial pressure damages the endothelium. Independently, angiotensin induces contraction of endothelial walls, allowing plasma to leak through interendothelial spaces. Eventually, deposition of plasma constituents in the vessel wall causes medial necrosis. Hypertensive vascular disease may progress to occlusion, aneurysm, or rupture of large vessels.

Pathophysiology of chronic hypertension

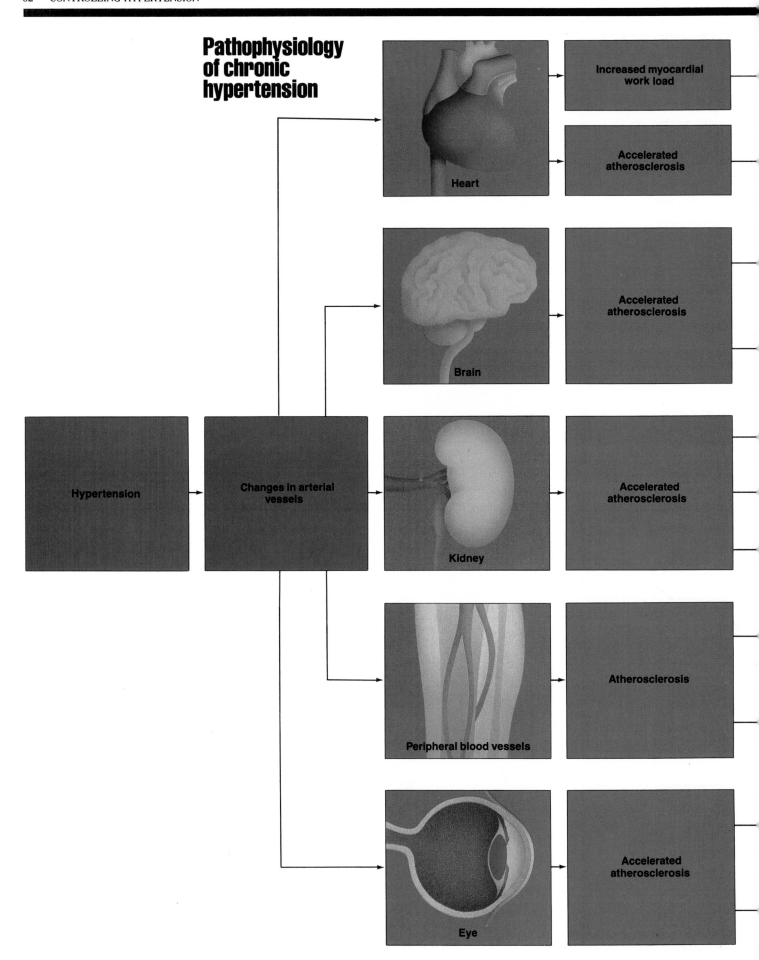

Hypertension

Changes in arterial vessels

Heart

Increased myocardial work load

Accelerated atherosclerosis

Brain

Accelerated atherosclerosis

Kidney

Accelerated atherosclerosis

Peripheral blood vessels

Atherosclerosis

Eye

Accelerated atherosclerosis

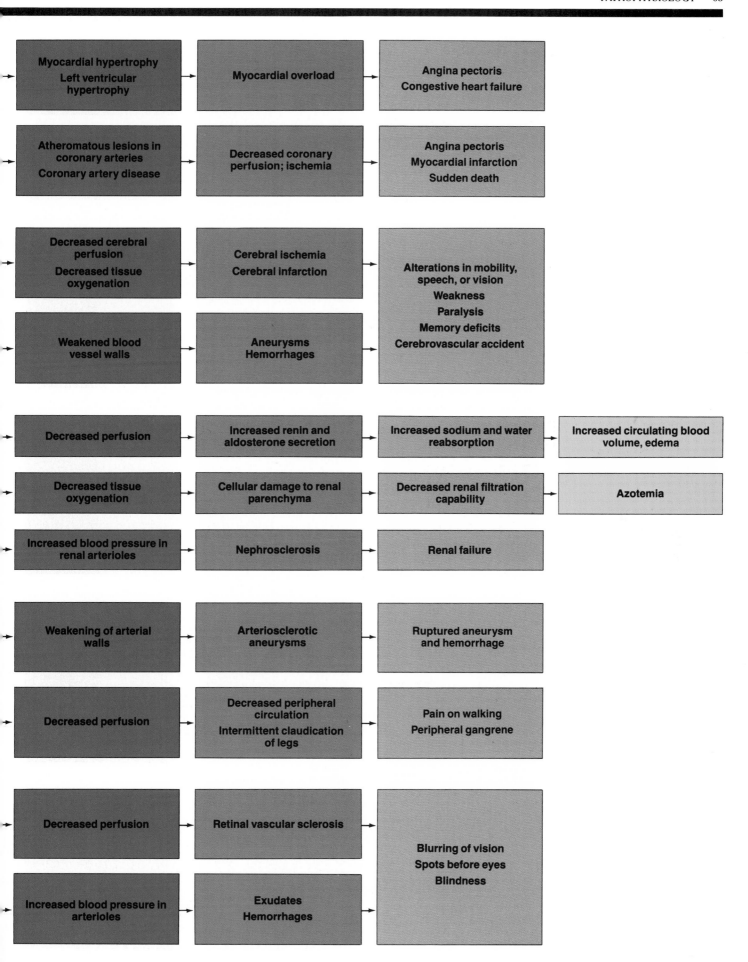

Retinal changes in hypertension

Normal

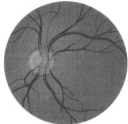

Because the retina is the only site where arteries are visible without invasive techniques, examination of the eyegrounds reliably indicates severity of hypertension. Evidence of blood vessel damage in the retina reliably indicates similar damage elsewhere in the vascular system.

The most commonly used system for grading the retinal effects of hypertensive vascular disease is the Keith, Wagener, and Barker (KWB) method, shown at right.

Grade I: Mild sclerosis or mild narrowing of the arterioles. This retinal change is associated with mild elevation of blood pressure.

Grade II

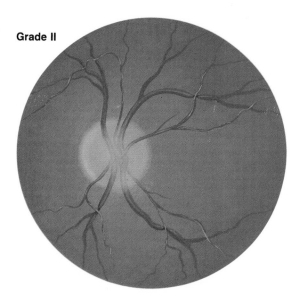

Grade III: Angiospastic retinitis with sclerotic changes in the arterioles, possibly with edema. This condition indicates severe and sustained hypertension that may be associated with the following evidence of cardiac and renal complications: dyspnea on exertion, EKG changes, nocturia, proteinuria, hematuria, headache, and vertigo.

Grade IV

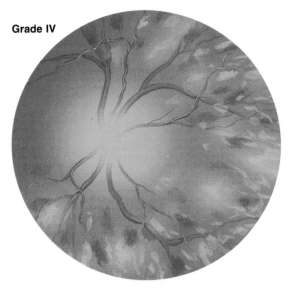

Grade I

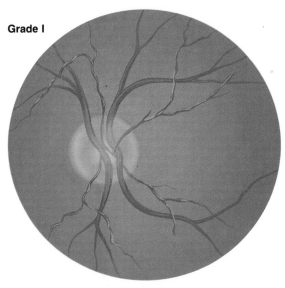

Grade II: Marked retinal changes with increased light reflexes and compression of veins at crossings. These changes indicate progressive and sustained hypertension, but are not associated with overt cardiac or renal complications.

Grade III

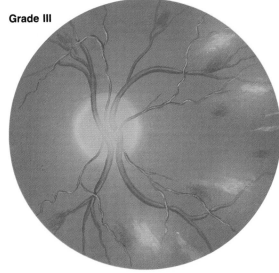

Grade IV: Papilledema with exudates and extensive hemorrhages. The characteristic retinal change is edema of the discs associated with severe narrowing of the arterioles and diffuse retinitis. This condition indicates malignant hypertension associated with marked renal and cardiac complications.

renal disease (protein excretion in the urine measured over a 24-hour period shouldn't total more than 0.2 to 0.4 g); serum analyses to determine impact on target organs—including BUN, serum creatinine, and serum electrolytes (especially potassium, which inversely denotes secretion of aldosterone); and establishment of baseline data for later evaluation of drug therapy. Medical evaluation should also include a chest X-ray to show cardiac size and pulmonary vasculature and an EKG to check for left ventricular hypertrophy and ischemia. Of course, the special diagnostic tests performed depend on the individual patient's age, health history, severity and duration of the hypertension, and probability of a secondary cause.

As the severity of hypertension progresses, overt clinical signs—as evidenced by organ involvement—aid medical diagnosis. For example, dyspnea, orthopnea, or chest pain in a person with sustained hypertension often points clearly to cardiovascular dysfunction. Leg edema suggests failure of venous return, probably from right-sided heart decompensation. Auscultation of heart sounds is likely to reveal S_4 and S_3. S_4 (atrial gallop) results from the rigorous left atrial contraction needed to eject blood into an already hypertrophied left ventricle. S_3 (ventricular gallop) indicates rapid filling of a dilated and incompetent ventricle.

Sustained hypertension rarely causes obvious signs of cerebral involvement. However, in advanced stages, such as hypertensive crisis, cerebral involvement may escalate to the classic signs and symptoms of encephalopathy: headache, nausea, vomiting, blurred vision, drowsiness, confusion, fleeting numbness or tingling in the limbs, convulsions, and coma. Because these same signs can also point to cerebrovascular accident (CVA), distinguishing between them is important, but not always possible. It's helpful to remember that CVA sometimes shows focal or lateral neurologic signs. Also, in CVA the neurologic deficits (such as one-sided weakness or paralysis) are progressive. In contrast, hypertensive encephalopathy often comes on suddenly and unexpectedly.

Current therapy
The overall goal of therapy is to minimize the patient's risk of end organ damage. The specific goal is to achieve and maintain diastolic blood pressure below 90 mm Hg or the lowest possible level above that without causing adverse effects. Additional goals of therapy are promoting long-term compliance and ensuring that the complications and expense of therapy do not outweigh its benefits.

In persons with mild hypertension, conservative management aims to reduce the risk of hypertensive heart disease by changing the life-style to reduce risk factors. Such management controls risk factors by emphasizing weight reduction, salt and cholesterol restriction, an exercise program, and efforts to reduce smoking and stress. If these measures fail to reduce blood pressure after 6 months and if one or more unmodifiable risk factors are present, the patient should probably receive drug therapy.

Drug therapy controls hypertension in two fundamental ways: by using renal control mechanisms to initially induce diuresis and lower total body sodium levels, and by influencing neural control mechanisms with large doses of adrenergic blockers. (See appendix for summary of antihypertensive drugs.)

The *stepped-care* approach is a simplified practical scheme for the medical management of hypertension (see *Understanding stepped-care,* page 66). It is recommended by The Joint National Committee on Detection, Evaluation and Treatment of High Blood Pressure. The stepped-care approach uses small doses of the fewest possible drugs.

Severe hypertension always requires vigorous drug therapy, usually with oral drugs. However, if the blood pressure reading and clinical signs confirm *hypertensive crisis,* such therapy requires parenteral administration to quickly lower blood pressure from life-threatening levels and then slowly restore it to normal range. Usually, a potent antihypertensive drug is administered by intravenous infusion and titrated according to the patient's response. However, some doctors now combine parenteral and oral drugs as an initial treatment for hypertensive crisis. The benefits of such combinations include a more effective reduction of blood pressure and earlier transition to long-term oral therapy.

Surgery sometimes
In a few patients (0.5% to 3%), hypertension requires surgical management. This is so, for example, in patients with more than 50% stenosis of one or more major renal arteries and a diastolic pressure that exceeds 100 mm Hg. Surgery is most effective in patients who:
• are under age 50 and have no generalized vascular abnormalities

• have discrete fibromuscular hyperplasia as opposed to atheromatous plaques
• do not have a coexisting nonvascular illness, such as insulin-dependent diabetes or advanced obstructive pulmonary disease.

Patients with terminal renal failure or severely elevated blood pressure that persists despite maximal tolerable doses of potent antihypertensive drugs and dialysis are candidates for bilateral nephrectomy. Another indication for surgical treatment of hypertension is pheochromocytoma (which requires excision of the adrenal tumor to reduce norepinephrine secretion).

Surgical procedures used to control hypertension include bypass with saphenous vein or Dacron grafts, endarterectomy, arteriotomy and patch-grafting; dilation of fibromuscular lesions; closed angioplasty (transfemoral dilation of involved arteries with a balloon catheter); nephrectomy; and excision of tumors.

NURSING MANAGEMENT
Whether you are dealing with acute or chronic hypertension, you can use the nursing process to approach patient care in a logical and practical way. It involves four stages: assessment, planning, intervention, and evaluation.

Begin assessment with the nursing history
Perform a nursing assessment by collecting

relevant data during the nursing history and physical examination. When taking the patient's history, be sure to ask the following questions:
• At what age was the patient's elevated blood pressure first noted?
• Has anyone in the patient's family had high blood pressure?
• Has the patient ever had renal or cardiovascular disease?
• Has the patient had a sudden weight loss (sign of pheochromocytoma) or sudden weight gain (edema)?
• Has the patient recently experienced severe headaches or drenching sweats (signs of pheochromocytoma)?

Ask specifically about characteristic symptoms indicating end organ damage—morning headaches, nausea, vomiting, blurred vision, drowsiness, shortness of breath, numbness or tingling, chest pain, swollen ankles, and any significant change in urine output—all may be indicative of end organ damage (complications) associated with severe hypertension. For each of these symptoms reported by the patient, determine its severity, onset, and duration.

Ask about previous diagnosis and treatment for hypertension, including past and present drug therapy, and determine how faithfully the patient followed and tolerated the pre-

Understanding stepped care

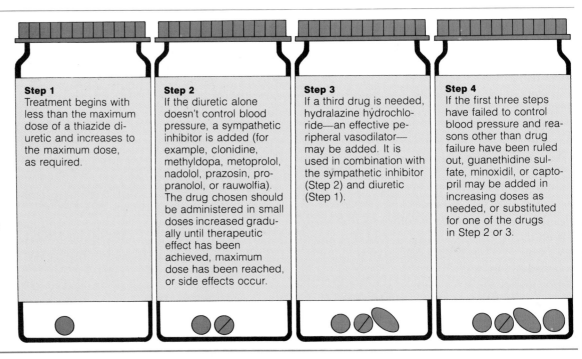

The stepped-care approach takes advantage of synergistic interaction of multiple antihypertensive agents which may permit effective treatment with smaller doses of individual drugs. Each drug should be administered in gradually increasing doses until goal blood pressure is achieved, side effects become intolerable, or the maximum dose is reached. Before moving from one step to the next, the doctor must rule out other causes of treatment failure, including poor adherence to therapy; excessive sodium intake or weight gain; and concomitant use of interfering drugs, such as oral contraceptives and vasopressor agents.

Step 1
Treatment begins with less than the maximum dose of a thiazide diuretic and increases to the maximum dose, as required.

Step 2
If the diuretic alone doesn't control blood pressure, a sympathetic inhibitor is added (for example, clonidine, methyldopa, metoprolol, nadolol, prazosin, propranolol, or rauwolfia). The drug chosen should be administered in small doses increased gradually until therapeutic effect has been achieved, maximum dose has been reached, or side effects occur.

Step 3
If a third drug is needed, hydralazine hydrochloride—an effective peripheral vasodilator—may be added. It is used in combination with the sympathetic inhibitor (Step 2) and diuretic (Step 1).

Step 4
If the first three steps have failed to control blood pressure and reasons other than drug failure have been ruled out, guanethidine sulfate, minoxidil, or captopril may be added in increasing doses as needed, or substituted for one of the drugs in Step 2 or 3.

scribed treatment. If the patient did not follow prescribed treatment, try to find out why.

Assess the patient's level of understanding about hypertension:
• Does he accept the fact that he has a lifelong condition requiring continuing treatment?
• Does he know the significance of blood pressure readings and when to report changes?
• Does he know how to take his blood pressure, and does he take it regularly?

Evaluate the patient's problems with compliance. Did the patient keep medical appointments? Did he lose time at work because of treatment? Did he have trouble remembering his dosage and schedule? Was he able to refill his prescriptions as needed? Can he afford the cost of drugs and medical visits?

Evaluate the patient's nutritional status. Note if the patient is overweight or obese. Ask about eating habits. Has the patient followed a low-sodium, weight-control diet? How has he reduced sodium intake? Does he use alcohol? Evaluate attitudes toward food, cooking, seasonings, and meal times to gauge his motivation to learn new eating patterns and to plan more effective teaching.

Ask about smoking habits. Cigarettes, cigars, pipe? How many per day? Has he tried to eliminate or decrease smoking?

Ask about exercise tolerance and interest. Does he engage in some form of exercise daily? Is he afraid to exercise? Does he become short of breath with minimal exertion?

Assess biopsychosocial adjustment through answers to the following questions:
• What are his hobbies and methods of relaxation? Is he having any sleep disturbances? Is he satisfied with his sexual patterns? What is his usual sexual activity? (It is important to document this before antihypertensive therapy begins.) What are his sources of social support? Who are the significant people in his life?
• How does the patient deal with stress and tension in his life?
• What are his fears and anxieties? Does he fear death, stroke, missing too much work or failing to get a promotion because of repeated doctor appointments, or having an altered body image or life-style from limitations imposed by disease?

As you talk with the patient during the nursing history, watch for clues to indicate whether the patient is ready to make the necessary changes in life-style to achieve blood pressure control.

Physical assessment next
After you have recorded this detailed nursing history, continue with physical assessment, using *inspection, palpation, auscultation, and percussion* to identify systemic abnormalities. (See also Chapter 2.) During physical examination, you can continue a close inspection.

Notice overall appearance. Does the patient have the moon facies and peculiar distribution of fat characteristic of Cushing syndrome? If the patient's a woman, is hirsutism present? Does the patient look flushed and anxious, characteristic of pheochromocytoma?

Notice overall skin color and condition, as well as perfusion. The funduscopic examination is an important part of assessment of the hypertensive patient. It is the only way to directly visualize arterioles. Look for arteriolar narrowing, exudates, hemorrhages, and papilledema. Observe the rate and quality of respirations. Is the patient dyspneic or tachypneic? Make sure your inspection also includes checking all extremities, especially the feet and ankles, for edema.

Using palpation, carefully evaluate the rate, amplitude, symmetry, and regularity of peripheral pulsations. Check for edema and evaluate its severity—pitting vs. nonpitting.

The results of auscultation are especially significant for determining the severity of hypertension. Listen carefully for the S_4 heart sound, an atrial gallop, that's likely to be present in a severely hypertensive patient. You may also hear an S_3 (called ventricular gallop) early in diastole, which indicates a dilated and incompetent ventricle filling rapidly. Both S_4 and S_3 indicate a deteriorating cardiovascular status. Also listen for abdominal bruits, which may signal renal arterial stenosis. Listen for bruits over all peripheral arteries where palpation was uneven.

Accurate BP measurement crucial
Of course, accurate evaluation of severity of hypertension requires accurate measurement of blood pressure. To ensure accurate measurement, take the patient's blood pressure in a quiet environment that provides privacy. Use equipment that's functioning perfectly and is calibrated regularly. Prepare the patient for measurement and encourage him to rest quietly for a few minutes before you begin.

Measure blood pressure (in both arms, if the initial evaluation), carefully using accurate technique, including the correct cuff size (see also Chapter 2).

Complete and accurate assessment data

Assessment for severe atherosclerosis and hypertension

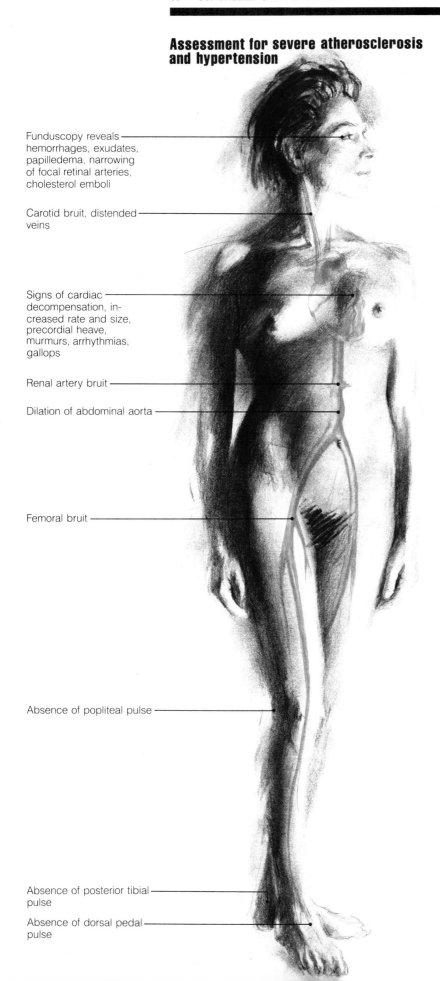

Funduscopy reveals hemorrhages, exudates, papilledema, narrowing of focal retinal arteries, cholesterol emboli

Carotid bruit, distended veins

Signs of cardiac decompensation, increased rate and size, precordial heave, murmurs, arrhythmias, gallops

Renal artery bruit

Dilation of abdominal aorta

Femoral bruit

Absence of popliteal pulse

Absence of posterior tibial pulse

Absence of dorsal pedal pulse

(including appropriate laboratory results) lead you to an accurate nursing diagnosis (examples: alteration in fluid volume related to sodium and water retention; alteration in heart rate and rhythm). Your list of nursing diagnoses may be brief or extensive. Although certain diagnoses have been generally accepted, don't limit your assessment solely to these. Include among your nursing diagnoses any aspect of the patient's condition that requires nursing care.

Plan for chronic care

Your role in managing chronic care of hypertension has been defined by the National Task Force on the Role of Nursing in High Blood Pressure Control. This group defined the following goals of nursing care:
• to help the patient and family recognize behaviors that promote health and so maintain stable blood pressure at the desired level with minimal target organ damage
• to assist the patient and family to comply with the demands of therapy by supporting successful adjustments to diagnosis and therapy and by monitoring drug therapy to minimize side effects
• to instruct, guide, and support patients in achieving and maintaining self-care so they can understand hypertension and prescribed therapy, assume responsibility for self-care, and maintain stable blood pressure at the desired level.

Intervene to promote health

Far more desirable than correctly treating established hypertension is prevention in the first place. Hypertension may not develop unless a predisposing environmental factor—such as high salt or cholesterol intake, stress, smoking, or weight gain—makes it possible. Primary and secondary prevention are areas of great promise and challenge.

Teach weight control. Many studies indicate a direct relationship between hypertension and obesity, defined as a weight 20% above the body-mass index (weight/height). This relationship has been explained physiologically as a disproportion between aortic capacity and increased cardiac output. As body mass increases, cardiac output increases. But the aorta cannot increase its capacity. The result: hypertension.

Thus, counseling overweight patients about a weight-reduction program is a good way to begin blood pressure control. It's a method of control that, correctly used, should have no side effects. To help the patient establish good dietary habits and weight control, explain the effects of excess weight on the heart's work load, hypertension, and general health. Emphasize that losing just 5 lb (2.3 kg) can measurably reduce blood pressure. Give the patient written dietary instructions, including recipes and menus to reinforce instructions.

You'll know you've effectively taught weight control if the patient can state his desired weight, recognize the need and express desire to lose weight, actively plan appropriate next steps, and show signs of progressing toward desirable weight during follow-up visits (as defined in the U.S. Department of Health and Human Services' "Report of the Working Group on Critical Patient Behaviors in the Dietary Management of High Blood Pressure").

Teach sodium restriction. Although excessive consumption of sodium (salt) leads to hypertension only in susceptible persons, failure to restrict salt is a common problem among hypertensive patients. Overcoming it requires an intense teaching program.

Assess understanding of sodium and its relation to fluid retention and high blood pressure. Explain how salt affects blood pressure. Gather data on the patient's diet history and cultural patterns to establish a practical diet plan. Determine possible effects of salt restriction on family members. Formulate a diet plan that fits the patient's cultural preferences, his financial means, and seasonal variations. A 2-g sodium diet allows no added table salt and only slight salting during cooking. It also requires avoidance of obviously salty foods and reduced consumption of canned and fast foods. Give the patient and family a list of foods and nonprescription drugs that contain sodium. Teach the patient to avoid foods high in sodium: milk products, processed foods, prepared foods, canned foods, and fast foods. Instruct the patient in reading labels and recognizing sodium-containing products. Tell the patient where to obtain specific product information. Warn patients to read labels carefully when using salt substitutes; many contain sodium.

After effective teaching, the patient should be able to explain the rationale for maintaining a low-sodium diet; identify favorite foods from a list of foods with high, moderate, and low sodium content; list common food groups to avoid or minimize consumption of; actively plan next steps; and report reduced salt intake at the next visit.

Discourage smoking. Counsel patients to quit smoking or reduce the number of cigarettes they smoke. Explain the importance of eliminating or decreasing smoking to reduce the risk of cardiovascular disease. Discuss a plan to help him quit. Inform the patient of counseling and support available through local clinics of the American Heart Association and the American Cancer Society. Encourage the patient to significantly reduce the number of cigarettes or eliminate smoking entirely within a few months.

Warn about alcohol intake. Explain alcohol's high caloric content and its vasodilatory and depressant effects. Check for interactions with prescribed medication and inform the patient about this verbally and in writing. The patient should be able to explain the effects of alcohol on the body and on the drugs he is taking.

Encourage exercise. Explain the importance of a regular, moderate exercise program, unless contraindicated. Determine what activities the patient enjoys and encourage them, if practical. Instruct the patient to increase daily exercise. The patient should be able to explain the importance of an activity program. He should be able to walk briskly for 30 minutes a day without fatigue or pain.

Teach effective stress management. Encourage the patient to verbalize his feelings. Help him to identify the stressors in his own environment. Explore ways to help him cope with stress, such as taking leisurely meals or spacing activities to avoid hurrying. Help him to distinguish avoidable stressors from unavoidable ones. Teach relaxation techniques, if desired and appropriate. Recommend counseling to help him change a stressful life-style.

You've helped the patient manage stress if he can identify two specific stressors, show some progress in eliminating at least one of them, express willingness to learn a relaxation technique, and accept counseling if necessary.

Promote compliance with drug therapy. The patient's active participation in his own care has been described as crucial for control of high blood pressure. Such control requires four critical patient behaviors:
• making the decision to control blood pressure
• taking medication as prescribed
• maintaining progress toward a blood pressure goal
• resolving problems that block control.

To help the hypertensive patient, you must

Critical patient behaviors for dietary control of hypertension

To achieve dietary control of hypertension, the patient must:

1. Acknowledge that he has hypertension and be able to state:
• what hypertension is, and its consequences if left untreated
• his actual and goal blood pressures
• that high blood pressure is treatable, not curable.

2. Consider diet modification as a potentially effective treatment and express willingness to try it. The patient must:
• understand that high blood pressure can be related to diet
• believe that diet modification might work for him
• understand that changing dietary habits takes time and effort
• understand his role in making dietary changes
• understand what kind of changes are required and the importance of family and social support.

3. Assess his current dietary pattern and develop a list of food-related behaviors and situations that need to be changed.

4. Acknowledge that successful modification of diet will take a long time and express realistic expectations, recognizing that setbacks are common and are not excuses for giving up; and dietary control must be maintained for life.

5. Develop an overall strategy and set goals for blood pressure, weight, and sodium intake. To develop such a strategy, the patient must:
• learn the facts about reducing sodium intake and reducing weight and apply these facts to his own life situation
• identify obstacles in his life and surroundings that might block this goal.

6. Plan for each dietary change.

7. Act to make each dietary change.

8. Assess the success of each planned change.

9. Assess attainment of his blood pressure goal.

EMERGENCY MANAGEMENT

Hypertensive crisis

Because the treatment for hypertensive crisis is lifesaving but in itself dangerous if inappropriately applied, your pivotal role in detection and management depends on the ability to distinguish between severe hypertension that is relatively stable and its fulminant, immediately life-threatening counterpart. Making this distinction requires that you recognize that hypertensive crisis is never just a blood pressure reading—however high—but a condition of rapidly progressive and critical deterioration of cerebral, cardiovascular, and renal function.

Watch for hypertensive crisis in patients with predisposing conditions. Common ones include essential or renovascular hypertension, glomerulonephritis, preeclampsia, eclampsia, and food or drug interaction with a monoamine oxidase inhibitor. Rare ones include withdrawal from antihypertensive drug, severe burns, head injury, acute left ventricular hypertrophy, intracranial hemorrhage, acute dissecting aortic aneurysm, and leaking abdominal aortic aneurysm.

Identify hypertensive crisis by its devastating cerebral, cardiovascular, and renal effects; specifically, hypertensive encephalopathy, acute left ventricular failure and pulmonary edema, and progressive renal insuffi-

ciency. Be prepared to treat it promptly and precisely.

Planning intervention
In the patient with acute hypertension, the goals of your intervention are:
• stabilization of blood pressure, preferably with diastolic pressure below 90 mm Hg or at some other level considered therapeutically safe
• prevention or correction of life-threatening compromise of renal, cerebral, and cardiovascular function. It requires prompt treatment to lower blood pressure, maintaining the lowest diastolic pressure consistent with safety and tolerance.

Generally, you should proceed as follows:
• If you have found severely elevated blood pressure, immediately remeasure blood pressure in both arms.
• Have the patient lie down in a comfortable position, and if possible, away from any commotion. Report your findings to the doctor.
• Prepare to obtain a chest X-ray and electrocardiogram.
• Prepare to collect blood and urine samples for laboratory studies. Appropriate blood studies usually include a complete blood cell count, a creatinine level, an electrolyte profile, and a plasma catecholamine

value. Urine studies usually require a single sample for red blood cells, protein and metanephrine, and a 24-hour sample for vanillylmandelic acid.
• Continue to monitor and record all findings. Watch the blood pressure carefully (it will probably decline somewhat with rest). Measure fluid intake and output and check for neurologic changes.

If you suspect hypertensive crisis, keep in mind the importance of distinguishing between hypertensive encephalopathy and cerebrovascular accident (CVA). If you suspect CVA, notify the doctor. In a patient with CVA, lowering the blood pressure rapidly can be dangerous.
• Prepare for transfer to the intensive care unit (ICU) if the patient needs treatment with nitroprusside sodium (Nipride).
• Prepare for antihypertensive drug infusion if the patient is not being transferred to the ICU. Prepare to start an intravenous line and be sure the appropriate antihypertensive drugs are available. Also prepare an infusion pump or a microdrip unit for accurate dose titration. The doctor starts treatment with a low dose of a parenteral drug, then increases it gradually until the blood pressure starts to drop. While the blood pressure is dropping, the dose is held

view your role as patient advocate as he learns these behaviors and struggles to achieve control.

In considering ways to encourage compliance with treatment, you must keep in mind that the greater its impact on the person's life-style, the less likely he is to comply. Thus, the duration and complexity of therapy and the expense and side effects of medication are all factors that can impair compliance. Absence of symptoms can also impair compliance, as it lets the patient deny that his illness is serious.

Before beginning counseling, find out if the patient has a history of hypertension and whether therapy was successful. Adjust your teaching to the patient's knowledge and expe-

rience. If appropriate, offer printed material to reinforce teaching (available from the National High Blood Pressure Education Program, the American Heart Association, the American Red Cross, and other health agencies).

Be sure to counsel the patient in detail about the expected effects of drug therapy. Help the patient understand and accept the *permanent,* lifetime need for drug therapy. Emphasize that because any drug reduces blood pressure only temporarily, it can't be discontinued. Help the patient develop a practical dosage schedule that fits his daily activities and needs. Verify his understanding by asking him to describe his drug and the prescribed schedule. Give written instructions for dosage and schedule and encourage mark-

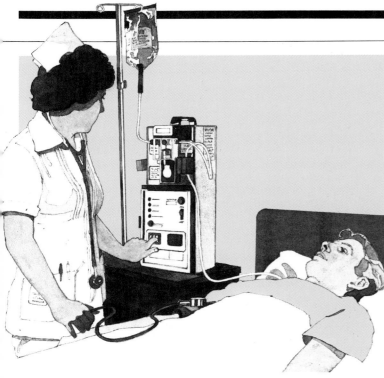

depends on the drug used: with nitroprusside sodium or trimethaphan camsylate, check blood pressure every 5 to 10 minutes; with hydralazine hydrochloride or methyldopa, check less frequently; for example, every hour.

• Carefully watch I.V. infusions of antihypertensive drugs. Be sure the I.V. site is always patent. Letting an I.V. infusion of such potent drugs infiltrate can have disastrous results.

• When using an infusion pump, be sure it's operating optimally at all times. Its failure can give the patient a hazardous bolus—risking catastrophic hypotension—or prevent effective dosage. Make sure every change in dosage is preceded and followed by careful measurement of blood pressure.

• To assure the necessary precision, blood pressure is usually taken with an arterial monitor and double-checked with a pressure cuff. (Remember, arterial-line readings tend to be higher and more accurate than cuff readings.)

• Keep checking cerebral, cardiovascular, and renal functions into transitional and maintenance-therapy stages.

• Keep a flow sheet showing minute-to-minute management. This flow sheet should contain the blood pressure, time and dosage of all medications, and the patient's condition (especially level of consciousness, heart rate, urine output, and the results of all laboratory tests).

Nitroprusside precautions

Because nitroprusside is unstable in solution and deteriorates rapidly when exposed to light, prepare this solution only when you're ready to administer it, and don't keep or infuse it for longer than 24 hours. If the solution changes from its characteristic brown to blue, green, or dark red, it has deteriorated and must be replaced. To protect the solution from light, cover the I.V. bottle with aluminum foil or the manufacturer-supplied opaque covering. Don't wrap the tubing, though; keep it uncovered so you can detect any color changes in the solution. As added protection for this unstable solution, don't add any other drugs to it, and keep the nitroprusside drip out of direct sunlight during the infusion. Normal room light is acceptable.

constant to avoid hypotension. If the blood pressure levels off but is still dangerously high, the dose is increased. Once the blood pressure reaches an acceptable level, the parenteral dose is slowly reduced in preparation for oral antihypertensive therapy.

Monitor drug therapy
Before giving a drug, check its dosage. Then check the patient's blood pressure. Even if you've checked it recently, check it again *immediately* before giving the drug.

• Also check blood pressure *after* giving the drug—how often

ing doses on a calendar to prevent forgotten doses. Emphasize the need to renew a prescription before exhausting the present supply. Encourage the patient to seek advice about financial assistance to cover the cost of drugs, as appropriate. If the patient has failed to follow prescribed drug treatment, find out why. Then help the patient to change circumstances that cause noncompliance.

Warn the patient appropriately about side effects and strongly warn against sudden discontinuation of drug treatment. Be sure to explain that sudden discontinuation can cause hypertensive rebound and that drug treatment should always be stopped slowly under the doctor's supervision. Provide a written list of the most common side effects

and what he should do about them. Recognize that the patient who feels fine before treatment may be annoyed by side effects. Encourage him to verbalize his feelings and offer sympathy and understanding. But emphasize that taking a drug is easier than treating complications.

Verify that the patient knows the important side effects of drugs prescribed for him and what he should do about them. Encourage him to seek medical advice before taking any nonprescription drugs.

Anticipate hypokalemia. Explain that certain diuretics may cause potassium deficit. To minimize potassium loss, teach the patient who must take these diuretics about the symptoms of potassium deficit and how to

Four steps to control hypertension

Your role in detecting and controlling hypertension is more important now than ever. A four-step program can help you make the most of it.

1 Extend your role in detection
• Participate in health-education activities that help develop screening and referral services and outreach programs to groups with undetected hypertension.
• Keep your knowledge up-to-date, using the latest national standards for measurement and detection.
• When dealing with hospitalized patients, consider the admission blood pressure an integral part of the nursing data base, regardless of the reason for admission. Blood pressure normally decreases during hospitalization as a result of bed rest, so don't disregard earlier elevations. Consider any elevations of arterial pressure—even isolated ones—worth discussing with the patient's doctor. Use the information gained to develop a plan for follow-up care after discharge.

2 Promote understanding and education
• Make an effort to understand the causes and underlying mechanisms of hypertension so you can knowledgeably support treatment and anticipate and identify complications.
• Encourage preventive health behavior and support decisions to seek screening, accept referral for care, and continue therapy to maintain blood pressure control.
• Promote public education about hypertension directly by acting as a role model for your family and community.

3 Assist with treatment
• Be prepared to assist with every phase of treatment, from providing acute care of a patient with severe hypertension or its complications to encouraging compliance in a patient with no symptoms.
• Support nurse-managed hypertension treatment programs.
• Understand the stepped-care approach to treatment and be ready to explain it to the patient.
• Know the current drug treatments and their usual effects and complications.
• When caring for patients known to be hypertensive before admission, use the time of hospitalization as an opportunity to reassess blood pressure control. Always consider this diagnosis so you can include antihypertensive drug therapy in your discharge planning.

4 Promote maintenance treatment
• Continue to express your interest and concern about the patient's progress toward an appropriate blood pressure goal in a way that encourages, motivates, and supports consistent compliance with treatment.
• Identify potential problems related to drug therapy: fear of drug therapy, scheduling of doses, and financial costs.
• Stress the importance of remaining under care.

prevent it. Consider that the patient may need an adjustment of dosage or substitution of a potassium-sparing diuretic. Tell the patient to watch for fatigue, leg cramps, and other symptoms of hypokalemia (provide a written list of the common ones). Also provide a list of foods high in potassium. Inform the patient that potassium deficit needs treatment with a supplement when the potassium level in the blood drops below 3 mEq/liter or causes symptoms. Be sure to inform such a patient that replacing potassium deficit from dietary sources alone is very difficult. Instruct him to mix the prescribed potassium supplement in chilled fruit juice, preferably orange juice to make it more palatable, and to take it after meals to minimize gastric irritation. Teach the patient that normal dietary intake of potassium should be 50 to 100 mEq/day (four glasses of orange juice or seven bananas contain 60 mEq of potassium).

Verify that the patient can state the symptoms of potassium deficit and can select foods that are high in potassium.

Explain postural hypotension. Because some patients receiving certain drugs may experience postural hypotension, explain why he may feel dizzy or faint when he stands suddenly from a lying position. Warn him to sit for a few minutes before standing up. If dizziness persists longer than 1 to 2 minutes, the patient should sit or lie down and either decrease or omit his next scheduled dose; he should notify his doctor if dizziness continues. Encourage the patient to sleep with his head elevated; to avoid prolonged standing, especially in the sun; and to avoid alcohol because of its vasodilatory effects. Tell him that taking the drug at bedtime may minimize postural effects.

Verify that the patient can explain why dizziness occurs and knows what to do about it.

Consider sexual dysfunction. If the patient complains of sexual dysfunction after taking an antihypertensive drug, consider that this may be a drug-related effect. However, remind the patient that such dysfunction can result from other causes, including alcohol, diabetes, stress, and marital difficulties. Initiate careful evaluation if the problem persists. This problem may require a change in drug therapy or referral for counseling.

Encourage self-care

Emphasize that the patient himself has the greatest responsibility for long-term control. Help the patient to deal effectively with this responsibility by explaining the fundamental pathology of hypertension.

Explain normal and abnormal blood pressure. Define blood pressure and the concepts of arterial circulation, systolic and diastolic pressure, and peripheral resistance. Assess his readiness to learn and his level of understanding regarding blood pressure. Explain that blood pressure is measured by sounds that result from the vibration of blood against the arterial wall. Explain that all blood pressures vary normally. Explain the meaning of systolic and diastolic pressure. With visual aids, explain how vasoconstriction and vasodilation influence pressure in the blood vessels.

Define *high* blood pressure. Explain that hypertension is not the same as anxiety or tension and that high blood pressure isn't the opposite of anemia.

After effective teaching, the patient should be able to define and state the limits of normal blood pressure, distinguish systolic from diastolic pressure, and tell what happens during increased or decreased peripheral resistance. The patient should be able to define high blood pressure accurately and distinguish between normal and abnormal blood pressure.

Explain causes and contributing factors in the onset of high blood pressure. Explain that the higher the blood pressure, the greater the likelihood of organ damage. Explain that hypertension usually causes no symptoms until it has progressed to a severe stage. Outline the devastating consequences of high blood pressure on blood vessels and vital organs in the body: heart failure, kidney failure, and stroke.

Make sure the patient understands the difference between control and cure. Inform the patient of what the desired blood pressure (goal) is for him. Avoid describing this goal as "normal" blood pressure. Instead, reinforce

the term "well controlled" when the patient reaches the desired goal.

The patient should be able to explain the most likely factors that contributed to his own hypertension, state that high blood pressure can exist without symptoms, and state effects of high blood pressure on the heart, blood vessels, kidneys, and brain.

Teach self-measurement of blood pressure. Some doctors ask their patients to record their blood pressure at home to detect patterns of variation, to compare home pressures to office pressures, and to monitor response to therapy. Even without their doctors' instructions, many patients and their families wish to learn how to measure blood pressure. When selecting patients for such teaching, be sure to take into account their physical (visual, auditory, manual) and intellectual abilities.

Evaluate your care plan

You can be sure your teaching has been successful when the patient:
• understands the what, why, and when of his total antihypertensive treatment program
• expresses willingness to assume responsibility for controlling his own blood pressure and makes a commitment to follow the prescribed treatment faithfully
• has received, read, and understood written dietary instructions; can plan an acceptable menu; and tell what is and isn't permitted
• knows the purpose, dosage schedule, and reportable side effects for each drug prescribed, and knows that drugs will control blood pressure only when taken regularly
• has received at least one descriptive pamphlet on hypertension and has the name and telephone number of at least one community-health resource person for further help and information (in addition to his doctor)
• can take his own blood pressure accurately and knows when to notify his doctor of the results
• has a follow-up appointment and promises (or contracts) to keep it.

Continue working with the patient until you have accomplished all these goals. For some patients, not all of these goals are appropriate or attainable, so you'll have to modify them to meet individual needs.

We are now certain that vigorous treatment of hypertension *does* save lives. Helping the patient to maintain control of high blood pressure is one of the most important services you can render. It's also one of the most challenging, but unquestionably worth the effort.

Points to remember

• Hypertension, in all grades of severity, has devastating effects on vital functions, primarily the cardiovascular, neurologic, and renal systems.
• Prompt and continuous treatment to control risk factors and reduce blood pressure with antihypertensive drugs prevents these harmful effects.
• The stepped-care approach to treatment effectively reduces morbidity and mortality related to hypertension.
• Consistent compliance with prescribed treatment is the key to control of hypertension.
• Nurses can promote compliance through patient education, especially by helping the patient to understand and accept necessary therapy.

5 COMPENSATING FOR CARDIAC FAILURE

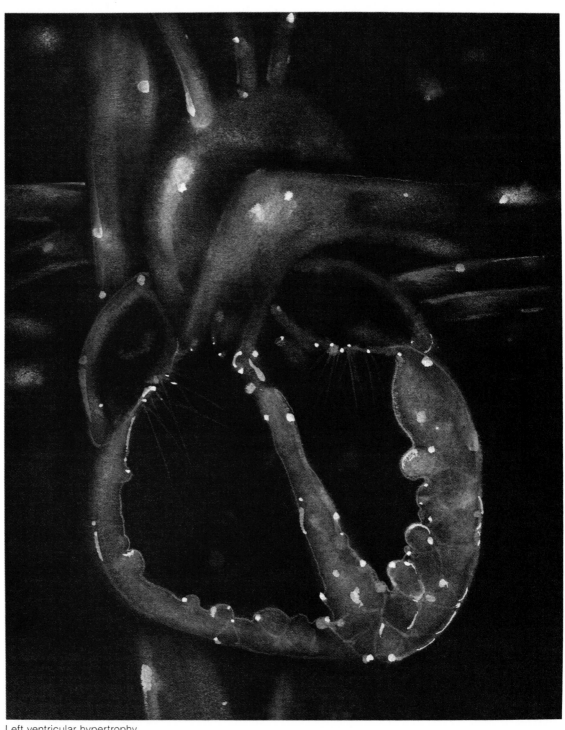

Left ventricular hypertrophy

Congestive heart failure (CHF) is becoming ever more common as more patients survive cardiac damage or live long enough to develop cardiac weakness. In fact, patients with CHF account for 10% to 15% of all hospital admissions. This disorder has pervasive physiologic effects that challenge your nursing skills. In its early stages, its subtle and almost imperceptible signs challenge your skills of observation and assessment. In its most severe stage, pulmonary edema, its life-threatening complications challenge your skill in providing emergency care.

The prognosis for survival in patients with CHF is usually 5 to 8 years—depending on the underlying causes, and on patient compliance and response to treatment. Because compliance is so important, careful teaching is your primary obligation in managing such patients. As you know, many patients with CHF are elderly—typically, they may miss medical appointments, forget to take prescribed medication, and fail to adhere to dietary restrictions. You can't guarantee such patients' compliance with treatment, but you can improve it by helping them to understand CHF and to correct the underlying reasons for noncompliance. To achieve these goals, you'll need to understand the pathophysiology and medical management of CHF. You'll also need to accurately assess the patient's condition to plan interventions that support effective cardiac compensation and to ease the effects of decompensation.

What is congestive heart failure?
Congestive heart failure is a syndrome characterized by myocardial dysfunction that leads to impaired pump performance (decreased cardiac output) or to frank heart failure and abnormal circulatory congestion. This syndrome can result from left ventricular failure (left heart failure), which primarily causes pulmonary congestion, or from right ventricular failure (right heart failure), which primarily causes congestion of the peripheral tissues and viscera. Because a properly functioning heart depends on both ventricles, failure of one ventricle almost always leads to failure of the other.

PATHOPHYSIOLOGY
In both right and left heart failure, a serious imbalance develops among the three essential factors that influence cardiac output—ejection fraction, preload, and afterload (see Chapter 1

for a review of these concepts). Even a healthy heart can falter when faced with a serious imbalance among these factors. For example, when a healthy heart is subjected to massive volume overload, preload can increase to such an extent that the ventricle can no longer meet pumping demands.

If even a healthy heart can develop signs of CHF, preexisting cardiac disease can deteriorate into CHF even more readily. After myocardial infarction, for instance, the heart cannot dilate normally in response to increased preload. As a result, afterload increases and may ultimately lead to decreased cardiac output. In coronary artery disease, the heart fails to achieve adequate contractility when oxygen demands increase.

Often, a patient with CHF develops cumulative imbalances. When the heart fails to respond to increased preload and cardiac output fails to rise appropriately, the sympathetic nervous system reacts to constrict the peripheral vessels, thereby maintaining blood pressure and blood flow to vital organs. But peripheral vasoconstriction also causes increased afterload, forcing the ventricle to work harder and to demand more oxygen—oxygen that may not be available because of an obstructed coronary artery or poor blood oxygenation. Thus, a destructive cycle emerges that threatens cardiac function.

Compensating for CHF
A patient with CHF may still manage to live a relatively normal life. How? By developing compensatory mechanisms. His heart rate increases, especially during mild exercise, to compensate for decreased stroke volume and to maintain adequate cardiac output. His kidneys conserve sodium and water to increase circulating blood volume, thereby increasing preload. Even during rest, his tissues extract more than the usual 40% of oxygen from their available blood supply, putting off—at least temporarily—the need for increased cardiac output.

But these compensatory mechanisms are a mixed blessing for the patient with CHF. They also make him more vulnerable to complications stemming from any disease that secondarily affects the cardiovascular system—renal disorders and emphysema, for example, can dangerously compromise his cardiac output. Similarly, increased activity can quickly produce fatigue, dyspnea, and tachycardia in such a patient. Infection, anemia, dysrhythmia, the use of alcoholic beverages, and overeating

Classifying congestive heart failure

Although CHF is usually classified by site of heart failure (left heart, right heart, or both), it may also be classified by level of cardiac output, stage, and direction. However, these varying classifications simply represent different clinical aspects of CHF, not distinct diseases.

Low- and high-output failure
Achieving a precise definition of low and high cardiac output is difficult since the normal range is wide. In some patients with low-output failure, cardiac output may be normal during periods of rest but fails to rise during exertion. In some patients with high-output failure, it may settle near the upper limit of normal.

In both low- and high-output failure, the heart is unable to deliver the precise amount of oxygenated blood to the tissues.

Low-output failure occurs in coronary artery disease, hypertension, primary myocardial disease, and valvular disease. High-output failure occurs in arteriovenous fistula, hyperthyroidism, anemia, sickle cell anemia, beriberi, Paget's disease, and thyrotoxicosis.

Acute and chronic heart failure
Frequently, acute and chronic heart failure overlap. For example, a patient with chronic heart failure may experience acute heart failure from myocardial infarction. Acute heart failure may also occur in valvular rupture or any condition that places stress on an already diseased heart. Chronic heart failure may occur in multivalvular heart disease, cardiomyopathy, and a healed, extensive myocardial infarction.

Backward and forward heart failure
Backward and forward failure can't be clearly separated, since both types are present in most patients with chronic heart failure. In *backward heart failure,*

one ventricle fails to expel blood, causing elevated ventricular end-diastolic volume and elevated pressure and volume in the atrium and venous system behind the failing ventricle. Such elevations, along with increased renal tubular reabsorption from increased renal venous pressure, cause retention of sodium and water, thereby increasing circulating blood volume.

In *forward heart failure,* the ventricles fail to expel enough blood into the arterial system. Retention of sodium and water then results from decreased renal perfusion and/or increased renal tubular absorption. As in backward failure, circulating blood volume increases, making the expulsion of blood even more difficult for the weakened ventricles.

**Normal
levels of cardiac output**
2.6 to 3.6 liters per min./sq. meter of body surface

Low-output failure
< 2.6 liters per min./sq. meter of body surface

High-output failure
> 3.6 liters per min./sq. meter of body surface (can be normal in athletic heart syndrome or pregnancy)

can overload an already weakened heart. Fluid retention can so increase preload that the ventricular muscle bundles no longer snap back. Instead, they become permanently distended, requiring additional oxygen to contract adequately; if that oxygen isn't available, the threat of cardiac ischemia mounts.

When compensation fails: Left heart failure
In left heart failure, the type most likely to occur after myocardial infarction when com-

pensatory mechanisms fail, a large volume of blood remains in the dilated left ventricle. This residual blood reduces the ventricle's capacity to accept blood from the left atrium. Because the left atrium is unable to eject all of its blood, it dilates from increased left ventricular pressure and is unable to receive the full volume of blood from the pulmonary veins. Pulmonary congestion results, characterized by increased pulmonary venous and pulmonary capillary pressures.

Pulmonary congestion causes the key sign

of left heart failure—dyspnea. Dyspnea varies greatly in severity and includes many forms—paroxysmal nocturnal dyspnea, Cheyne-Stokes respirations, and orthopnea. Usually, dyspnea first accompanies moderate to severe exertion that the patient once tolerated easily. As cardiac reserve progressively declines, smaller and smaller levels of exertion evoke dyspnea. Paroxysmal nocturnal dyspnea, respiratory distress that awakens the patient, varies in severity from nocturnal restlessness or anxiety to extreme respiratory distress. Cheyne-Stokes respirations, alternating periods of apnea and deep breathing, result from severe left ventricular failure or central nervous system disorders and may be secondary to respiratory alkalosis, a common condition in patients with CHF. Orthopnea, breathing difficulty when the patient is in the supine position, results from increased blood flow to the heart, increased pulmonary congestion, and decreased pulmonary capacity.

Since dyspnea is a subjective complaint, its severity doesn't always correlate with the severity of congestive heart failure. An apprehensive patient with moderate dyspnea might report more difficulty than a stoic patient with severe dyspnea. Still, orthopnea and Cheyne-Stokes respirations do correlate with the severity of heart failure.

Other signs and symptoms of left heart failure include tachycardia (a compensatory sympathetic response), fatigue, muscle weakness, decreased renal function, edema and weight gain, irritability, restlessness, and a shortened attention span.

Right heart failure

Right heart failure often follows left heart failure because the right heart must pump against increased resistance in the pulmonary system. Signs of right heart failure vary according to the presence and extent of left heart failure but typically include dependent edema. Usually, such edema begins in the ankles; after 5 to 10 lb of edema accumulates, pitting occurs. Edema may progress to the severe generalized form called anasarca. Edema results from retention of sodium and water from low cardiac output.

Another telltale sign of right heart failure is neck-vein distention when the patient is upright. Neck veins may show abnormal pulsations, appear distended, and feel rigid—all signs of high venous pressure.

Other signs and symptoms of right heart failure include hepatomegaly, which, in turn,

Cellular changes in CHF

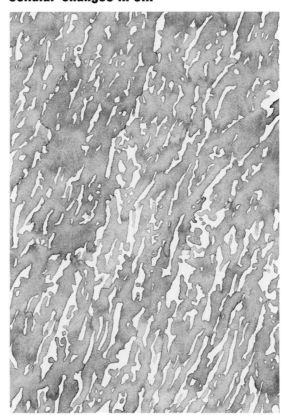

In the normal heart, cells are arranged in an orderly pattern.

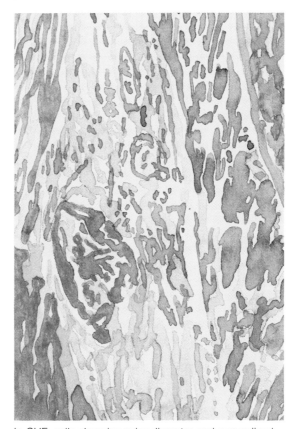

In CHF, cells show irregular diameter and generalized enlargement.

Staging pulmonary edema

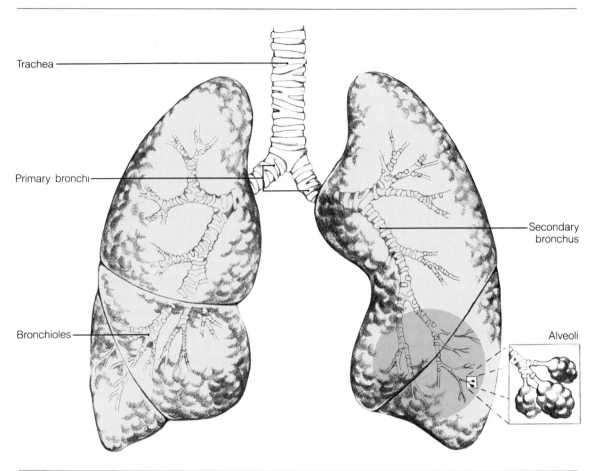

Trachea

Primary bronchi

Bronchioles

Secondary bronchus

Alveoli

Stage	Pathophysiology	Signs and symptoms
Initial	Usually, left ventricular failure increases pulmonary vascular bed pressure, forcing fluid and solutes from the intravascular compartment into the interstitium of the lungs. As the interstitium overloads with fluid, fluid enters the peripheral alveoli, impairing adequate gas exchange.	Persistent cough—patient feels like he has "a cold coming on" Slight dyspnea/orthopnea Exercise intolerance Restlessness Anxiety Crepitant rales may be heard over the dependent portion of the lungs Diastolic gallop
Acute	Fluid accumulation throughout pulmonary vasculature and further filling of the alveoli.	Acute shortness of breath Respirations—rapid, noisy (audible wheeze, rales) Cough more intense, producing frothy, blood-tinged sputum Cyanosis Diaphoresis, cold and clammy skin Tachycardia, dysrhythmias Hypotension
Advanced	Patient's condition rapidly deteriorates as the bronchial tree fills with fluid.	Decreased level of consciousness Ventricular dysrhythmias Shock Diminished breath sounds

Initial stage

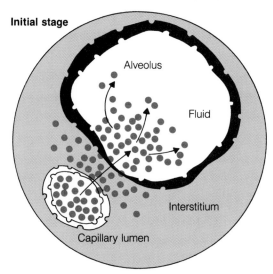

Fluid overloads interstitium and enters alveolus.

Acute stage

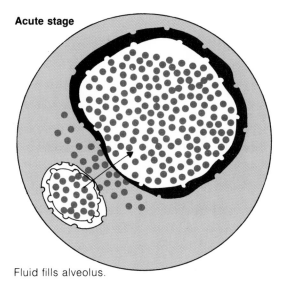

Fluid fills alveolus.

Advanced stage

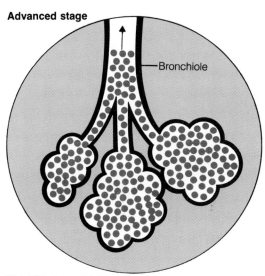

Fluid fills bronchial tree.

represses splenic drainage and leads to splenomegaly; anorexia, nausea, and vague abdominal pain from congestion of the viscera; fatigue from low cardiac output; and occasionally, ascites from high systemic venous pressure or hepatic dysfunction.

Sometimes, right heart failure can result from cor pulmonale—hypertrophy of the right ventricle caused by primary pulmonary hypertension. Cor pulmonale begins with chronic cough, exertional dyspnea, fatigue, wheezing, and weakness. As it progresses, edema, hepatomegaly and other signs of right heart failure develop.

Simultaneous right and left failure

In many elderly patients, who tend to have both arteriosclerosis and age-related degenerative changes, both ventricles may begin to falter simultaneously in their capacity to pump blood. Consequently, signs of left and right heart failure develop simultaneously, so their pattern may not be clear-cut and onset may be insidious.

MEDICAL MANAGEMENT

Medical management varies according to the severity and cause of heart failure. However, its goals are always the same: to identify or prevent precipitating or aggravating factors; to reduce cardiac work load and to improve contractility and pumping efficiency; and to treat the effects and complications of congestion.

Standard treatments

The cornerstones of standard treatment are bed rest, diet modification, hemodynamic monitoring, and drug therapy. Bed rest, which may be complete or partial depending on the patient's condition, reduces the heart's work load, improves the efficiency of heart pumping, promotes diuresis, decreases circulating blood volume and pulmonary congestion, and eases dyspnea. Diet modification consists of restricting sodium intake and providing smaller, more frequent meals. Concomitant hemodynamic monitoring allows evaluation of the severity of CHF and the patient's response to treatment.

Traditional drug therapy includes use of digitalis or related cardiotonic glycosides to increase the force of contractions, and diuretics to reduce circulating blood volume and vascular congestion. In acute pump failure requiring hemodynamic monitoring, a positive inotropic agent, such as intravenous dopamine

Diagnostic findings in congestive heart failure

Various invasive and noninvasive tests provide important information in the diagnosis of CHF. *Pulmonary artery catheterization* shows elevated pulmonary artery and capillary wedge pressures, reflecting elevated left ventricular end-diastolic pressure in left heart failure and elevated right atrial pressure in right heart failure. *Cardiac catheterization* may show ventricular dilatation, coronary artery occlusion, and valvular disorders (such as aortic stenosis) in both left and right heart failure.

Central venous pressure monitoring shows elevated readings as left heart failure progresses to right heart failure or as hypervolemia results from increased retention of sodium and water.

Electrocardiography may show ischemia in both left and right heart failure. In left heart failure, it may also show heart strain, left ventricular hypertrophy, or dysrhythmias.

The *chest X-ray* may show cardiomegaly and pulmonary congestion in both left and right heart failure.

Cardiac blood pool imaging shows a decreased ejection fraction in left heart failure.

Echocardiography may show ventricular hypertrophy, decreased contractility, and valvular disorders (such as aortic stenosis) in both left and right heart failure. Serial echocardiograms may help assess the patient's response to therapy.

Echocardiogram results

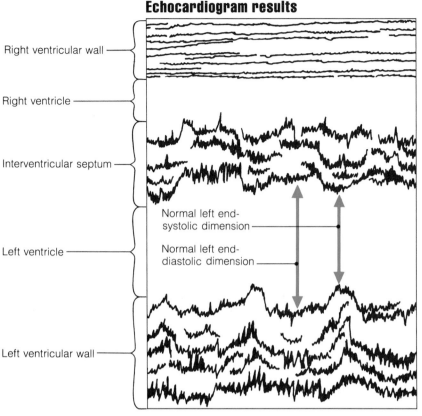

Right ventricular wall

Right ventricle

Interventricular septum

Left ventricle

Normal left end-systolic dimension

Normal left end-diastolic dimension

Left ventricular wall

In a normal echocardiogram, end-diastolic dimension is 3.5 to 5.6 cm.

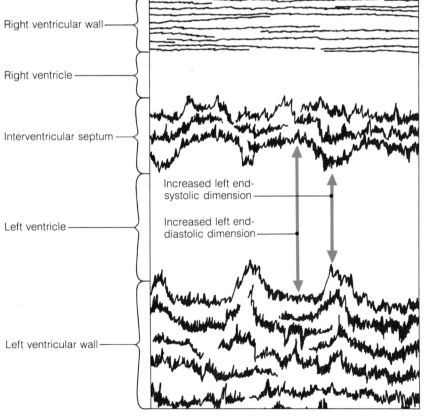

Right ventricular wall

Right ventricle

Interventricular septum

Increased left end-systolic dimension

Increased left end-diastolic dimension

Left ventricle

Left ventricular wall

In left ventricular failure, the muscle wall thickens and the left ventricular cavity increases, so end-diastolic dimension increases.

or dobutamine, may replace digitalis because of its rapid action and short half-life; diuretic therapy begins with fast-acting, potent agents—furosemide and ethacrynic acid. Once the patient's condition stabilizes, less potent drugs—usually thiazides, triamterene, amiloride and spironolactone—provide maintenance diuresis.

Supplementary treatments commonly include administration of oxygen, especially in a patient with dyspnea complicated by pulmonary disease or coronary thrombosis; and anticoagulant therapy and application of anti-embolism stockings to prevent venostasis and thromboembolism. Other treatments can correct underlying causes. Surgery, for example, may be required to correct valvular dysfunction; antihypertensive drugs may be required to lower blood pressure.

New treatments offer new hope
Treatment with unloading agents and new positive inotropic agents offer new hope for patients with refractory heart failure who fail to respond to maximal dosage of digitalis and diuretics. Even with these new treatments, severe refractory heart failure may also require fluid restriction and, rarely, paracentesis or thoracentesis to relieve abdominal distention or dyspnea.

Unloading agents. Venous and arterial vasodilators and angiotensin II inhibitors decrease cardiac work load by restoring efficient preload and afterload. Although unloading agents are not new, they're newly indicated for treatment of CHF. *Venous vasodilators,* such as nitrates, reduce ventricular volume and preload by pooling blood in the peripheral veins. *Arterial vasodilators,* such as hydralazine and minoxidil, decrease arterial resistance, reducing afterload so the ventricle can increase its output and decrease its work load. Some unloading agents, such as prazosin and nitroprusside, combine the effects of venous and arterial vasodilators. *Angiotensin II inhibitors,* such as captopril and teprotide, decrease arterial resistance and afterload. In addition, angiotensin II inhibitors promote decreased secretion of aldosterone, thereby decreasing fluid retention.

Positive inotropic agents. In some institutions, salbutamol, pirbuterol, milrinone, or amrinone may be used with or instead of unloading agents. These drugs are more potent than digitalis in their effects on myocardial contractility—and are less likely to cause cardiotoxicity. Amrinone, however, causes thrombocytopenia in 15% of patients.

Digitalis toxicity: Its causes and signs

igitalis is the most commonly used drug for treating congestive heart failure. But because of the narrow range between therapeutic and toxic blood levels, digitalis toxicity occurs in nearly one third of the patients taking this drug. Toxicity may result from overdosage or from accumulation of digitalis glycosides in the myocardium after changes in the patient's condition or treatment. For example, gastrointestinal disorders may cause potassium loss and so increase the heart's sensitivity to digitalis. Hypothyroidism and acid-base and electrolyte disturbances can also increase sensitivity to digitalis. Hepatic and renal disorders may decrease excretion of digitalis.

Treatment, such as cardioversion, can influence the patient's response to digitalis. For elective cardioversion, digitalis is typically withheld for 1 to 2 days before the procedure and the dosage is adjusted after it. Concurrent drug treatment with amphotericin B, intravenous calcium, intravenous glucose, potassium-wasting diuretics, propantheline or quinidine predisposes the patient to digitalis toxicity.

To detect digitalis toxicity, watch first for extracardiac signs: anorexia, nausea, vomiting, diarrhea, abdominal pain, fatigue, headache, generalized muscle weakness, malaise and visual disturbances (blurred, yellow-green halo or double vision). Then watch for cardiac signs: heart failure or such dysrhythmias as ventricular premature beats, atrial fibrillation, tachycardia, accelerated junctional nodal rhythm, supraventricular tachycardia, atrioventricular dissociation, heart block, or bradycardia with a pulse rate below 60.

To confirm digitalis toxicity, the doctor will order measurement of serum electrolyte and digitalis levels. Typically, serum digitalis levels are measured 6 to 12 hours after an oral dose; serum levels over 2.3 ng/ml suggest digitalis toxicity, and levels under 1.6 ng/ml tend to rule out toxicity. However, patients with sensitivity to digitalis may develop signs of toxicity with normally therapeutic serum levels.

NURSING MANAGEMENT
A thorough understanding of the pathophysiology and medical management of CHF prepares you for effective history-taking and assessment; for establishment of appropriate nursing diagnoses, goals, and interventions; and for correct evaluation of the patient's response to treatment.

Detailed patient history
Your first aim in history-taking is to define the progression of CHF in a detailed interview. However, you'll have to modify the interview according to the patient's condition. If the patient is in distress upon admission, keep the initial history brief and to the point, and avoid repeating questions the doctor already asked. If you can't complete a satisfactory interview at admission, you can continue it later, when the patient is more comfortable.

Be sure to ask the patient these questions:
• Has he had a previous myocardial infarction or dysrhythmia, recent hemorrhage, anemia, respiratory infection, chronic respiratory disease, pulmonary embolism, thyrotoxicosis, fever, hypoxia, or any other problem that could cause or aggravate congestive heart failure?
• What drugs is he currently taking? Does he take the current dosage according to the prescribed schedule? If not, find out why not.

• Has he recently experienced shortness of breath? Try to pinpoint when. Does he become breathless with slight exertion, with heavy exertion, or at night?
• Has he recently experienced fatigue, muscle weakness, decreased urination, weight gain, anorexia, bloated feelings, depression, or anxiety? For each reported symptom, determine its severity, onset, and duration.
• Has he recently experienced any severely stressful events?
• Has he ever been treated for CHF with medication or any dietary, fluid, and activity restrictions? If so, has he followed the prescribed treatment? If not, why not?
• What effect does CHF have on his life-style? What support systems does he have?

During your interview with the patient, form an overall impression. Does he appear edematous? Is he overweight? Is he breathless when he speaks?

Perform a cardiovascular assessment
After completing the history and forming your overall impression, you're ready to begin a complete cardiovascular assessment. Remember, though, that a patient with acute CHF is likely to be extremely anxious, which intensifies signs and symptoms. Consequently, you'll need to reassess the patient later when his condition is stable and he's more comfortable.

Your initial assessment, though, remains critically important since early recognition of CHF promotes prompt treatment and possible prevention of serious complications. Typically, your cardiovascular assessment of a patient with CHF reveals:

• *pale, cool, moist extremities and dusky-colored nail beds.* Depress nail beds to test capillary refill, which probably will be poor.

• *dependent edema.* If the patient is ambulatory or often sits erect in a chair, check his ankles and calves. If he is bedridden or often sits in a reclining chair with his feet elevated, check the sacral area or the back of his thighs.

Describe his edema, noting the extent and severity—including pitting—and the location of the body surface involved. Describe the degree of pitting in terms of depth: 0″ to ¼″ is mild (1 +); ¼″ to ½″, moderate (2 +); and ½″ to 1″, severe (3 +). A typical description might read: "bilateral, symmetrical, lower-leg edema extending from the toes to 4″ (10 cm) below the knees; with 3 + pitting."

• *peripheral edema.* Check the patient's hands and ankles. Describe peripheral edema the same way as dependent edema.

• *jugular vein distention.* Position the patient at a 45° angle to detect pulsation and, consequently, distention of the jugular veins.

• *tachycardia or pulsus alternans.* Take the patient's pulse to detect tachycardia or pulsus alternans (a pattern of alternating strong and weak beats). Keep in mind that tachycardia is one of the most reliable clues to heart failure.

• *decreased peripheral pulses.* On palpation, peripheral pulses may be fleeting or absent because of poor left ventricular pumping or because of chronically diminished arterial flow from atherosclerosis. However, peripheral pulses may be normal if the patient has slight left ventricular compromise or atherosclerosis.

• *abnormal apical impulse.* Locate the apical impulse at the left midclavicular line and fifth intercostal space. In left heart failure, cardiomegaly displaces the apical impulse to the sixth or seventh intercostal space and laterally away from the midclavicular line; also, normally localized tapping of the apical impulse may be diffuse. Since the apical impulse defines the left lateral and inferior cardiac border, locating it helps determine the extent of the heart's enlargement.

• *ventricular heave.* Warm your palm, and palpate the precordium along the parasternal

Characteristic findings in CHF

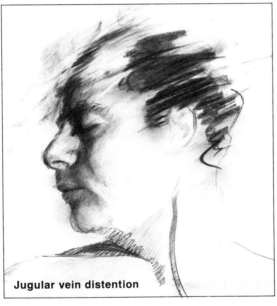
Jugular vein distention

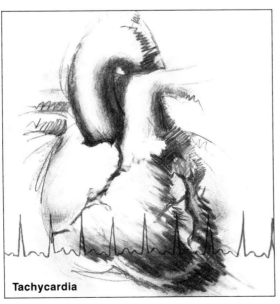
Tachycardia

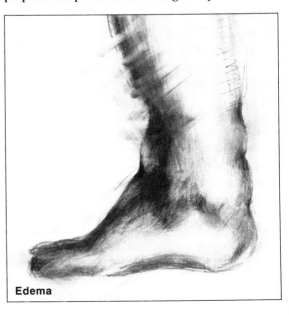
Edema

borders. In right ventricular failure, you'll feel a lifting sensation.

• *softened S_1 and S_2*. Listen for S_1 and S_2. These sounds may be normal or may soften as the heart's pumping action diminishes.

• *murmurs*. Listen for systolic murmurs that soften. Consider any murmur of grade IV to VI intensity that softens to a grade II as a sign of cardiovascular deterioration. Such softening occurs when blood flows over the abnormal valve with diminished force, creating less turbulence than normal.

• *extra heart sounds*. Auscultate for extra heart sounds produced as blood flows into a compliant ventricle. You may hear S_3 (also called ventricular gallop), one of the early signs of congestive heart failure. In left heart failure, you may hear S_3 over the apex; in right heart failure, over the left sternal border. Remember that a physiologic S_3 occurs in many children and young adults. However, physiologic S_3 disappears when the patient sits erect. Pathologic S_3 doesn't disappear. Sometimes in CHF, you may hear a brief, low-pitched fourth heart sound just before S_1.

• *altered heart rate and rhythm*. The patient's medical history is usually the best baseline for determining changes in heart rate and rhythm. However, if the history is incomplete, establish a baseline in your initial assessment and monitor for changes.

• *bibasilar rales*. Check both lungs for this early sign of CHF. Failure to check both lungs in a patient positioned laterally can lead to inaccurate findings, because fluid may shift to one lung.

• *hepatomegaly*. Palpate and percuss the upper right quadrant of the abdomen. Palpation will probably reveal tenderness and a palpable liver. Percussion may reveal fluid in the abdominal cavity.

• *reduced urinary output and dark, concentrated urine*. Record fluid intake and output and observe urine color.

• *neurologic abnormalities*. Usually, the patient shows no neurologic abnormalities, but you may observe a shortened attention span, memory impairment, depression, and anxiety.

Plan and implement nursing care

Integrate the subjective data from the patient history and the objective data from the cardiovascular assessment to formulate a nursing diagnosis. Your nursing diagnosis should consider the severity of congestive heart failure,

Characteristic findings in CHF (continued)

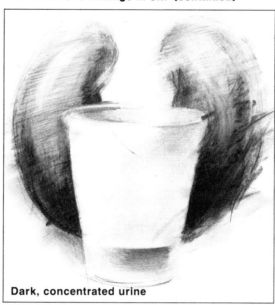

Dark, concentrated urine

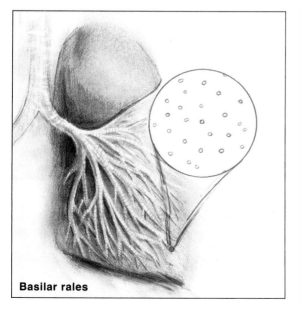

Basilar rales

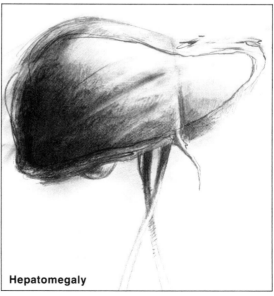

Hepatomegaly

EMERGENCY MANAGEMENT

Treating pulmonary edema

A patient is rushed to the emergency room. His skin is cold and clammy; his blood pressure is elevated and he's cyanotic. His respirations sound bubbly, with moist rales over both lungs, and he has frothy, blood-tinged secretions in the corners of his mouth. Every sign points to an advanced stage of pulmonary edema, in which fluid has accumulated in the extravascular spaces of the lung. Without immediate treatment, to reduce extravascular fluid and improve gas exchange and myocardial function, the patient will die.

Here are the priorities that you should follow in this life-threatening emergency.

Relieve respiratory distress

Your first priority is to relieve respiratory difficulties. Begin by checking the patient's airway. If it's obstructed, instruct the patient to cough and expectorate. If coughing and expectoration fail to clear the obstruction, begin to suction the patient. If suctioning fails, prepare to assist the doctor with intubation, which facilitates aspiration of thick secretions and the use of intermittent positive pressure breathing.

If the patient's airway isn't obstructed, assist him to a sitting position in bed and, if possible, allow his legs to dangle over the sides to decrease venous return and to relieve dyspnea. Also, give a high concentration of oxygen by mask using intermittent or continuous pressure. This method of oxygen administration overcomes the pressure barrier caused by fluid accumulation and ensures adequate blood oxygenation. To monitor oxygen administration, draw arterial blood samples for laboratory analysis.

Watch for dysrhythmias

First, connect the patient to a cardiac monitor. Then, monitor the EKG waveforms on the oscilloscope screen and be alert for dysrhythmias. Be sure to have resuscitation equipment ready.

Monitor response to drug administration

To remove the excess alveolar fluid, the doctor will probably order a rapid-acting I.V. diuretic, such as furosemide or ethacrynic acid. Since diuretics increase excretion of water and electrolytes, carefully monitor urinary output and serum electrolyte levels.

Along with an I.V. diuretic, the doctor will probably order morphine, unless the patient has a history of cerebrovascular accidents or chronic obstructive pulmonary disease, or is in cardiogenic shock. Morphine alleviates anxiety and promotes blood flow from the pulmonary circulation to the periphery. However, because morphine can severely depress respiration, have naloxone hydrochloride and intubation equipment within easy reach.

The doctor may also order administration of aminophylline and an inotropic agent, such as digitalis, to improve cardiac output. Aminophylline relieves severe bronchospasm and increases cardiac output, renal flow and urinary output of sodium and water. Be sure to administer aminophylline slowly to prevent a sudden—and possibly fatal—drop in blood pressure. Also, be alert for tachydysrhythmias because aminophylline may increase heart rate. If the doctor orders digitalis, watch for signs of toxicity.

the patient's emotional state and ability to comply with treatment, and the effects of decreased cardiac output on various body systems and on the patient's life-style. Typically, your nursing diagnosis of a patient with CHF may include altered cardiac output, potential deterioration of the patient's condition, potential electroconductive alteration, ineffective breathing patterns, sleep pattern disturbances and various emotional and cognitive problems.

Altered cardiac output. Such alteration causes changes in thought processes and reduces activity tolerance. With this diagnosis, your goal is *to maintain hemodynamic stability.* Hemodynamic monitoring—measurement of pulmonary artery end-diastolic pressure (PAEDP), mean pulmonary capillary wedge pressure (PCWP), and cardiac output—is a useful tool for assessing the patient's response

to treatment and maintaining hemodynamic stability. PCWP is probably the most accurate indicator of impending heart failure, but measurement of cardiac output is also useful. CHF always reduces cardiac output, causing hypoperfusion.

In acute failure, if nitroprusside and a positive inotropic agent have failed to restore hemodynamic stability, the doctor may insert an intraaortic balloon pump (IABP) until the patient's condition stabilizes or until valve replacement. If appropriate, prepare the patient for this procedure, assist during insertion of the IABP, and monitor the pressure readings.

Position the patient properly. Correct positioning helps maintain hemodynamic stability. Unless an IABP has been inserted, place the patient in a semirecumbent position in bed or in an armchair to decrease venous return. If the patient is in bed, elevate the head of the bed on 20 cm to 30 cm (8″ to 12″) blocks. Support the arms with pillows. If the patient is orthopneic, have him sit on the side of the bed, supporting his head and arms on an over-the-bed table. Place a pillow under the lumbosacral spine, and support the feet.

Promote rest. Provide supportive care to reduce cardiac work load. Provide a bedside commode to prevent overexertion. Make sure the patient's room is quiet, cool, and well ventilated. Also limit the number of visitors, eliminate unnecessary physical exams, and allow the patient to rest between care procedures, before and after meals, and at several intervals during the day.

To promote sound sleep, administer oxygen, as ordered, to decrease respiratory effort and increase comfort. Provide a night light to help prevent disorientation for the patient who wakens at night. If the dyspneic patient insists on leaving his bed at night, position him comfortably in an armchair. Avoid using restraints. Instead, administer a mild sedative, as ordered—but do so carefully to prevent respiratory depression. Also, realize that because of poor hepatic and renal function, drugs will clear more slowly.

Potential for deterioration. Such deterioration may result from inadequate gas exchange and impaired arterial and venous peripheral circulation. With this diagnosis, your goal in planning interventions is *to prevent complications:* pulmonary and systemic congestion, infection, skin breakdown, thromboembolism, and cardiogenic shock.

Prevent pulmonary and systemic congestion. Check for fluid retention and weigh the patient daily. If his weight increases more than 500 g/day, promptly notify the doctor. Monitor fluid intake and output and test urine specific gravity every 2 hours. To minimize fluid retention, avoid rapid or excessive hydration. When administering I.V. fluids or drugs, use a microdrip or infusion pump. If the patient requires oxygen, give volumes that don't depress his stimulus to breathe.

Monitor drug therapy. Since systemic congestion may inhibit drug metabolism and even low doses may cause toxic effects, be alert for signs of drug toxicity and watch for effectiveness. If a drug doesn't seem to be achieving its desired effect, discuss with the doctor the possible need for an increased dose. Watch carefully for drug side effects that affect fluid balance. If the patient retains fluid, give diuretics, as ordered, but observe for hypokalemia. If the patient is taking digitalis and

develops hypokalemia, observe closely for signs of digitalis toxicity. Give potassium supplements for hypokalemia, as ordered.

Prevent infection. Maintain strict aseptic technique when inserting I.V. lines or a Foley catheter. If the patient develops an infection, take his temperature regularly and try to pinpoint the source of the infection.

Avoid skin breakdown. Assess the patient frequently for reddened or marked areas, especially if he has edema. Change his position every 2 hours. Slowly increase the patient's activity level, as ordered and as tolerated. Check blood pressure, pulse, respirations, and EKG (if monitored) just before and after each increase in activity level. Watch the patient for signs of activity intolerance, such as decreased blood pressure.

Prevent thromboembolism. While the patient is confined to bed, apply antiembolism stockings to help maintain venous pressure in the legs and prevent blood pooling, which may cause blood clot formation. Encourage him to slowly increase his activity and, if ordered, perform passive range-of-motion exercises.

Try to prevent cardiogenic shock. Continuously observe for signs of cardiogenic shock,

Critical end-diastolic pressure values

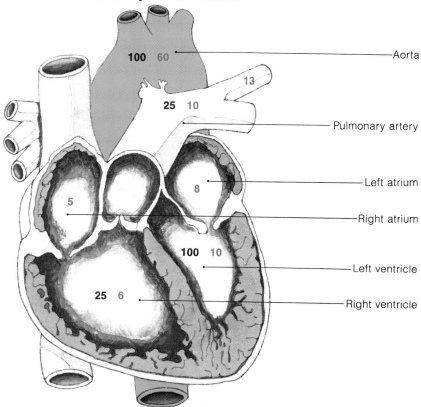

Black numbers indicate systolic pressures. Red numbers indicate end-diastolic pressures above which failure begins.

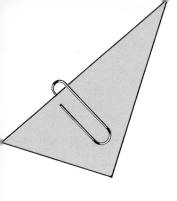

PATIENT-TEACHING AID

Living with congestive heart failure

Dear _____

You have congestive heart failure, a condition which impairs your heart's ability to pump blood. Because overexertion places a tremendous strain on your heart, you'll need to modify your life-style to decrease your heart's work load and minimize symptoms.

Take digitalis, as prescribed, to strengthen your heart and improve its pumping ability. Do not substitute one brand of digitalis for another without first consulting your doctor. Check your pulse rate daily before taking digitalis, and call your doctor immediately if it's less than 60 or more than 120 beats per minute. Also report promptly any loss of appetite, nausea and vomiting, diarrhea, fatigue, visual disturbances, headache, muscle weakness, or apathy.

Take a diuretic, if prescribed, to reduce your body's total volume of water and salt. Because a diuretic can cause loss of potassium, promptly report dizziness, nausea and vomiting, loss of appetite, abdominal distention, muscle weakness and fatigue, leg cramps, malaise, confusion, or headache. Because these symptoms may intensify if you become dehydrated, notify your doctor if you cannot eat or drink normally. Do not, however, stop taking any prescribed drug without first consulting your doctor.

Before taking any over-the-counter drugs, such as cold remedies, be sure to ask your doctor.

Restrict sodium intake to decrease retention of fluid, thereby decreasing your heart's work load. Don't add salt to your food. Avoid salted "snack" foods, canned soups and vegetables, prepared foods (such as TV dinners), luncheon meats, cheeses, or pickles and any other foods preserved in brine. Check food labels for sodium content. And finally, be sure to

Check pulse rate before taking digitalis.

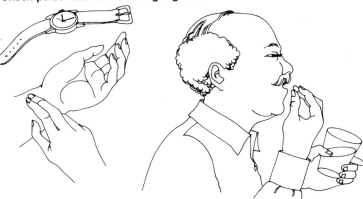

Get adequate rest.

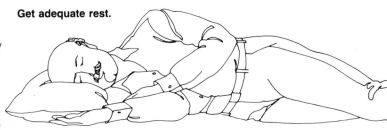

Avoid salt.

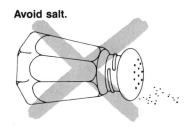

Watch for weight gain.

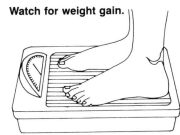

adhere to the diet plan provided by your doctor.

Make sure to get adequate rest. If possible, shorten your work day and set aside a daily rest period. Also, try to avoid emotional stress.

Gradually increase walking and other physical activities to your capacity. Continue at whatever activity level you can maintain without developing shortness of breath, palpitations, or severe fatigue. Also, notify your doctor if these symptoms increase. He may be able to adjust your medication dosage to allow increased activity.

Try to avoid temperature extremes. When possible, stay in a

cool, comfortable environment. In hot weather, perform your activities in the cooler part of the day. In cold weather, dress warmly but avoid restrictive clothing, which interferes with circulation. Wrap a scarf over your nose and mouth to warm the air and make breathing easier.

Watch for and report signs and symptoms of recurring congestive heart failure. These include weight gain, loss of appetite, shortness of breath upon activity, persistent cough, frequent urination at night, and swelling of the ankles, feet or abdomen.

Keep your regular doctor appointments.

particularly if the patient is over age 65 or has had a previous myocardial infarction or CHF. These signs include altered mental status, decreased urinary output (less than 20 ml/hour), decreased blood pressure, and respiratory distress. Report any of these signs immediately.

Potential electroconductive alteration. With this diagnosis, your goal is to *maintain electrophysiologic stability.* If needed, continuously monitor the patient's EKG. Also, check the pulse for atrial fibrillation, a common dysrhythmia in CHF. This dysrhythmia may result from atrial dilatation and distention or from digitalis toxicity. (Realize that administration of digitalis, the drug of choice for atrial fibrillation, and emergency cardioversion are contraindicated if the patient shows signs of digitalis toxicity.) Report any dysrhythmias to the doctor immediately. Be prepared to treat a life-threatening dysrhythmia: check emergency resuscitation equipment every shift for proper functioning and availability.

Emotional disturbances and knowledge deficit. The patient may experience fear of heart failure, of life-style changes, of powerlessness or death; may express anger and hostility as a result of his illness; or may lack the knowledge necessary for full compliance. If you see these problems, your goal is *to reduce the patient's anxiety level.* This is essential since anxiety produces vasoconstriction, increases arterial pressure and heart rate, and, according to some evidence, reduces urine output. Teach the patient relaxation techniques, and play soft music or read to him. Encourage the patient and his family to verbalize their fears.

Teach the patient about the treatment. Begin your teaching on the day of admission. Tell the patient to stay in bed most of the time at first, getting up just to use the bathroom and to sit in a chair for meals. Advise him to change positions slowly to prevent dizziness. Explain that you'll perform passive range-of-motion exercises 3 times a day, and will evaluate the effects of these exercises on his respirations, energy level, and heart rate.

Explain any dietary and fluid restrictions. Tell him that you'll record intake and output and weigh him once daily.

Help the patient accept realistic limitations. The patient with CHF frequently feels torn between what he wants to do and what his weakened heart allows him to do. In resolving this dilemma, the patient can easily overreact: the cautious patient may restrict activity un-

necessarily, whereas the stoic patient may overexert himself. Help your patient steer clear of these extremes by giving him a thorough explanation of CHF and the limitations appropriate for his condition.

Discuss specific changes in life-style, but avoid frightening him. Negotiate changes that don't involve his self-image. If he objects strongly to eliminating an activity, explore the reasons with him. When possible, suggest that he continue a favored activity at a less strenuous level.

Before discharge, assess the patient's ability to comply with treatment and make referrals for follow-up care as needed. If the patient fails to understand his treatment regimen, clarify his role. Also, refer him to the American Heart Association for information and, if necessary, to psychologic and social services to promote and ease necessary adjustments in life-style.

Evaluate response to treatment

Look for signs of a positive response to treatment: signs of decreased congestion, improved cardiac output, and decreased anxiety. Signs of decreased congestion include decreased pitting edema, weight loss, normal urinary output, and absence of neck vein distention, rales, and dyspnea. Diagnostic test results that confirm decreased congestion include decreased pulmonary congestion on the chest X-ray, shorter circulation time (measured by the cardiac index), and decreased central venous pressure and pulmonary capillary wedge pressure. Signs of improved cardiac output include decreased heart rate, diuresis, increased activity tolerance, and absence of any earlier confusion and dizziness supported by an improved cardiac output or cardiac index. Signs of decreased anxiety include relaxed verbal and nonverbal behavior.

Evaluate your patient's knowledge of CHF. Was your teaching program successful? Make sure the patient and his family know the risk factors of CHF and how to modify or avoid them, the necessary discharge regimen (activity modification, diet, drugs), and details of follow-up care. Evaluate their ability to check pulse rate and their knowledge of the symptoms that require prompt medical attention.

Although you can't ever guarantee the patient's compliance with treatment, you can improve it with effective teaching and thus help prolong effective cardiac compensation for as long as possible.

Points to remember

- Congestive heart failure is becoming increasingly common as more people survive cardiac damage or live long enough to develop cardiac weakness.
- Congestive heart failure can result from left ventricular failure, which primarily causes pulmonary congestion, or from right ventricular failure, which primarily causes systemic congestion. Failure of one ventricle almost always causes failure of the other ventricle.
- Traditional drug therapies are being replaced by new, more effective drugs, such as unloading agents and positive inotropic agents. These drugs offer new hope for the patient with refractory heart failure whose symptoms continue after maximal dosages of digitalis and diuretics.
- Because compliance with treatment is critically important for the CHF patient, thorough patient teaching is your primary responsibility.

6 FORESTALLING CORONARY CRISIS

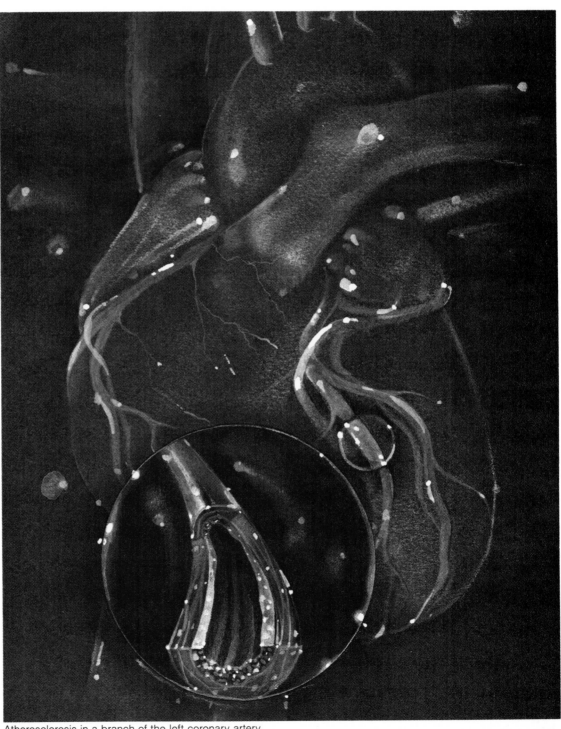

Atherosclerosis in a branch of the left coronary artery

Coronary artery disease (CAD) is near-epidemic in the Western world. Although researchers have made tremendous strides in treating its severe forms, with streptokinase therapy and percutaneous transluminal coronary angioplasty, to name just two, managing CAD is still an enormous challenge. For you, first of all, that means learning to identify CAD in all its stages by mastering cardiovascular assessment. It means being able to distinguish the chest pain of angina from that of acute myocardial infarction (MI) and many other disorders. It means recognizing characteristic—and, at times, ominous—EKG changes and knowing what emergency and supportive care they require. And it means helping the patient and his family cope effectively with their fears and anxieties.

To successfully meet the nursing challenge of CAD, you'll need a thorough understanding of its pathophysiology and its traditional and experimental treatments.

What is CAD?
Coronary artery disease is an umbrella term for various diseases that reduce or halt blood flow in the coronary arteries. Atherosclerosis accounts for more than 90% of the cases of CAD; arteriosclerosis, arteritis, coronary artery spasm, embolism, thrombosis, and certain infectious diseases account for the remainder.

What causes CAD?
Although CAD claims more lives each year than any other disease, its causes are poorly understood. Consider atherosclerosis. For many obscure reasons, the cells lining the coronary arteries of susceptible persons begin to change. Gradually, over a period of years, fatty or calcified deposits accumulate on the walls of the coronary arteries, thereby reducing the heart's blood supply. These deposits, called *plaques,* can eventually clog an artery. Typically, the patient receives a warning—the chest discomfort of angina. Angina indicates that a portion of the heart muscle is being deprived of its needed supply of oxygen—the result of arterial narrowing, arterial spasm, or both.

Usually, patients do not experience angina until the lumen of the artery is narrowed by 70% to 75%. If the artery does close, the part of the heart this artery serves becomes necrotic—a myocardial infarction, the end stage of coronary artery disease, has taken place.

Although all the causes of CAD aren't known, investigators have identified some significant risk factors, many of them controllable. These risk factors include a family history of heart disease, obesity, smoking, a high-fat and high-carbohydrate diet, a sedentary life-style, a "Type A" personality, diabetes, hypertension, and hereditary hyperlipoproteinemias. If both genetic and acquired risk factors are present in the same person, the risk of developing CAD increases markedly.

Besides the risk factors, investigators know the demographic data. Typically, CAD strikes more whites than blacks, and more men than women. It's more prevalent in industrial than in underdeveloped nations, and affects more affluent than poor people. Its characteristic atherosclerotic changes may occur as early as age 10, but usually occur after age 30.

PATHOPHYSIOLOGY OF ATHEROSCLEROSIS
Atherosclerosis is believed to involve three mechanisms: lipoprotein abnormalities, arterial wall injury, and platelet dysfunction.

Lipoprotein abnormalities are caused by a class of hyperlipidemias known as *hyperlipoproteinemias,* which are defects of lipoprotein metabolism. Such abnormalities may be genetically determined or acquired. Acquired lipoprotein abnormalities may result from other disorders, such as nephrotic syndrome and hypothyroidism, or from dietary or environmental factors. Two important hyperlipoproteinemias are hypercholesterolemia and hypertriglyceridemia.

In *hypercholesterolemia,* the liver is unable to remove cholesterol from low-density lipoproteins (LDLs) in the plasma. An unknown factor allows the LDLs to infiltrate the intima (the innermost layer) of the arterial walls, leading to plaque formation. In North America, studies report that cholesterol levels above 220 mg/dl pose an increased risk of atherosclerotic heart disease in patients under age 50. However, some patients with hereditary atherosclerosis may have normal blood cholesterol levels.

In *hypertriglyceridemia,* the increased levels of triglycerides are closely related to increased levels of very low-density lipoproteins (VLDLs). An increase in either level correlates with increased incidence of atherosclerosis in patients under age 50.

Arterial wall injury is thought to encourage plaque formation after injury to the intima. Initially, injury disrupts the endothelial layer,

Fat facts: Lipids and lipoproteins

Key:

- Protein
- Cholesterol
- Phospholipid
- Triglyceride

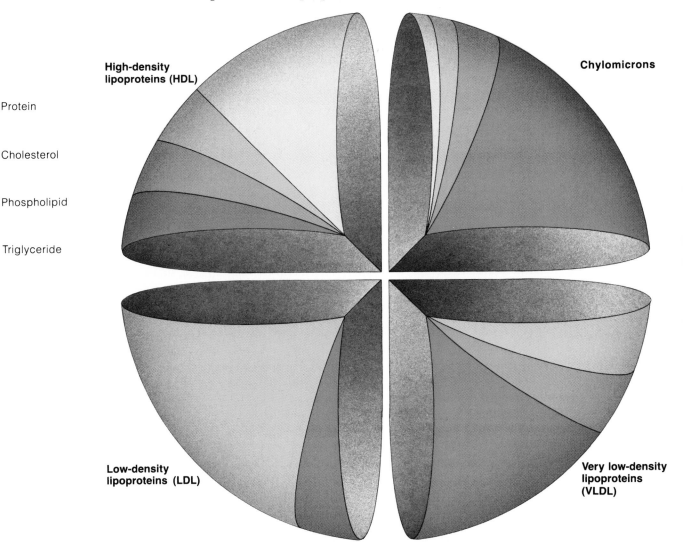

High-density lipoproteins (HDL)

Chylomicrons

Low-density lipoproteins (LDL)

Very low-density lipoproteins (VLDL)

Lipids are fats or fatlike substances, insoluble in water and stored in the body as an energy source. They're also important constituents of cell membranes and other cellular structures. Four kinds of lipids occur naturally in the body: triglycerides, phospholipids, cholesterol, and apoproteins.

Triglycerides are the main storage form of lipids, and constitute about 95% of fatty tissue. They consist of one molecule of glycerol bonded to three molecules of fatty acids. Together with carbohydrates and protein, these compounds furnish energy for metabolism.

Phospholipids, which are lipid soluble, contain glycerol, fatty acids, phosphate, and a nitrogenous compound. Although formed in most cells, phospholipids typically enter the circulation as lipoproteins synthesized by the liver. They form part of the cell membrane and help to lower interfacial tension between the membrane and surrounding fluids.

Cholesterol, a structural component of cell membranes and plasma lipoproteins, is a precursor of glucocorticoids, sex hormones, and bile salts. It's absorbed from food in the gastrointestinal tract and also synthesized in the liver.

Apoproteins are water-soluble proteins that combine with most lipids to form lipoproteins. Apoproteins are being studied as diagnostic tools.

Before lipids can be transported through the body, they must combine with plasma proteins to form *lipoproteins.* Four classes of lipoproteins contain varying amounts of the four naturally occurring lipids.

Chylomicrons, the lowest density lipoproteins, consist mostly of triglycerides, with small amounts of lipids and protein. They're the form in which long-chain and cholesterol fats move from the intestine to the blood.

Very low-density lipoproteins (VLDL) consist mostly of triglycerides, with moderate concentrations of phospholipids and cholesterol.

Low-density lipoproteins (LDL) consist mostly of cholesterol, with relatively few triglycerides.

High-density lipoproteins (HDL) are approximately half protein and half phospholipids, cholesterol, and triglycerides.

exposing underlying collagen of the arterial wall. Then, according to current theory, platelets may gather at the site of injury and release *thromboxane,* a prostaglandin that promotes platelet aggregation and vasoconstriction. At the same time, the exposed intima releases its own prostaglandin, called *prostacyclin,* which counteracts thromboxane by retarding platelet aggregation and causing vasodilation. According to theory, if intimal injury is minor, the two prostaglandins cancel each other's effects and the injury heals. However, if intimal injury is severe, the intimal layer begins to deteriorate; it releases less prostacyclin, favoring the clotting effect of thromboxane.

Plaque development
Once established, atheromatous plaques evolve through three types of lesions: fatty streaks, fibrous plaques, and complicated lesions. As plaques become more extensive, the arterial wall degenerates (see *Four Stages of Atherosclerosis,* page 97).

Fatty streaks—soft, yellow, raised lesions—are the first obvious evidence of atherosclerosis, but they don't cause vascular obstruction. These streaks may regress, remain static, or progress to plaques, but the mechanism involved is not well understood.

Fibrous plaques may develop from fatty streaks, but may also occur spontaneously. These grayish-white plaques thicken and extend into the lumen of the artery, interfering with blood flow. Progressive sclerosis of the artery occurs as fibroblasts penetrate the areas of degeneration.

Complicated lesions develop from the continued accumulation of fat, connective tissue, and cells, and these lesions may become vascularized. As they extend into the lumen, blood clots develop and form thrombi. Continued deterioration of the arterial wall may lead to rupture and hemorrhage.

Calcified plaques may form when calcium precipitates out of the blood and lipids, such as cholesterol, and are released from mononuclear cells in the arterial wall into the plaque. This type of arterial wall degeneration progresses to arteriosclerosis, in which the vessels lose their elasticity and eventually rupture.

Coronary artery narrowing, with resulting ischemia, can also result from simple embolic occlusion, bacterial endocarditis of the aortic or mitral valves, formation of calcified emboli, and after surgery for a stenosed valve.

Ischemia: When circulation fails
Myocardial ischemia results from the reduction or occlusion of arterial blood flow by atherosclerotic plaques, or from arterial spasm. Reduced or occluded blood flow forces the myocardium to shift to anaerobic metabolism, which produces lactic acid as a byproduct. Localized accumulation of lactic acid is thought to irritate nerve endings in the affected area, causing pain. In addition, hypoxia leads to reduced energy availability and acidosis, which reduces myocardial contractility and depresses left ventricular function. The ischemic heart wall becomes hypokinetic and contracts less effectively during systole, which reduces cardiac efficiency.

The hemodynamic effects of reduced contractility and impaired wall motion vary, depending on the extent of ischemic involvement and the response of autonomic reflex compensatory mechanisms. Depressed left ventricular function may lower cardiac output by decreasing stroke volume. As ventricular volume increases, left ventricular end-diastolic pressure and pulmonary capillary wedge pressure increase. Continued ischemia aggravates these increases in pressure, and reduced compliance further increases pressure for a given ventricular volume.

The hemodynamic pattern during ischemia usually consists of slight increases in heart rate and blood pressure before the onset of pain. This may be a sympathetic compensatory response to depressed myocardial function rather than a response to the pain and anxiety caused by an attack. Depressed blood pressure may mean that ischemia has affected a large part of the myocardium.

Ischemic attacks usually subside within minutes if the imbalance between oxygen supply and demand is corrected and the metabolic, functional, hemodynamic, and electrocardiographic changes are reversed. During an ischemic or anginal attack, the patient may report pressure under the breastbone that radiates to an arm (usually, the inner aspect of the left arm), the neck, the jaw, or other parts of the upper body. Frequently, the patient grinds a clenched fist against his breastbone—a classic clue to anginal pain. However, many patients never report characteristic anginal pain, since their discomfort may mimic indigestion or even a toothache. Angina caused by coronary artery spasm may be triggered by cold; smoking or caffeine consumption; or exercise. Some patients become dyspneic on exertion, without chest pain.

The pathway to infarction

If ischemia is prolonged, it causes irreversible tissue necrosis. This area of necrotic myocardium is called an *infarct,* or a *myocardial infarction.* The infarct may occur in the anterior, septal, lateral, and/or diaphragmatic or inferior heart walls, depending on which coronary artery is occluded. It may be *transmural,* damaging the full thickness of the heart wall, or *nontransmural (subendocardial),* damaging only a partial thickness.

An ischemic zone usually surrounds an infarction. If effective treatment begins immediately, necrosis can be minimized and the ischemic zone can recover. If not, this zone can also become necrotic, extending the infarction and further depressing myocardial function.

If an infarction isn't fatal, the myocardium begins to heal. Within 24 hours, leukocytes infiltrate the infarcted area, beginning at its periphery. The injured myocardial cells release characteristic enzymes that can be measured in the serum to help gauge the extent of tissue damage. Within 24 hours, degradation and removal of necrotic tissue begins. After 3 weeks, scar tissue begins to form; tissue removal causes thinning of the heart wall, which may cause rupture if it occurs too rapidly. After 4 to 6 weeks, scar tissue is completely formed. This nonelastic tissue can impair the heart's performance in several ways: it reduces contractility, changes ventricular wall compliance, reduces stroke volume and ejection fraction, and raises ventricular end-systolic and end-diastolic pressures.

The extent of functional impairment and the patient's prognosis depend on the size and location of the infarct, the condition of the uninvolved myocardium, the potential for collateral circulation, and the effectiveness of compensatory mechanisms. Collateral circulation may develop in response to impaired perfusion and ischemia, thereby eventually improving blood flow to the affected area.

Several reflex compensatory mechanisms help sustain cardiac output and peripheral perfusion. After an MI, sympathetic nervous enhancement of contractility can improve ventricular function. Vasoconstriction increases total peripheral resistance and mean arterial pressure. It also reduces venous capacity, which enhances venous return to the heart. Increased ventricular filling increases ventricular volume and diastolic filling pressure; this stretches the myocardial fibers, which increase their force of contraction proportionately, according to Starling's law. Decreased cardiac output causes the kidneys to retain sodium and water, which further increases circulating blood volume, adding to the heart's work load.

After an MI, the hemodynamic response varies. Cardiac output may be normal or decreased, and heart rate usually doesn't remain elevated unless there is extensive myocardial depression. However, persistent tachycardia decreases the diastolic filling time of the coronary arteries. Decreased heart rate and blood pressure can result from stimulation of parasympathetic ganglia in the myocardium. This vasovagal response diminishes cardiac output and peripheral perfusion.

Complications of myocardial infarction

The size and location of infarction may affect far more than ventricular integrity and performance. A severely damaged ventricle or other cardiac structure can cause serious and sometimes fatal complications.

Sudden death most commonly results from the rapid onset of ventricular fibrillation, but may also result from ventricular standstill. Other dysrhythmias, such as idioventricular rhythm, marked sinus bradycardia, or complete atrioventricular heart block, may encourage ectopic mechanisms that can lead to ventricular tachycardia and fibrillation. Rarely, death may result from rupture of the ventricular wall. Such rupture may occur before scar formation, releasing blood into the pericardial sac. The accumulating blood compresses the heart and causes cardiac tamponade, which impairs venous return and cardiac output. Ventricular rupture is commonly heralded by sudden tachycardia, followed by marked bracycardia with electromechanical dissociation (EMD)—electrical activity without peripheral pulses.

Cardiogenic shock affects 10% to 15% of patients with MI, with mortality of 80% to 90%. This condition is marked by a circular pattern of progressive hemodynamic deterioration: falling cardiac output causes hypotension, which triggers compensatory mechanisms. If compensation fails to maintain arterial blood pressure or perfusion of vital organs, blood pressure falls below a critical level, resulting in ischemia of all organs.

Congestive heart failure (CHF) and *pulmonary edema* may result if the damaged left ventricle fails to adequately expel blood at systole. This causes increased ventricular

Danger signals: EKG changes in myocardial infarction

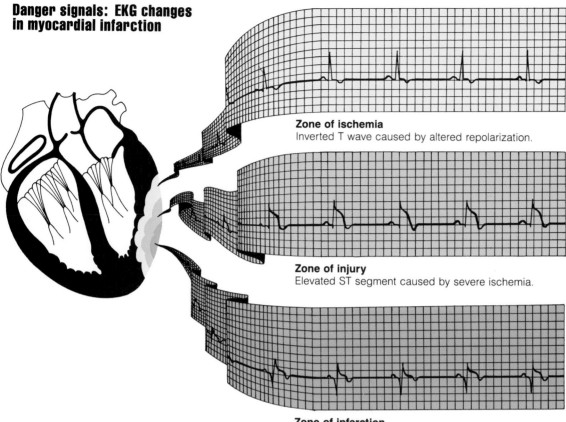

Zone of ischemia
Inverted T wave caused by altered repolarization.

Zone of injury
Elevated ST segment caused by severe ischemia.

Zone of infarction
Deepened Q wave caused by lack of depolarization in necrotic tissue.

Myocardial infarction (MI) produces characteristic EKG changes in several leads at once, enabling the doctor to determine accurately the location and extent of tissue damage. Three pathologic changes occur during MI: development of an area of necrotic tissue (the infarction), surrounded by a zone of injury, bounded in turn by an outer zone of ischemia. The zone of ischemia produces characteristic T-wave inversions. The zone of injury produces characteristic ST-segment elevations. The zone of infarction produces pathologic Q waves, indicating developing myocardial necrosis—a true infarction. (Diagnostic Q waves should be larger than one of the small squares on the chart: 0.04 second by 0.1 millivolt. They're also usually one third the height of the R wave.) The infarction can be located by studying characteristic wave changes in various lead combinations.

volume and pressure, leading to pulmonary congestion. Fluid escapes into the interstitial spaces and alveoli, impairing gas exchange.

Ventricular septal defect may occur when necrosis of the interventricular septum causes rupture of the septal wall. Such rupture indicates extensive CAD, because the septum receives blood from arteries descending from the anterior and posterior surface of the interventricular groove. The rupture shunts blood from the left to the right ventricle, reducing left ventricular output. This greatly reduces cardiac output and increases right ventricular work load and pulmonary congestion.

Ventricular aneurysm, a bulging of the ischemic heart wall, may develop in about 25% of patients. Such an aneurysm usually is associated with transmural infarction and involves the anterior or apical wall in 80% of cases. Ventricular aneurysm may cause ventricular dysrhythmias, chronic congestive heart failure, and release of mural thrombi into the systemic circulation. An EKG may suggest aneurysm if persistent elevated ST segments appear.

Rupture of the papillary muscles, which ensure normal mitral valve closure, may cause mitral regurgitation. Depending on the severity of regurgitated blood flow, this can lead to diminished forward aortic flow and increased left atrial and pulmonary pressures.

Thromboembolism may occur when thrombi form on the roughened endothelium. If thrombi form in the systemic venous system, right atrium, or right ventricle, venous embolization can cause pulmonary embolism.

Pericarditis may result when MI extends to the pericardial surface, producing localized or occasionally extensive fibrinous pericarditis. Typically, pericarditis occurs within a week of acute MI, causing chest pain that often radiates to left shoulder and is aggravated by deep inspiration. Pain may abate when patient sits up and leans forward. Auscultation may reveal pericardial friction rub.

Dysrhythmias result from ischemia, hypoxemia, autonomic nervous system influences, metabolic and electrolyte imbalances, hemodynamic abnormalities, and digitalis therapy.

Dressler's syndrome (post-MI syndrome) is pericardial inflammation of unknown etiology. It's thought to be an autoimmune reaction. The syndrome appears a few weeks or months after MI and is characterized by fever, pleuropericardial chest pain, pericardial friction rub, and left pleural effusion.

Thallium scans identify the ischemic heart

After exercise

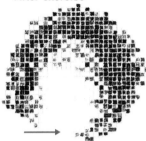

At rest

This thallium scan of a patient with coronary artery disease shows a "cold spot" (arrow), indicating stress-induced ischemia after treadmill exercise. The second scan shows the same heart at rest after the test; the spot has disappeared.

MEDICAL MANAGEMENT

Successful medical management of CAD depends on early diagnosis and aggressive treatment with drugs and, at times, surgery. Although diagnosis of uncomplicated CAD primarily depends on the patient's history and characteristic pattern of pain, diagnostic tests help determine the extent of disease and provide baseline data.

Diagnosis: The critical first step

Typically, the first diagnostic tests include the 12-lead EKG, the chest X-ray, and various blood studies. After these tests provide baseline information about the patient's condition, more sophisticated tests—nuclear medicine scans, coronary angiography, and echocardiography—may be performed to pinpoint the diagnosis (see also Chapter 3, Updating Diagnostic Concepts).

The 12-lead EKG. Performed at rest or during exercise, the 12-lead EKG distinguishes three pathophysiologic events: ischemia, injury, and infarction. Unless the patient experiences anginal pain during the resting EKG, this test isn't usually helpful for diagnosing CAD. However, it may reveal an old or recent myocardial infarction. The exercise EKG allows evaluation of the myocardium under increased oxygen demand. Ischemia is indicated by ST segment depression. The exercise EKG is also valuable for evaluating dysrhythmias and the heart's exercise capacity.

The chest X-ray. This test may reveal abnormalities resulting from atherosclerosis or its complications. Possible findings include cardiac enlargement (resulting from chronic heart failure and/or hypertension), congestive heart failure, ventricular aneurysm, and pulmonary congestion (resulting from left ventricular dysfunction).

Blood studies. Cardiac enzyme analyses, complete blood count (CBC), and lipid analyses are used to evaluate risk factors for CAD in stable patients, or to rule out MI. Cardiac enzyme analyses—especially, creatine phosphokinase (CPK), serum glutamic-oxaloacetic transaminase (SGOT), and lactic dehydrogenase (LDH)—help detect acute MI by measuring the levels of the enzymes released into the blood from necrotic heart muscle.

Creatine phosphokinase, which is present in heart muscle as well as in skeletal muscle and brain tissue, increases after MI. However, CPK levels also increase in skeletal muscle disease, chronic alcoholism, and hypothyroidism. Consequently, measurement of elevated levels of CPK-MB, an isoenzyme found primarily in heart muscle, reliably indicates cardiac damage.

Serum glutamic-oxaloacetic acid—an enzyme found primarily in the heart, liver, kidneys, pancreas, and skeletal muscles—increases after MI, returning to normal levels in 4 to 5 days.

Lactic dehydrogenase—an enzyme found in almost all body tissues—increases in many disorders. However, two LDH isoenzymes, LDH_1 and LDH_2, appear primarily in the heart. Measuring their levels helps support CPK isoenzyme test results or promotes diagnosis when CPK isoenzymes weren't measured within 24 hours of an acute MI.

The complete blood count (CBC) also helps confirm myocardial necrosis and inflammation. The CBC includes determinations of hemoglobin concentration, hematocrit, red and white cell counts, differential white cell counts, and stained red cell examination. This battery of tests may reveal anemia, or polycythemia, which increases blood viscosity and the heart's work load.

Various lipid analyses may be performed to detect and classify hyperlipoproteinemias and to monitor patients after an MI. Lipoprotein phenotyping is a useful screening test for younger patients with a family history of CAD that suggests a need for early preventive therapy (primarily dietary adjustments). Lipoprotein-cholesterol fractionation tests, which isolate and measure the major lipids in serum—chylomicrons, very low-density lipoproteins (VLDL), low-density lipoproteins (LDL), and high-density lipoproteins (HDL)—help to assess the risk of CAD. The cholesterol in LDL and HDL fractions is most significant: the higher the HDL level, the lower the incidence of CAD; the higher the LDL level, the higher the incidence of CAD.

Nuclear medicine scans. Three nuclear medicine scans are used to diagnose CAD. *Thallium imaging* evaluates myocardial blood flow and the status of myocardial cells after I.V. injection of the radioisotope thallium-201. Although healthy myocardial tissue absorbs the radioisotope, ischemic tissue does not, and appears as a "cold spot" on a thallium scan. Resting thallium imaging can detect the location and size of recent MI or suspected ischemia. Stress thallium imaging, performed after treadmill exercise, can assess known or suspected CAD: a cold spot appears during peak exercise but disappears at rest.

Unlike thallium imaging, *technetium pyro-*

phosphate scanning reveals ischemic myocardial tissue as a "hot spot"—an area where the radioisotope technetium pyrophosphate accumulates after I.V. injection. Used to detect the acute phase of a suspected MI and to determine its extent, this test can detect ischemic myocardial tissue within 12 hours after infarction. Typically, hot spots are most apparent up to 48 to 72 hours, and disappear after 1 week.

Cardiac blood pool imaging, in which the radioisotope technetium-99m pertechnetate is tagged to red blood cells and injected I.V., outlines the heart cavity to detect myocardial wall-motion abnormalities, and to calculate the ejection fraction. In first-pass imaging, a scintillation camera records the radioactivity emitted by the radioisotope in its initial pass through the left ventricle.

Gated cardiac blood pool imaging, performed after first-pass imaging or as a separate test, has several forms. In multiple-gated acquisition (MUGA) scanning, the camera records 14 to 64 points of a single cardiac cycle, yielding sequential images that can be studied like motion picture films to evaluate regional wall motion and determine the ejection fraction. In the stress MUGA test, the same test is performed at rest and after exercise to detect changes in ejection fraction and cardiac output. In the nitro MUGA test, the scintillation camera records points in the cardiac cycle after sublingual administration of nitroglycerin, to assess its effect on ventricular function.

Coronary angiography. This radiographic test involves cineangiographic visualization of the coronary arteries. It allows the doctor to detect and gauge the extent of CAD and to evaluate left ventricular function. It also verifies the extent of coronary arterial narrowing or occlusion before treatment.

Echocardiography. This widely used noninvasive test uses ultrahigh-frequency sound waves to study heart chamber size, wall thickness, contractility, and valvular motion and structures. Two techniques, M-mode (motion) and two-dimensional, are commonly used. An M-mode echocardiogram provides an "ice-pick" view of the heart, in which a narrow ultrasonic beam reflects off the various heart structures to a recording device. A two-dimensional echocardiogram is a live-motion study; the ultrasonic beam sweeps rapidly through an arc, producing a fan-shaped image of cardiac structures that is videotaped for later analysis.

A boost for the ailing heart

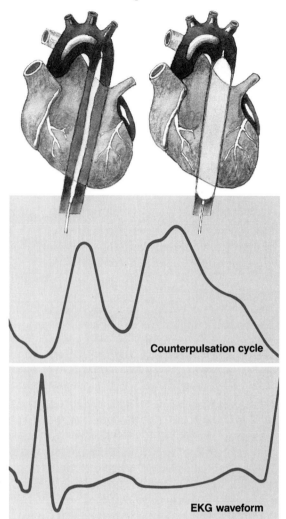

Counterpulsation cycle

EKG waveform

When the left ventricle fails to support adequate circulation and perfusion, insertion of an intra-aortic balloon pump (IABP) can be critically important to your patient's recovery. The device consists of a polyethylene balloon that's inserted via the femoral artery into the descending thoracic aorta distal to the left subclavian artery, and connected to an external pump.

The pump inflates the balloon with helium or carbon dioxide during diastole, and deflates it during systole. This inflation-deflation cycle is triggered by the patient's EKG. The IABP makes ejection easier and reduces the ventricular work load. Because it helps increase coronary artery perfusion and aids left ventricular ejection, it's an effective way to treat complications of myocardial infarction, including low-output heart failure; cardiogenic shock; severe angina pectoris; and severe ventricular damage that precludes discontinuing cardiopulmonary bypass measures during open-heart surgery.

Treatment: Speed is vital
Once diagnostic tests have detected CAD, treatment should begin promptly, since CAD's mortality rises with delay. Controlling pain, providing physical and emotional rest, and correcting the imbalance between myocardial oxygen supply and demand are immediate priorities. Treatment may include drugs, percutaneous transluminal coronary angioplasty (PTCA), coronary artery bypass grafting (CABG), or streptokinase therapy.

Standard medical treatment depends on the patient's history and condition. For dysrhythmias, treatment includes antiarrhythmic drugs and/or artificial pacing, and electrical cardioversion. For left ventricular failure, treatment includes diuretics, vasodilators, and cardiotonics (especially digitalis). For low cardiac output, it may include fluids, vasodilators, and cardiotonics, and insertion of an intra-aortic balloon pump (see *A boost for the ailing heart,* above). For thromboembolism, it includes anticoagulants, antiembolism stockings, and passive range-of-motion exercises.

Drug therapy. Current therapy for CAD includes nitrates, beta blockers, calcium antagonists, inotropic agents, and anticoagulants.

Nitrates are indicated to relieve or prevent an acute anginal attack. Their major effect in the overall management of angina seems to be coronary and peripheral vasodilation. By decreasing venous preload, nitrates reduce the volume of the blood returning to the heart, thereby reducing the heart's work load and demand for oxygen. Nitrates also dilate normal coronary arteries and may cause redistribution of coronary blood flow to ischemic areas. They may decrease arteriolar resistance (afterload). Sublingual or chewable nitroglycerin helps relieve acute attacks of angina; topical or oral nitroglycerin provides prophylactic treatment.

Beta blockers, such as propranolol, nadolol, metoprolol, pindolol, atenolol, and timolol maleate, inhibit the beta receptors of the sympathetic nervous system. They reduce heart rate, decrease cardiac contractility, and lower systolic blood pressure—all of which reduce myocardial oxygen demand. They can be given alone or in combination with nitrates to prevent anginal attacks. (However, if myocardial contractility is impaired, beta blockers may be contraindicated because they have a negative inotropic effect on the myocardium.) Since some beta blockers cause vasoconstriction in the lungs, they're usually contraindicated in patients with chronic obstructive pulmonary disease (COPD). Also, because of their peripheral vasoconstriction, they may be contraindicated in patients with vascular disorders, such as Raynaud's disease.

When used with other drugs, beta blockers may help reduce mortality in post-infarction patients by preventing secretion of catecholamines. After an MI, secretion of catecholamines is thought to cause dysrhythmias, and to increase inotropic and chronotropic activity. Because sudden discontinuation of beta blockers may cause rebound angina, the patient should be weaned off these drugs.

Calcium blockers, such as nifedipine, verapamil, and diltiazem, prevent the influx of calcium ions into arterial smooth muscle and myocardial cells. Also called calcium antagonists and slow-channel blockers, these drugs are vasodilators, helpful in treating angina caused by vasospasm of the coronary artery. In other forms of angina, they're used to dilate coronary arteries, increase coronary blood

flow, and encourage collateral circulation. Of the three drugs, verapamil has the most negative inotropic effect. In clinical dosages, verapamil and diltiazem have anti-arrthythmic properties, but nifedipine does not.

A relatively new inotropic drug, *dobutamine,* is used to treat reduced myocardial contractility. In severe decompensation, it acts to increase cardiac output and, to a lesser extent, blood pressure.

The use of anticoagulants in treating acute MI is controversial. Their effectiveness in reducing post-infarction mortality is now disputed, and their primary indications are for prevention of venous thromboses, pulmonary emboli, and reocclusion of arteries opened by surgery.

Restoring coronary circulation. If drug therapy alone fails to relieve angina, the patient may undergo a new technique called percutaneous transluminal coronary angioplasty (PTCA). Or, depending on the severity and location of coronary arterial stenosis, he may undergo coronary artery bypass grafting (CABG), or streptokinase therapy.

Percutaneous transluminal coronary angioplasty is a radiologic technique used to dilate an obstructed coronary artery without opening the chest. Performed under fluoroscopic guidance, it involves passing a tiny catheter through a guiding catheter into the narrowed section of artery and there inflating the catheter's balloon tip. The inflated balloon compresses the obstruction against the arterial walls to allow increased blood flow.

PTCA requires three catheters: an introducer catheter, to lead the guiding catheter into the peripheral artery; a guiding catheter, which is positioned in the ascending aorta at the coronary ostium, or opening of the obstructed coronary artery; and a balloon catheter, which is advanced to the obstruction. Once the balloon is positioned, the doctor inflates it with saline solution and contrast medium for several seconds, one or more times, while observing the fluoroscope. He measures pressures at the distal and proximal ends of the lesions to determine the pressure gradient. As the obstruction is compressed, the pressure gradient decreases.

After successful dilation, the doctor removes the balloon. He leaves the introducer sheath in place for several hours after the procedure to maintain access for intravenous drug administration or reintroduction of the dilating catheter if the artery reoccludes.

Not every patient with CAD is a candidate

Four stages of atherosclerosis

Although development of an arterial occlusion doesn't always follow an obvious sequence, these illustrations show the general stages of plaque development, growth, and eventual occlusion of blood flow in an artery.

Atherosclerosis begins when an injury to the endothelial lining of the artery (the intima), or some other pathologic event, makes it permeable to circulating lipoproteins.

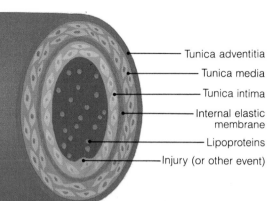

Tunica adventitia
Tunica media
Tunica intima
Internal elastic membrane
Lipoproteins
Injury (or other event)

Lipoproteins penetrate the smooth muscle cells in the intimal layer, producing a nonobstructive lesion called a "fatty streak."

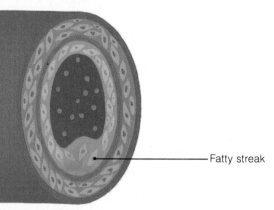

Fatty streak

A fibrous plaque eventually develops, made up of lipoprotein-filled smooth muscle cells, collagen, and muscle fibers. It's large enough to impede blood flow through the artery.

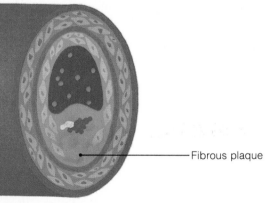

Fibrous plaque

Calcification or rupture of the fibrous plaque into the arterial lumen marks the final stage of atherosclerosis. Thrombosis is now likely, with near-total occlusion of the lumen.

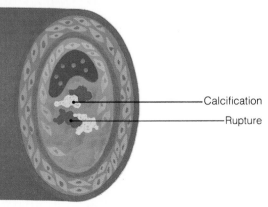

Calcification
Rupture

Cardiogenic shock: Cycle of decompensation

After myocardial infarction, even slight reduction of arterial pressure can set off a cycle of cardiac deterioration due to diminished coronary blood flow. As the damaged ventricle fails to eject its blood, stroke volume and, consequently, cardiac output fall. Then, sympathetic and neurohormonal compensatory mechanisms attempt to prevent further deterioration. If they fail, decompensation progresses.

Next, falling arterial pressure leads to tissue hypoxia, simultaneously increasing vascular deterioration and myocardial damage. Vascular deterioration allows fluid to shift from plasma to the interstitial space, thereby decreasing venous return and further decreasing cardiac output. It also causes vasodilation, which decreases peripheral resistance and causes a further decline in arterial pressure. Together, these events produce multiple interwoven cycles of falling cardiac output, falling arterial pressure, diminishing tissue perfusion, and ever increasing myocardial damage.

The resulting signs and symptoms of cardiogenic shock include: weak, rapid pulse; decreased arterial pressure; increased central venous and pulmonary capillary wedge pressures; rapid breathing; pallor; cold, clammy skin; weakness; and oliguria. In cardiogenic shock, central venous pressure and pulmonary wedge pressure are usually increased; pulse is often irregular; and mental function is often impaired.

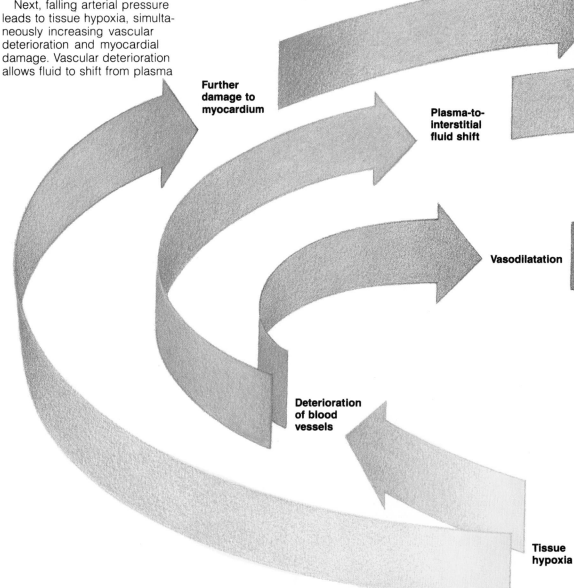

Further damage to myocardium

Plasma-to-interstitial fluid shift

Vasodilatation

Deterioration of blood vessels

Tissue hypoxia

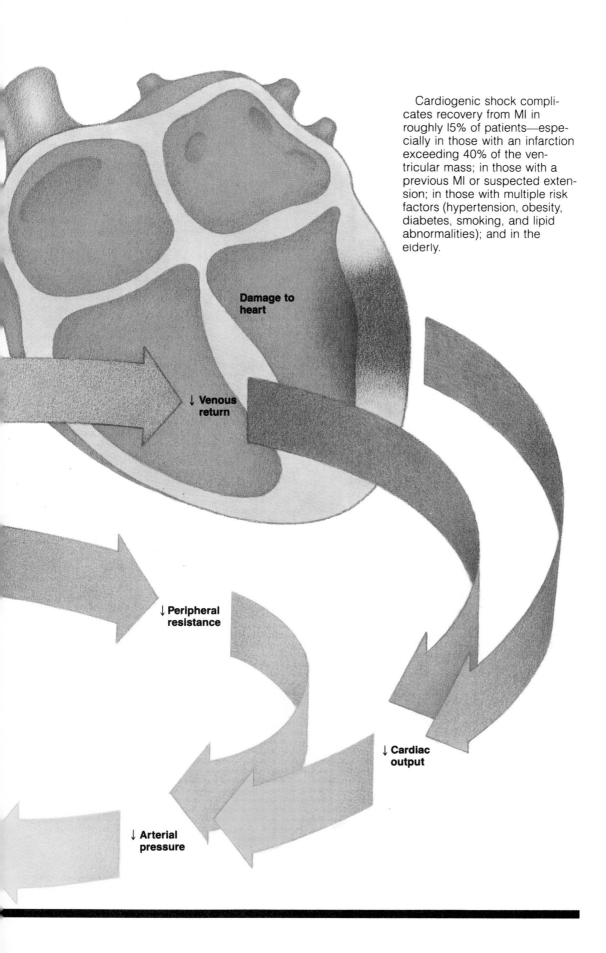

Damage to
heart

↓ Venous
return

Cardiogenic shock compli-
cates recovery from MI in
roughly 15% of patients—especially in those with an infarction
exceeding 40% of the ven-
tricular mass; in those with a
previous MI or suspected extension; in those with multiple risk
factors (hypertension, obesity,
diabetes, smoking, and lipid
abnormalities); and in the
elderly.

↓ Peripheral
resistance

↓ Cardiac
output

↓ Arterial
pressure

To help the failing heart— or to replace it?

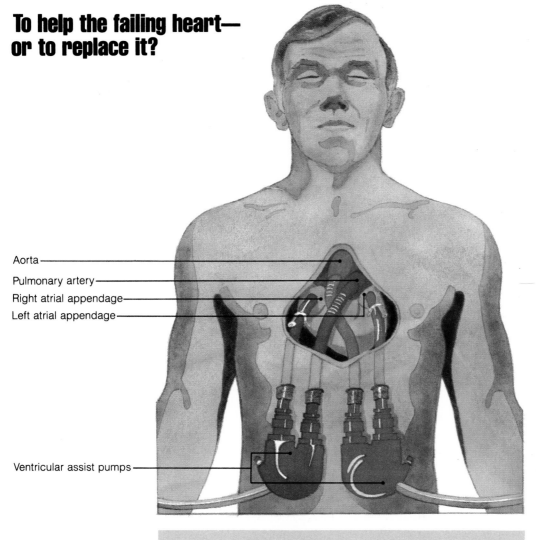

Aorta

Pulmonary artery

Right atrial appendage

Left atrial appendage

Ventricular assist pumps

Aorta

Pulmonary artery

Left atrium

Right atrium

Left ventricle

Right ventricle

Velcro patch

Connectors to drive unit

When a patient's heart fails or undergoes cardiogenic shock after open-heart surgery, it may not respond to drug therapy or insertion of an intra-aortic balloon pump. In such instances, two experimental devices may be available to surgeons: the ventricular assist pump and the artificial heart.

The Pierce ventricular assist pump (left), one of several current designs, is being used in some centers to support the circulation in patients who can't be weaned from cardiopulmonary bypass after open-heart surgery. The sac-type pump is fitted with tilting disc valves and powered pneumatically by periodic compression of the flexible sac. One or both ventricles may be assisted at one time. In the diagram at left, a cannula inserted into each atrial appendage drains blood from the atria into the pumps. One pump propels blood into the pulmonary artery; the other propels it into the aorta.

An alternative to ventricular assist pumping is heart transplantation, in which an irreparably diseased heart is replaced by a donor heart from a brain-dead patient. However, although about 75,000 patients a year need new hearts, only 1,000 to 2,000 potential donors are available each year.

An obvious solution is to implant an artificial heart, and one of the latest designs is shown at left. Designed by Dr. Robert Jarvik of the University of Utah, the device consists of a pair of mechanical ventricles that are attached to Dacron sleeves stitched to the patient's aorta, pulmonary artery, and atria. The heart is powered by compressed air, which activates internal diaphragms and valves to pump blood. Once it's successfully implanted, the artificial heart must function for the rest of the patient's life without malfunctioning or causing blood clots.

for PTCA. To qualify for PTCA, the patient's obstruction can be in the distal or proximal part of one or more major arteries, discrete, less than 2 cm long, uncalcified, not totally occluded, and not located at a bifurcation. Also, the affected artery shouldn't be tortuous or sharply angled. Ideally, the patient should have a history of angina for less than 2 years. Since PTCA may cause acute arterial occlusion, the patient must also be a candidate for immediate emergency CABG.

PTCA has an overall mortality of 1%—lower in patients with single vessel disease; higher in those with multivessel disease because of decreased myocardial reserve; and still higher in those who've had previous bypass surgery. Only 3% to 6% of patients require emergency bypass surgery after the procedure. About 10% of dilated arterial lesions become stenotic (roughly the same percentage as after bypass surgery), but they can be reopened. Current records suggest that a vessel that remains open for 6 months after dilation is likely to remain open indefinitely.

After PTCA, the patient requires careful follow-up, including monitoring of anticoagulant therapy. An exercise EKG is performed during hospitalization, and again after 4 months, with or without a thallium scan, to confirm successful arterial clearance.

Coronary artery bypass grafting. Although some patients with CAD are treated medically with diet, exercise and drugs, about 50,000 patients a year turn to coronary artery bypass graft (CABG) surgery. This makes the procedure one of the most frequently performed cardiac surgeries today. The operation relieves angina in many patients with two- or three-vessel obstruction. Its potential benefits—improved life expectancy and quality—make it an appealing choice for CAD patients. It may also be used to prevent myocardial infarction in patients who have angina but who have not yet had an MI.

Although surgery does reduce symptoms in over 80% of patients, objective evidence that bypass surgery halts CAD and actually prolongs life is scanty. Many doctors prefer to recommend surgery only for symptomatic patients who fail to respond to medical treatment.

In CABG, a cardiopulmonary bypass ("heart-lung") machine, moderate to total hypothermia, myocardial hypothermia (surrounding the heart with ice and cold saline solution), and intracoronary infusion of potassium at 4° C are employed to temporarily reduce cardiac metabolism and allow surgery to progress with a stable heart and permit careful grafting. Typically, the saphenous vein from the patient's leg is grafted in place in reverse to allow blood to flow in the direction of the valves. The length of vein needed depends on the number of arteries to be bypassed, but the incision itself usually extends from the knee to the ankle. If the vein isn't suitable for grafting, an incision is made in the other leg. After a suitable donor vein is "harvested," the doctor performs a midline sternotomy to expose the heart. Blood is then diverted to the heart-lung machine (see pages 102 and 103). With blood flow diverted from the immediate operative site, the saphenous vein segments are grafted into place. Proximally, the veins are anastomosed to the ascending aorta; distally, to the coronary arteries beyond the occluded areas.

After CABG, some patients can't be weaned from the heart-lung machine because of ventricular failure that won't respond to volume loading, catecholamines, or insertion of an intra-aortic balloon pump. In the past, many of these patients died from cardiogenic shock. Today, some of them may be helped by a ventricular-assist pump, which has been used experimentally to support circulation and restore ventricular function after coronary bypass. A few others may be helped by a heart transplant or implantation of an artificial heart. (See opposite page.)

Streptokinase therapy. This promising therapy offers increased hope for reopening a totally occluded artery and restoring myocardial perfusion in the early hours of acute MI. A thrombolytic agent derived from streptococci, streptokinase is being used for intracoronary infusion. When infused at the site of an arterial occlusion, streptokinase hastens fibrinolysis. It joins with plasminogen to form a complex that then reacts with additional plasminogen to form plasmin, a proteolytic enzyme that dissolves the clot and relieves the occlusion (see page 107). After successful streptokinase therapy, the suddenly improved perfusion causes cardiac enzymes to be released into the blood, raising their serum levels above normal. Also, ST segments of the EKG return to baseline more quickly.

Streptokinase infusion is carried out in a catheterization laboratory. After coronary artery catheterization confirms occlusion, coronary vasodilating drugs may be administered to rule out occlusion due to spasm. If the occlusion persists despite pharmacologic va-

Laser phototherapy vaporizes plaques safely

Laser beams, already used for cauterization and excision of tissues, are now being tested experimentally to clear occluded arteries in animals and cadavers. So far, lipoid, fibrous, and calcified plaques have been safely vaporized without damaging adjacent vessel walls; the pulse of laser energy can be adjusted to the size of the occlusion.

In a typical procedure, an angina patient would report to an outpatient clinic or a cardiac catheterization laboratory, where a doctor would insert a fiberoptic catheter through the femoral artery and thread it through the aortic arch to the occlusion site in a coronary artery. Once the catheter is in position, the doctor would trigger a burst of laser light through the fiberoptic scope to vaporize the plaque, a few millimeters at a time. The restored coronary artery perfusion would free the patient of pain and greatly reduce the risk of an MI.

Bypassing coronary artery disease

The heart-lung machine provides cardiopulmonary bypass to an extracorporeal circuit during open-heart surgery, with a minimum of hemolysis and trauma. As shown in this simplified diagram, cannulas inserted in the inferior and superior venae cavae divert blood into the machine from its normal path to the right atrium. Also, when the heart is opened, blood is continuously aspirated and returned to the heart-lung machine along with venous blood.

The circuit returns filtered, oxygenated blood to the arterial system through an arterial cannula, which usually is placed in the ascending aorta.

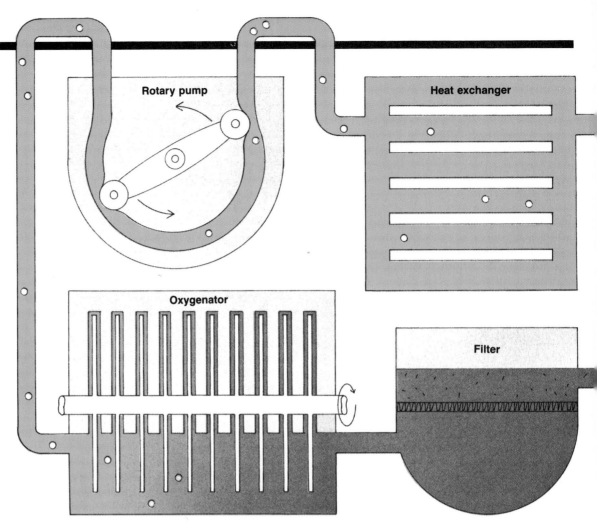

sodilatation, a streptokinase infusion follows. After a bolus dose of 10,000 to 20,000 units, the dosage of streptokinase ranges from 2,000 to 6,000 units/minute. Successful therapy is determined by angiography; small amounts of dye are injected into the artery during the procedure to check on arterial patency.

Dissolving a clot in an occluded coronary artery without surgery has obvious benefits, but it also has drawbacks. Because streptokinase alters the natural clotting mechanisms, it can lead to hemorrhage. This occurs most frequently at the site of recent surgery, needle puncture, or trauma. Close monitoring of clotting factors, hemoglobin, and hematocrit, as well as meticulous care of the infusion site, can reduce the risk of hemorrhage. Although controversial, streptokinase can be administered into a peripheral vein after an acute MI is diagnosed.

NURSING MANAGEMENT
Successful nursing management of the patient with CAD requires a thorough history and accurate assessment. After collecting this subjective and objective data, you'll be ready to form a nursing diagnosis, set goals, and plan and evaluate your interventions.

Collect subjective data
During the initial patient interview, find out the patient's chief complaint. If he reports chest discomfort, encourage him to describe it as specifically as possible. Ask about the time of onset, possible causes, duration, frequency, location, radiation, quality, quantity, setting, concurrent symptoms, and any alleviating or aggravating factors. *Possible causes* include exertion, emotional upset, exposure to excessive heat or cold, or no specific event. *Duration* and *frequency* should be stated in terms such as, "My chest pain usually lasts from 2 to 10 minutes and occurs 3 times a week." The exact *location* and *radiation pattern* can be determined by having the patient point with his fingers. *Quality* refers to the unique characteristics of the pain, such as sharp, dull, stabbing, crushing, aching, burning, and so on. *Quantity* refers to severity of the pain. The *setting* refers to the environment where the pain usually occurs (at home, at work, and so on). *Concurrent symptoms* may include dyspnea, dizziness, diaphoresis, nausea, vomiting, and palpitations. *Alleviating or aggravating factors* may include rest, position changes, use of nitroglycerin, a heavy meal, or exercise. If nitroglycerin relieves the pain,

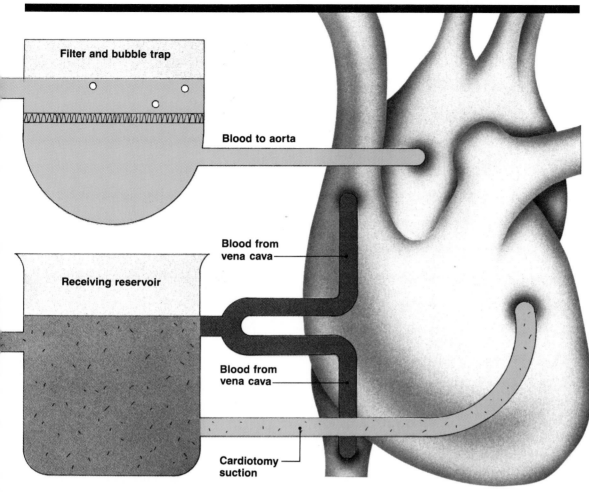

Filter and bubble trap

Blood to aorta

Blood from vena cava

Receiving reservoir

Blood from vena cava

Cardiotomy suction

find out how soon after taking it relief begins and whether it's partial or complete.

The patient's description of chest pain, as well as your observations during the interview, will help you distinguish angina from MI. In an acute MI, the patient may describe the pain as the worst he's ever experienced—deep, visceral, vise-like, or crushing. Or he may report a burning sensation, a dull ache, indigestion, or slight discomfort. Unlike the pain of angina, the pain of an acute MI is usually more severe, lasts much longer, and isn't relieved by nitroglycerin. It's not necessarily related to exertion or emotional upset and doesn't subside with rest. Typically, it originates in the central part of the chest and epigastrium, and sometimes radiates to the arm. Occasionally, it radiates to the abdomen, back, jaw, and neck; usually, it doesn't radiate above the jaw or below the umbilicus. It's often accompanied by weakness, diaphoresis, nausea, vomiting, dyspnea, palpitations, and obvious anxiety.

Unlike the angina patient, who tries to guard against a recurrence of pain by remaining immobile, the MI patient characteristically moves about, trying to find the most comfortable position. He's anxious and rest-

less, squirms around in bed, and may vomit or belch in his attempts to relieve pain.

If the patient isn't in obvious distress, ask about previous episodes of chest pain and previous hospitalizations for angina pectoris, coronary insufficiency, MI, CHF, hypertension, diabetes, dysrhythmias, or other disorders. Ask about a family history of these conditions. Ask also about acquired risk factors, such as tobacco use, obesity, a high-carbohydrate and high-fat diet, and stress or emotional tension. Observe the patient's mental status and speech, which reflect the adequacy of cerebral perfusion. Look for signs of depression or denial of his condition, as well as for coping mechanisms.

Be aware of the patient's anxiety level, not only to put him at ease, but also to recognize its effect on the cardiovascular system. Because his willingness to learn about his condition and cooperate with tests and treatments depends greatly on reducing his anxiety, observe him carefully to identify one of these four generalized levels of anxiety:

• *No anxiety.* The patient may feel there's "nothing to worry about." This is a common denial tactic.

• *Mild anxiety.* The patient is concerned and

Angina's many guises

After angina has been diagnosed, accurate and complete documentation of your patient's attacks is crucial for correct treatment. As you evaluate the patient's attacks, keep in mind the following types of angina and their characteristics.

• *Chronic stable angina:* Chest pain occurs at a predictable level of physical or emotional stress, and responds promptly to sublingual nitroglycerin or rest; the pattern, duration, frequency, and severity of anginal attacks are stable; there's no pain while at rest.

• *Unstable angina:* An abrupt change occurs in the level and frequency of symptoms, or on- set of pain at rest; attacks last longer (up to 20 to 30 minutes); EKG obtained during pain shows reversible ST segment depression. (Also called inter- mediate coronary syndrome, crescendo angina, progressive angina, coronary insufficiency, or impending MI.)

• *Resting angina:* Recurrent pain, frequently at the same time every day, usually not brought on by exercise or re- lieved by rest; pain lasts longer and is more severe than with chronic stable angina and may lead to MI; EKG changes during pain frequently show ST seg- ment elevation. This angina is rare and may be caused by coronary artery spasm. (Also called variant angina or Prinz- metal's angina.)

• *New-onset angina:* Angina that has developed within the last 60 days.

• *Postinfarction angina:* Angina in a patient who's had MI.

• *Atypical angina:* Unusual symptoms, such as a toothache or earache, are related to physi- cal or emotional exertion and are relieved by rest or adminis- tration of nitroglycerin.

• *Nocturnal angina:* The patient awakens with chest pain, often after disturbing or exciting dreams. Nocturnal angina may be associated with sympathetic nervous activity, or with underly- ing congestive heart failure (an- gina decubitus).

---

nervous. He may have trouble sleeping. He asks questions about his condition and gains relief from reassurances by you or his family.

• *Moderate anxiety.* The patient asks questions, but doesn't pay attention to the answers. He's hyperactive.

• *Severe anxiety.* The patient may experience nausea, headache, and feelings of doom.

Ask about the patient's life-style, goals, and values. Such questions may lead to descrip- tion of a "Type A" personality, who may be predisposed to an acute MI. Although some recent studies suggest no direct correlation between a Type A personality and CAD, you should nevertheless be aware of the Type- A behavior pattern. Such a person might tell you some of these things about himself: he's chronically impatient—he talks, walks, and eats quickly; his mind is always active; he can converse only on topics that interest him; he is fiercely competitive and feels guilty for relaxing. He'll perform many activities at once to save time—like watching TV as he reads the newspaper during a meal.

At the conclusion of the patient interview, you'll be able to evaluate his knowledge of his disease as well as his ability to understand and carry out a prescribed treatment regimen.

Collect objective data
Now, you're ready to perform a systematic cardiovascular assessment, using the tech- niques of inspection, palpation, auscultation, and percussion described in Chapter 2. During this assessment, be sure to carefully inspect the skin, check vital signs, auscultate for abnormal heart sounds, and recognize signs of cardiogenic shock, congestive heart failure and pericarditis.

Inspect the skin. Note skin color and the presence of diaphoresis and edema. Pallor along with cold, clammy skin indicates hypo- tension resulting from an acute MI. The pres- ence of edema—especially in the extremities—indicates a decreased pumping ability of the heart.

Check vital signs. Heart rate and blood pressure may increase at the onset of isch- emia. However, prolonged myocardial ischemia eventually decreases blood pressure, since the damaged ventricles can't eject enough blood to maintain adequate cardiac output.

A low-grade fever occurs during the first few days after MI, the result of inflammation and leukocyte infiltration around the infarct. Usu- ally, temperature falls when myocardial in- flammation subsides, as fibroblasts replace leukocytes and scar tissue forms.

Listen for heart sounds. During auscultation, you may hear signs of ventricular dysfunc- tion, including atrial (S_4) and ventricular filling (S_3) gallops, and decreased intensity of heart sounds.

A transient apical systolic murmur, presumably the result of mitral regurgitation caused by papillary muscle dysfunction during acute MI, may occur in mid- to late systole. In many patients with transmural MI, you may occasionally hear a pericardial friction rub within a few days of infarction. A pericardial friction rub (a "grating" sound, heard at the apex or lower left sternal border) reliably indicates pericarditis.

Auscultation can also reveal rales in the lungs, resulting from impairment of the heart's pumping ability. As blood volume and pressure rise in the left heart, back pressure builds and causes fluid to shift from the blood vessels in the lungs to the alveoli.

Watch for signs of cardiogenic shock. Your assessment of the CAD patient must be continuous, since complications often occur quickly and without warning. Cardiogenic shock, a life-threatening complication, may occur in predisposed patients. Such patients may be over age 65 and have a history of three-vessel CAD, hypertension, diabetes, polycythemia, or cardiomegaly. Suspect cardiogenic shock if you detect signs of pulmonary edema, pulmonary capillary wedge pressure above 18 to 20 mm Hg; dysrhythmias; systolic pressure under 80 mm Hg or diastolic pressure under 55 mm Hg; and chest pain or gallop rhythm that persists longer than 24 hours. Watch for classic signs of hypoperfusion—cool, clammy, mottled skin and decreased or absent peripheral pulses. You may find that pulse, heart sounds, and breath sounds are all normal at first, but the ensuing hypotension causes rapid deterioration.

Also watch for other signs of hypoperfusion: clouded sensorium, altered mental state, hypoxemia, lactic acidosis, and urinary output that's less than 20 ml/hour. Be sure to consider other possible causes of shock, such as trauma, infection, or hypovolemia.

Formulate nursing diagnoses

After collecting subjective data from the patient interview and objective data from the cardiovascular assessment, you're ready to formulate nursing diagnoses that clearly explain the patient's problems and allow you to plan appropriate goals and interventions. Typically, your nursing diagnoses reflect the physiologic and psychologic consequences of acute MI, and the need for patient teaching about drug and surgical treatments during hospitalization and after discharge.

Altered hemodynamic status resulting from an acute MI. This diagnosis suggests the po-

tential for sudden death, congestive heart failure, cardiogenic shock, lethal dysrhythmias, and other life-threatening complications. Your goals are to provide constant patient monitoring, to promptly detect changes in the patient's condition, to prevent sudden death and complications, and to limit the size of the infarction. To achieve these goals, admit the patient to the coronary or intensive care unit for constant monitoring and early treatment of dysrhythmias. (Remember that the risk of ventricular fibrillation and death is greatest in the first few hours after an acute MI.) Position the patient comfortably in bed, and attach EKG electrodes to his chest to monitor heart rhythm.

Measure and record vital signs to detect impending complications, especially dysrhythmias, cardiogenic shock, and CHF. Be sure to take both apical and radial pulse rates simultaneously and characterize pulse quality as regular, bounding, or weak. Also note the strength of peripheral pulses.

Start and maintain an I.V. line for emergency drug administration. Know your unit's standing orders and have emergency cardiac drugs and resuscitation equipment on hand. Observe the cardiac monitor for premature ventricular beats, which may lead to ventricular tachycardia and ventricular fibrillation. If dysrhythmias occur, treat them according to standing orders or the doctor's orders, and run an EKG strip immediately.

If ordered, obtain arterial and venous blood samples. Provide continuing nursing assessment. Check skin color, moistness, and turgor to evaluate peripheral perfusion. Observe for neck vein distention, which may indicate ventricular dysfunction. Auscultate the lungs for adventitious breath sounds, and the heart for gallops, murmurs, or pericardial friction rub. Be alert for signs of deteriorating mental status (confusion, apathy, restlessness) resulting from inadequate cerebral perfusion. Administer oxygen with a nasal cannula or mask as needed.

Keep accurate intake/output records to anticipate early CHF or renal dysfunction. Note the presence, location, and extent of edema. Check the laboratory report for serum potassium levels, since hyperkalemia causes extrasystoles that may progress to more ominous dysrhythmias. Apply antiembolism stockings to increase venous return to the heart and prevent thrombus formation.

If the patient has difficulty breathing, place him in a sitting position, supported by a pil-

Nursing care after streptokinase therapy

• Don't give I.M. or I.V. injections for 24 hours.
• Maintain alignment and immobility of the involved extremity; don't raise the head of the bed more than 15°.
• Check the infusion site for bleeding every 15 minutes for 1 hour, every 30 minutes for the next 2 hours, then once every hour until the catheter is removed.
• When you check the site for bleeding, document pulse, color, temperature, and sensitivity of both extremities.
• After removal of the catheter, apply direct pressure to the infusion site for at least 30 minutes. Assess the involved extremity distal to the pressure point, as you did when the catheter was still in place. Keep the patient on bed rest for at least 6 hours; keep his leg straight and the head of the bed no higher than 15°.
• Observe for signs and symptoms of GI bleeding.

low, as needed. He may have to sleep in this position. Minimize his activities to reduce cardiac work load and oxygen demand. Avoid disturbing him and eliminate unnecessary noise or activity at bedside.

If the patient develops cardiogenic shock, watch central venous and pulmonary capillary wedge pressures for changes in fluid balance. Check arterial blood gases and pH to detect metabolic acidosis. Also check urine output, pulse pressure, and level of consciousness to help evaluate cardiac output.

Evaluate your interventions. Consider your nursing interventions effective when:
• No additional pathologic changes appear on the EKG.
• Hemodynamic measurements improve.
• All dysrhythmias have been treated and resolved.
• The patient looks comfortable, and his skin feels warm and dry.

Potential for severe chest pain resulting from an acute MI. After this nursing diagnosis, your goals are to relieve chest pain and promote rest. To achieve these goals, assess, document, and report to the doctor the locations, radiation, and duration of pain, and any factors that affect it. Also report the effect of chest pain on perfusion to the heart, brain, kidneys, and skin.

Obtain a 12-lead EKG during chest pain, as ordered, to determine variant angina or extension of infarction. Administer oxygen, as ordered. To relieve pain, first check vital signs and then give I.V. morphine or meperidine to decrease sympathetic activity and reduce myocardial oxygen demand. If vital signs remain within normal limits, repeat I.V. doses as needed until relief is obtained. Be alert for decreased blood pressure, which may herald shock and dysrhythmias.

If the patient continues to experience severe pain, stay with him and give emotional support. Persistent or recurring pain suggests an impending or extending infarction, and requires immediate, aggressive treatment. If the patient is quiet, watch for nonverbal signs of pain, since he may try to deny discomfort or may be afraid to ask for drugs.

To avoid undue strain during defecation, administer a stool softener, as ordered. Assist him to the bedside commode, and teach him to exhale with physical movement to avoid a Valsalva maneuver. During and after defecation, watch for decreased heart rate resulting from vagal stimulation.

To ensure comfort, provide back and arm

rests, and a liquid diet, if tolerated.

Evaluate your interventions. Consider your nursing interventions effective when:
• The patient reports relief of chest pain within 15 to 30 minutes.
• Vital signs return to normal levels.
• The patient appears restful and coherent.
• His skin feels warm and dry.

Knowledge deficit about streptokinase infusion. After reaching this diagnosis, your goals are to reduce anxiety in the patient and his family and to encourage their active participation in preparing for the procedure. Even though you may not have much time to prepare the patient and his family, be sure to convey a calm, reassuring attitude. First, ask about previous conditions that could contraindicate streptokinase therapy, such as cardiogenic shock, recent CVA, surgery within the past 10 days, recent serious trauma, recent severe GI bleeding, or severe arterial hypertension. Then, explain that blood samples will be collected to evaluate clotting factors and to determine levels of electrolytes, ABGs, BUN, creatinine, and cardiac enzymes. Tell the patient and his family that nitroglycerin will be infused to alleviate his chest pain. Show them a sample catheter and reinforce their knowledge of the purpose and goal of the procedure. Explain that the treatment will be given in the cardiac catheterization laboratory. Also explain all nursing actions performed before, during, and after the procedure to alleviate unnecessary anxiety. Make sure the patient and his family understand and sign a consent form.

Evaluate your interventions. Consider your preparation of the patient and his family effective if they will proceed with therapy and can verbalize its purpose and goals.

Anxiety and fear of death resulting from an acute MI. With this diagnosis, your goals are to reduce the patient's and family's anxiety and fear, to help prevent extension of the infarction, to encourage expression of feelings, and to promote effective coping mechanisms. To meet these goals, first assess, document, and report to the doctor the patient's and family's level of anxiety and their coping mechanisms. Anxiety and fear increase the heart rate, raise blood pressure, and cause the adrenal glands to release epinephrine, which may produce dysrhythmias.

As soon as the patient is receptive, explain all activity restrictions, care measures, use of equipment, and relevant hospital procedures. Answer his questions completely and

Treating acute MI with streptokinase

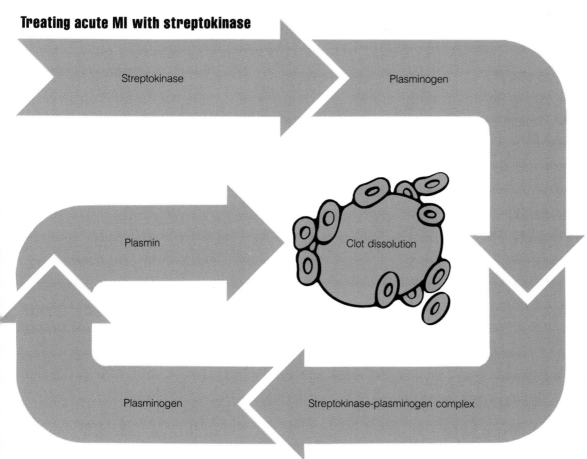

Streptokinase

Plasminogen

Plasmin

Clot dissolution

Plasminogen

Streptokinase-plasminogen complex

Prompt therapy with the thrombolytic drug streptokinase in the early stages of acute myocardial infarction may positively alter the outcome. How can this drug make a difference? Because streptokinase can dissolve the clot in an occluded artery, it restores perfusion and helps prevent or limit the size of an infarction.

If you have an MI patient scheduled for this procedure, explain to him that it's done in the cardiac catheterization laboratory. Explain that he'll have an arterial catheter threaded through major blood vessels to his heart, and that dye is injected to outline the coronary arteries to locate the occlusion. Then, streptokinase is infused through the catheter. The infusion lasts for several hours, to dissolve the clot as much as possible. During this time, angiograms are taken to assess the effectiveness of the treatment.

present a calm, supportive attitude. Allow the patient and his family to express anxiety and fear by showing genuine interest and concern. Remember that coping with the pain and emotional trauma of an acute MI is difficult for both the patient and his family. Expect that their natural defense mechanisms—shock, denial, and anger—will color their initial responses. However, recognize that the patient's anger may temporarily increase cardiac work load. Watch for signs of increased work load: jugular vein distention, pallor, cyanosis of the lips and nail beds, and EKG changes. Provide medication or oxygen, as ordered, and notify the doctor.

Assess the patient for maladaptive coping mechanisms, such as inappropriate denial, withdrawal, changes in his usual communication patterns, and destructive behavior. To counteract these, give the patient positive feelings about the progress of his treatment, if possible. After an acute MI, patients usually undergo a sequence of emotions—anxiety, denial, depression, and, finally, acceptance. It often helps to tell the patient that these emotions are perfectly normal. Help him focus on what he can do, not on what he can't do. Encourage his family to provide emotional support and, if possible, allow flexible visiting

hours. Also, assess the patient's need for spiritual counseling and, if appropriate, contact a clergyman.

Evaluate your interventions. Consider your nursing interventions effective when:
• The patient and his family can discuss their anxieties and fears about death, and appear less apprehensive.
• The patient looks comfortable at rest. His heart rate is less than 100 beats/minute. His blood pressure remains within the normal range, and his respiratory rate remains less than 16 breaths/minute. His skin feels warm and dry.

Impaired coronary blood flow. Such impairment results in angina and may cause MI. With this diagnosis, your goals are to prevent MI, to restore the balance between myocardial oxygen supply and demand, and to relieve pain. To achieve these goals, immediately restrict all physical activity. Assess, document, and report the characteristics of the patient's chest pain and its effect on hemodynamic status. Using a nasal cannula, administer oxygen.

Obtain a 12-lead EKG during chest pain and report marked changes to the doctor. If you suspect MI, collect blood samples for CPK isoenzyme analysis.

Nursing care after open-heart surgery

Your immediate priority after open-heart surgery is to transfer the patient to the recovery room and stabilize his condition. First, connect the endotracheal or nasotracheal tube to assisted or controlled mechanical ventilation. Then, connect all venous and arterial lines and drainage receptacles. Next, draw blood samples and check vital signs and hemodynamic pressures. Examine dressings and measure urine output.

Systematic assessment
After stabilizing the patient's condition, you're ready to begin a continuous, systematic assessment.

Respiratory status. Observe for signs of hypoxia, such as cyanosis of the extremities, restlessness, and hyperventilation. Check arterial blood gases as needed, to maintain pH, PCO_2, and PO_2 within the patient's physiological limits. Suction the endotracheal or nasotracheal tube as often as every 2 hours, and note the color of secretions. If they're red, rule out trauma; if pink, rule out pulmonary edema. Listen to breath sounds as needed; be especially alert for decreased breath sounds in the left lung, which could indicate that the endotracheal tube has slipped into the right mainstem bronchus. (If breath sounds decrease, order an immediate chest X-ray.) Take a chest X-ray daily to check for hemothorax, pleural effusion, atelectasis, pulmonary congestion, or widening of the mediastinum. Assess the patient's discomfort and administer analgesics as ordered.

To keep the patient's chest tubes patent, milk and strip them as needed. Measure chest drainage at least every 2 hours and check hemoglobin and hematocrit every 2 to 4 hours. Observe for excessive drainage, which may indicate cardiac tamponade. Replace drainage with blood, as ordered.

Cardiovascular status. Check vital signs every 15 minutes initially, every 30 minutes when the patient is stable, then every hour. Maintain systolic blood pressure at 90 to 120 mm Hg, diastolic at 70 to 80 mm Hg. Lower readings may impair cerebral and renal perfusion. Watch for dysrhythmias, which are usually associated with excessive bleeding, hypertension, ischemia, MI, acid-base imbalances, or abnormal serum potassium levels. Set the appropriate alarms on the cardiac monitor; if dysrhythmias develop, notify the doctor, and administer antiarrhythmics as ordered. Record an EKG daily, compare results with previous EKGs, and report any changes. Check cardiac enzyme levels daily for 3 days, since abnormally high levels may indicate MI. Watch for increased CVP, which suggests fluid overload, cardiac failure, or cardiac tamponade. After CABG, check pedal and femoral pulses frequently. Diminished pulse may indicate embolized or separated graft. Ensure that the elastic bandage on the donor leg allows adequate circulation.

Fluid status. If the patient excretes less than 30 ml of urine per hour for 2 consecutive hours, notify the doctor. (This may indicate inadequate cardiac output due to hypovolemia.) If brisk diuresis develops, test urine glucose frequently to rule out osmotic diuresis, which may cause hypokalemia. Keep intake below 2,000 ml for the first 24 hours to prevent cardiac overload. Check his weight daily to detect excessive fluid loss or retention.

Neurologic status. Regularly check pupil reactivity, general movement, strength of extremities, and level of consciousness. Evaluate for symptoms of postperfusion psychosis which may result from disturbances in cerebral circulation following cardiopulmonary bypass. Reassure the patient's family that this condition is usually transient.

Preparation for convalescence and discharge
During convalescence, encourage progressive ambulation, within the limits of the patient's cardiac capability. To prepare for discharge, discuss diet, exercise, medications, and reportable symptoms of angina with the patient and his family.

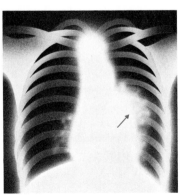
Atelectasis in left upper lobe

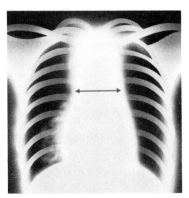
Widened mediastinum

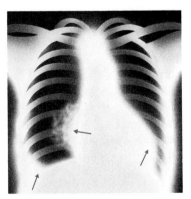
Pulmonary congestion, with pleural effusion and cardiomegaly

Administer nitroglycerin or other antianginal drugs, as ordered, and continuously evaluate the patient's response to therapy. Take blood pressure every 3 minutes (1 to 2 minutes after giving the drug) to evaluate drug effects; there should be a moderate decline in systolic pressure. Check blood pressure and heart rate with the patient in an upright position, and observe for dizziness and faintness. Caution the patient to take no more than two or three sublingual nitroglycerin tablets in any 15-minute period.

Don't let the patient become fatigued. Plan for him to rest for 20 to 30 minutes twice each day. Caution him to avoid sudden outbursts of activity or emotion. Be alert for situations that could provoke emotional upsets, and try to minimize or eliminate them. Tell the patient to rest for an hour after each meal. Also, plan rest periods between his activities. For example, when he washes, he should rest 5 to 10 minutes before he shaves.

Evaluate your interventions. Consider your nursing interventions effective when:
• Within 5 minutes after taking nitroglycerin, the patient reports relief of chest pain, and heart rate, systolic blood pressure, and respiratory rate return to normal levels.
• He appears comfortable and his skin feels warm and dry.
• ST segments and T waves on the EKG revert to the pattern before onset of chest pain.
• CPK isoenzymes are within normal limits.

Knowledge deficit about CABG. After this nursing diagnosis, your goal is to encourage active participation in preoperative teaching. To achieve these goals, you need to convey a calm, reassuring attitude to the patient and his family. First, find out what the patient knows about his heart condition. Then, answer his questions fully. Explain the preoperative procedures: the anesthetist's visit, shave, preparation, and administration of a sedative the night before surgery.

Next, explain the surgical procedure. Tell the patient that the doctor will make an incision in at least one arm or leg to remove a vein segment, and will make a second incision in the chest to connect this vein segment, or graft, to the aorta. Explain that the expected result is relief of his anginal pain.

Explain the postoperative procedures and, if possible, give the patient a tour of the coronary or intensive care unit. Tell the patient that he'll be connected to a mechanical ventilator for at least 1 day and, as a result, won't be able to talk. Also tell him that chest tubes, arterial and venous lines, and an indwelling catheter will be inserted. Reassure him that a nurse is present in the unit at all times, and that she'll monitor him closely.

Prepare the patient for convalescence. Explain and demonstrate IPPB treatment, use of blow bottles, and coughing and deep-breathing exercises.

Evaluate your interventions. Consider your nursing interventions effective when:
• The patient and his family can discuss or demonstrate the purpose of CABG, preoperative preparation, the purpose and use of ICU equipment, the use of IPPB and blow bottles, and coughing and deep-breathing techniques.
• The patient and his family appear less anxious about CABG.

Knowledge deficit about PTCA. With this nursing diagnosis, your goals are to reduce the patient's and family's anxiety about PTCA and to encourage active participation in preoperative teaching. To achieve these goals, you'll need to fully understand this new procedure before you can effectively deal with the patient and his family. Because PTCA is relatively new, the patient and his family will need to understand many new concepts before giving informed consent. Consider first what the doctor has told the patient and his family. Typically, he'll explain PTCA, its complications, and any alternative treatments.

Besides reinforcing the doctor's explanation, you should also discuss drug regimens, hospital procedures, and follow-up care. First, explain the dosage, action, and side effects of any prescribed drugs. Tell the patient that he'll usually require 2 days of medical evaluation before PTCA, bed rest afterward in the coronary or telemetry unit, and 1 to 2 days of post-test evaluation. Explain that he'll be awake during PTCA, that the procedure lasts 1 to 4 hours, and that he'll be asked to hold deep breaths periodically to allow fluoroscopic visualization of the balloon catheter. Mention that he may experience angina, especially during inflation of the balloon catheter. Tell him to report angina to the doctor.

Tell the patient that he'll receive anticoagulant therapy for 6 to 9 months after PTCA. Mention that a stress thallium imaging test will be performed 1 to 2 days after PTCA and will be repeated at 3- to 6-month intervals, and that cardiac catheterization will be performed 6 to 9 months after PTCA.

Evaluate your interventions. Consider your nursing interventions effective when:
• The patient and his family can understand

Preventing ischemia with PTCA

Percutaneous transluminal coronary angioplasty (PTCA)—an alternative to bypass surgery—is an investigational procedure that opens an occluded coronary artery without opening the chest. It's performed in the cardiac catheterization laboratory after coronary angiography confirms the presence and location of the occlusion. Once the occlusion is located, the doctor threads a guide catheter through the patient's femoral artery into the coronary artery under fluoroscopic guidance, as shown at right.

When the guide catheter's position at the occlusion site is confirmed by angiography, the doctor carefully introduces a smaller double-lumen balloon catheter through the guide catheter and directs the balloon through the lesion (lower left), where a marked pressure gradient will be obvious.

The doctor alternately inflates and deflates the balloon until an angiogram verifies successful arterial dilation (lower right) and the pressure gradient has decreased.

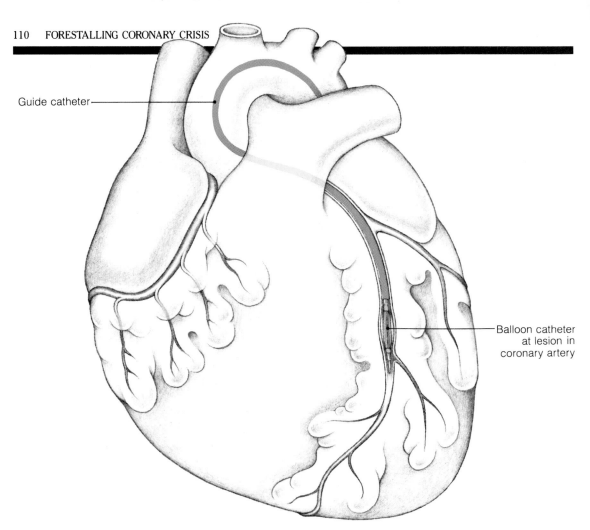

Guide catheter

Balloon catheter at lesion in coronary artery

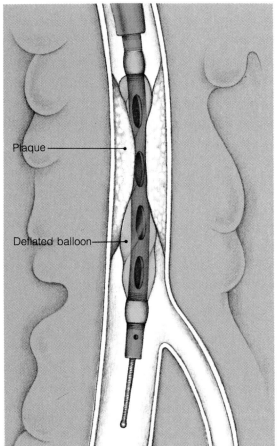

Plaque

Deflated balloon

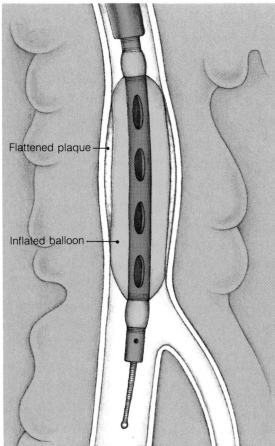

Flattened plaque

Inflated balloon

and discuss the important aspects of PTCA and follow-up care.
• The patient and his family report less anxiety after the teaching sessions.

Knowledge deficit about cardiac rehabilitation after discharge. After this diagnosis, your goal is to encourage active participation by the patient and his family in a cardiac rehabilitation program.

For the *MI patient,* assess the patient's and family's level of knowledge and readiness to learn. Explain normal heart function to them, and describe what happens in MI and how the heart heals itself. Relate this to the patient's symptoms.

Discuss the patient's risk factors, and explain the significance of adhering to dietary restrictions, abstention from smoking, control of stress, and so on. If the patient has a coexisting disease, such as hypertension or diabetes, explain ways to control it.

Discuss the relationship between the patient's daily activities and recovery. Suggest that he follow an exercise program at home, and provide opportunities for him to exercise before his discharge. Encourage him to exercise at home as much as he did while still hospitalized. Unless contraindicated, he should be encouraged to gradually increase his walking until he's up to 1 to 2 miles a day. Encourage him to walk outside on level ground in good weather.

Explore with the patient ways to simplify his work routine; tell him to avoid or modify activity after meals, stress, or exposure to temperature extremes. Discuss with the patient and his sexual partner the relation of sexual activity to his condition.

Discuss the meaning and significance of maximum heart rate, and teach the patient to count his pulse. Point out symptoms that require immediate medical attention. Provide information about drugs the patient will take after discharge. Include the name, purpose, dosage, and schedule for each drug. Stress the importance of not discontinuing any drug suddenly unless so advised by his doctor. (Many patients, when they run out of the prescribed drug, believe they don't have to take any more.)

If nitroglycerin is prescribed, explain its preventive use, side effects, and correct storage. To simplify dosage scheduling, group times of administration, when possible. Provide information on follow-up tests, such as exercise electrocardiography and cardiac catheterization.

Assess the patient's potential compliance with the discharge regimen. Inform him and his family to expect periods of depression and fatigue, especially during the first few weeks at home. Provide frequent opportunities for the patient and his family to ask questions and express their concerns and fears.

For the *angina patient,* stress the importance of identifying activities or emotions that precipitate anginal pain, such as dressing, showering, walking, and climbing stairs. Remind him to take nitroglycerin as a precaution before performing any activity that might provoke angina. Teach him to avoid strenuous lifting of grocery bags, suitcases, children, pets, and heavy objects. Instruct him to avoid extremes of temperature, since cold or hot, humid weather may cause angina. Tell him to wear a muffler to protect his face in cold weather, and to avoid physical exertion in hot, humid weather.

Teach the patient to respond immediately to anginal pain: he should stop whatever he's doing and sit down, take nitroglycerin as directed and expect prompt relief. Tell the patient and his family to contact the doctor immediately if the pain persists longer than 10 minutes after taking two doses of nitroglycerin.

Discuss the patient's risk factors, and explain the significance of adhering to dieting and tobacco restrictions and exercise and weight control programs. Teach stress management techniques. Make sure he has the number of the local hospital, his doctor and/or cardiac rehabilitation unit.

Evaluate your interventions. Consider your nursing interventions effective when:
• The patient and his family understand MI or angina.
• The patient asks pertinent questions about self-care, identifies risk factors, and discusses how he plans to modify or eliminate them.
• The patient recognizes and describes symptoms requiring medical attention and repeats information needed to comply with his drug regimen and follow-up care.

A final word

Coronary artery disease presents a formidable nursing challenge. But it's a challenge that you can successfully meet by understanding its pathophysiology and its traditional and experimental medical management—and, of course, by polishing your skills of history-taking, assessment, planning, intervention, and evaluation.

 Points to remember

• Coronary artery disease (CAD) is an umbrella term for many disorders that can decrease blood flow through the coronary arteries. Atherosclerosis accounts for more than 90% of all cases of CAD.
• Atherosclerosis is believed to involve three interdependent mechanisms: lipoprotein abnormalities, arterial wall injury, and coagulation and platelet dysfunction.
• After acute MI, the degree of functional impairment depends on the size and location of the infarction, ability of uninvolved myocardium, potential for collateral circulation, and on compensatory mechanisms.
• Successful medical management of CAD depends on early diagnosis and aggressive therapy.
• Percutaneous transluminal coronary angioplasty is a promising alternative to coronary artery bypass grafting.
• Successful nursing management of CAD requires a thorough patient history and accurate assessment to determine appropriate nursing diagnoses, goals, and interventions.

7 COPING WITH VASCULAR ABNORMALITIES

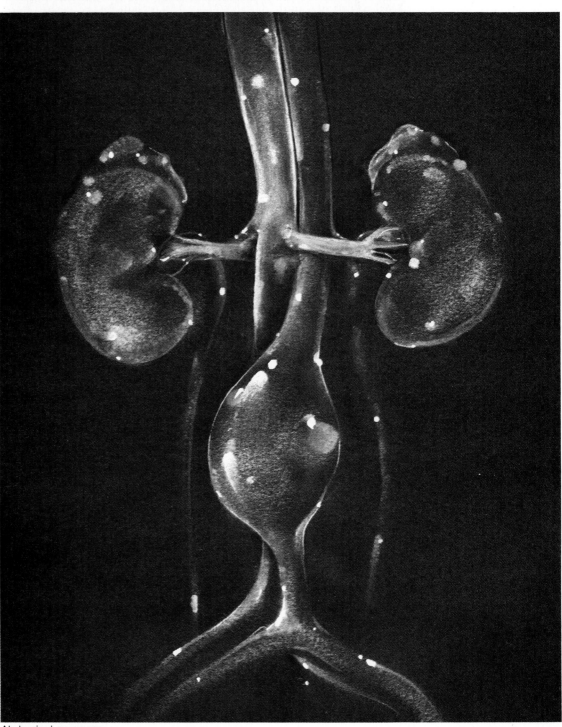

Abdominal aneurysm

Vascular disorders encompass various abnormalities of the blood vessels, and can affect the arteries, the veins, or both at once. These disorders, which are usually degenerative, are becoming more common as more people live longer. These disorders are most likely to develop in persons who show the same risk factors associated with other forms of cardiovascular disease—smoking, diabetes, obesity, and hypertension. They're sure to challenge your nursing skills in both acute and chronic forms and in routine and emergency situations. To meet these challenges, you need to understand how these disorders develop and how to recognize them.

PATHOPHYSIOLOGY

The major arterial disorders are aneurysms, which result from a weakening of the arterial wall; and arterial occlusive disease, which commonly results from atherosclerotic narrowing of the artery's lumen. Rarer arterial disorders, which may be linked to immunologic dysfunction, include polyarteritis, Raynaud's disease, and aortic arch syndrome.

The major venous disorders are varicose veins and thrombophlebitis. Varicose veins result from valve incompetence or dilatation of the affected vessel. Superficial and deep-vein thrombophlebitis result from inflammation or occlusion of the affected vessel.

Aneurysm

An aneurysm is an abnormal dilatation—commonly a saclike formation—in the weakened arterial wall. Such weakening can follow arteriosclerosis (in about 95% of abdominal aortic aneurysms); cystic medial necrosis; trauma; syphilis and other infections; congenital disorders; or hypertension with coexisting arterial occlusive disease. Aneurysms tend to favor certain sites. Thoracic aneurysms commonly involve the ascending, transverse, or descending portion of the aorta; abdominal aneurysms generally involve the aorta between the renal arteries and iliac branches; peripheral arterial aneurysms commonly involve the femoral and popliteal arteries.

At any of these sites, an aneurysm may be *saccular,* producing a unilateral bulge; *fusiform,* a spindle-shaped bulge that involves the entire vessel (most commonly an abdominal aneurysm); or it may be *dissecting,* most often a thoracic aneurysm that splits and penetrates the arterial wall. A fourth type, a *false aneurysm,* is a pulsating hematoma on the vessel wall. It results from trauma or disruption of arterial repair, and may be mistaken for a true aneurysm. (See *Types of aortic aneurysms* on page 114.)

How arteriosclerotic aneurysm develops

First, degenerative changes in the arterial wall produce a focal weakness. Then, blood pressure within the aorta progressively increases the tension and weakens the arterial wall, resulting in enlargment of the aneurysm. As an aneurysm develops, the roughened intimal surface of the artery becomes lined with a mural thrombus—an aggregate of blood cells, platelets, and cellular debris interlaced by fibrin—that decreases the diameter of the lumen. (See *Development of a mural thrombus* on page 115.)

The progressive weakening and distention of the arterial lumen at the aneurysm predisposes it to rupture. In fact, a large, untreated aneurysm progresses to fatal rupture—causing leakage of aortic blood from a large hole in the aneurysm wall—within 5 years of diagnosis in 85% of patients. Rupture is possible in both large and small aneurysms, but is more common in aneurysms that exceed 6 cm in diameter.

The direction of the rupture influences a patient's chances of survival. An intraperitoneal rupture is almost always fatal because there are no intervening structures to control the bleeding by tamponade. An aortic rupture usually occurs retroperitoneally. A retroperitoneal rupture carries the best prognosis: intervening structures, such as the peritoneum and kidneys, create a temporary tamponade, which allows time for transport and lifesaving surgery.

If the ruptured aneurysm extends into the inferior vena cava, a massive arteriovenous fistula forms, accompanied by shock and heart failure. Rupture of the aneurysm into the duodenum or rectum causes massive gastrointestinal bleeding.

What causes dissection?

Dissection, a hemorrhagic separation of the outer aortic wall, usually begins with an intimal tear. Such dissection may occur on the anterior or posterior ascending aorta. In the dissected area, turbulent blood flow may even split the aortic wall apart, sometimes for a considerable distance. For example, a thoracic dissecting aneurysm may rupture into the pericardium, with resulting tamponade.

Next, cystic medial necrosis weakens the

Types of aortic aneurysm

Saccular

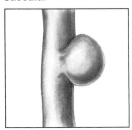

Unilateral pouchlike bulge with a narrow neck

Fusiform

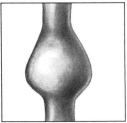

A spindle-shaped bulge encompassing the entire diameter of the vessel

Dissecting

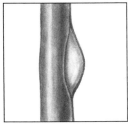

A hemorrhagic separation of the medial layer of the vessel wall, which creates a false lumen

False aneurysm

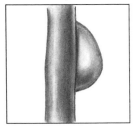

Pulsating hematoma resulting from trauma or anastomotic disruption and often mistaken for an abdominal aneurysm

tunica media. This degenerative process causes the loss of aortic elasticity and a weakening of the blood vessel. Then, stress from the resulting turbulent blood flow extends the dissection. Occurring most commonly in the region of the aortic arch, such dissection may extend toward the heart, involving circulation to the coronary arteries; or it may extend distally to include the arteries that supply the gastrointestinal tract, the kidneys, the spinal cord, and even the legs. Obviously, an acute dissecting aneurysm is a lethal emergency. Untreated, it is fatal within 48 hours in 35% of all patients; within 2 weeks in 75%.

Recognizing a dissecting or ruptured arteriosclerotic aneurysm in time for lifesaving surgery is critical but often difficult. For example, most abdominal aneurysms are asymptomatic until rupture is imminent. In some patients, an abdominal aneurysm may be palpable as a pulsating abdominal mass. Such patients may sense a "heart beat" when lying down. Unfortunately, the first real symptom of abdominal aneurysm is usually a dull ache in the midabdominal left flank or low back, which may signal impending rupture.

Thoracic aneurysms may cause varying clinical effects according to the size and location of the aneurysm as it compresses, distorts, or erodes surrounding structures such as the lungs, trachea, larynx, esophagus and spinal nerves. The most common symptom is pain, often sudden, with a tearing sensation in the chest. It may extend to the neck, shoulders, lower back or abdomen, but rarely to the joints and arms, which distinguishes it from myocardial infarction.

Arterial occlusive disease
The atherosclerotic accumulation of fatty, fibrous plaques usually causes arterial occlusive disease. These accumulating plaques progressively narrow or obstruct the arterial lumen and eventually interrupt the flow of blood of the aorta and its major branches—the carotid, vertebral, innominate, subclavian, mesenteric, and iliac arteries. Such plaques commonly develop in the arteries of the legs and feet, causing signs and symptoms of arterial insufficiency in the lower extremities.

Arterial occlusion causes varying clinical effects, depending on the severity and site of occlusion. For example, a single mild stenosis in the aortoiliac or superficial femoral segment may have no obvious effect on the legs. But a multiple-segment occlusion often causes severe ischemia, leading to intermittent claudication; severe burning pain in the toes, aggravated by elevating the extremity and sometimes relieved by keeping the extremity in a dependent position; and ulcers and gangrene. Other signs include dependent rubor, pallor on elevation, delayed capillary filling or blanching response, decreased temperature, hair loss, and trophic nail changes. Progressive arterial disease causes diminished or absent pedal pulses.

Progressive narrowing of the arterial lumen stimulates the development of collateral circulation in smaller surrounding blood vessels. Collateral vessels may develop further with a daily exercise program. These smaller, less efficient blood vessels may be able to maintain a useful extremity with tolerable symptoms. However, with insufficient collateral development, thrombosis or total occlusion may occur, severely jeopardizing the limb.

Prognosis for arterial occlusive disease depends on modification of risk factors (such as hypertension and smoking), the extent of the disease, the site of occlusion, the effectiveness of collateral circulation, and, in acute occlusion, the duration of interrupted blood flow.

Arterial immunity-linked disorders
Three arterial disorders may be linked to immune function: polyarteritis, Raynaud's disease, and aortic arch syndrome.

Polyarteritis. This relatively rare disorder produces randomly distributed inflammatory lesions in small and medium-sized arteries, often at bifurcations. Initially, polyarteritis produces focal lesions in the medial layer. Eventually, these medial lesions may extend into the adventitial and intimal layers as well, and may form palpable beadlike nodules along the affected artery. These lesions in the arterial wall may precipitate fibrosis; ultimately, they weaken the arterial wall, and may promote the formation of aneurysms. Polyarteritis characteristically causes widespread arterial damage throughout the body and frequently leads to aneurysmal rupture with hemorrhage. The prognosis depends on the severity and location of the arterial lesions, but is usually poor.

Symptoms of polyarteritis may appear abruptly, but more often follow illness, such as a respiratory infection, or drug reaction. Early symptoms are nonspecific and include fever, leukocytosis, general weakness, anorexia, and weight loss. Later symptoms

Development of a mural thrombus

Initial arterial dilatation

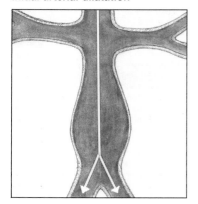

Dilatation increases the radius and decreases the thickness of an artery. As a result, arterial tension rises, enlarging the aneurysm.

Progressive arterial dilatation

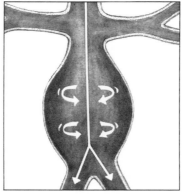

With progressive dilatation, the velocity of the blood flow near the arterial wall decreases, resulting in turbulence. This causes vibration and weakening of the arterial wall.

Mural thrombus formation

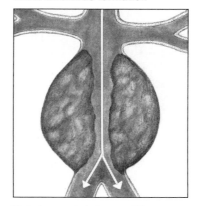

Turbulence and abnormalities on the lining of a damaged arterial wall promote formation of a mural thrombus—platelets, blood cells, and cellular debris interlaced by fibrin.

depend on the organ or body system affected and the severity of the lesions, but most often involve the muscles, kidneys, heart, liver, gastrointestinal tract, and the peripheral nerves.

Raynaud's disease. This condition is marked by a syndrome called Raynaud's phenomenon, which consists of episodic vasospasms in the small peripheral arteries and arterioles precipitated by exposure to cold or stress. It usually affects the hands, or, less often, the feet. Raynaud's phenomenon may exist as a primary disorder, called Raynaud's disease, or as a secondary manifestation of more serious vascular diseases, such as scleroderma, Buerger's disease, and other collagen diseases. Raynaud's disease is benign and occurs most often in females between puberty and age 40. Similar clinical features may occur in Raynaud's phenomenon, which may lead to ischemia, gangrene, and, ultimately, amputation. In some patients, several years of mild, chronic Raynaud's disease may precede overt connective tissue disease.

Symptoms of Raynaud's disease include skin color changes (such as pallor, cyanosis, and finally rubor), possible numbness, and tingling after exposure to cold or stress. Characteristically, Raynaud's disease is marked by bilateral involvement, absent or minimal cutaneous gangrene, normal arterial pulses, and a history of symptoms that have persisted longer than 2 years.

Aortic arch syndrome. This condition progressively occludes the ascending aorta and obliterates its branches. A rare disease, it occurs predominantly in Oriental women be-

tween age 18 and 40, and less often in women of other races. This disease produces nonspecific inflammation of the arterial wall (primarily the adventitia and media) and, later, scarring and thickening of the intima, which leads to thrombus formation and occlusion of the aortic arch branches. Because this condition interferes with the blood supply to the areas supplied by these branches, it can cause the loss of brachial and carotid pulses and tissue ischemia, especially of the nervous system.

Initially, symptoms are nonspecific and similar to those of collagen vascular disease, including malaise, pallor, nausea, night sweats, arthralgias, anorexia, and weight loss. As the disease progresses, variable cardiovascular symptoms follow extensive involvement of arch vessels. Aortic arch syndrome is usually fatal within 2 to 5 years after diagnosis, as a result of heart failure, hypertension, or neurologic complications.

Varicose veins: A common problem

Varicose veins are distended, tortuous superficial veins with incompetent valves. In normal veins, the wall of the vein is strong enough to withstand the lateral pressure of the blood. But in varicose veins, dilatation of the vein from long periods of pressure prevents complete closure of the valves. The resulting backflow of blood produces varicosity.

Varicose veins are most common in people of middle age and older. They can follow chronic thrombophlebitis or other conditions that impair venous outflow or cause valvular damage. However, a history of thrombophlebi-

Development of collateral circulation

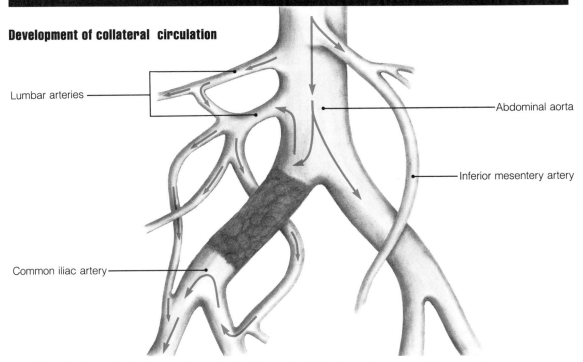

Lumbar arteries

Abdominal aorta

Inferior mesentery artery

Common iliac artery

Arterial occlusion results in the development of collateral circulation in smaller surrounding vessels.

tis is not usually obtainable in patients with varicosities. What *is* commonly associated with varicosities is a history of certain accelerating factors: pregnancy, ascites, abdominal tumors, obesity, or prolonged standing. These factors obviously increase pressure in the veins, cause venous distention, and ultimately lead to incompetence of the valves. However, they do not explain the fundamental predisposition to develop this disorder.

Some investigators explain this predisposition as the result of a generalized abnormality of the veins. They support this view by citing evidence of increased forearm vein distensibility and decreased amounts of collagen and hexosamine in the uninvolved veins of patients with leg varicosities. It's interesting to note, too, that such varicosities often coexist with hemorrhoids and diverticulosis. In light of these facts, and their prevalence in Western civilization, some investigators speculate that varicose veins may be associated with a low fiber diet.

Varicose veins may be asymptomatic or produce mild-to-severe leg symptoms, including a feeling of heaviness; nocturnal cramps; diffuse, dull aching during menses; easy fatigability; minimal skin discoloration; and palpable, distended nodules.

Thrombophlebitis
An acute venous disorder, thrombophlebitis is characterized by thrombus formation and inflammation. Thrombosis may begin in the

valve cusps where local venous stasis permits the accumulation of activated clotting factors that would normally be removed from the circulation. As a result, thrombin is generated and combines with platelets to form a platelet thrombus, which grows from a deposit composed of layers of fibrin and aggregated platelets.

When the propagating thrombus occludes the vein, retrograde thrombosis occurs. Most venous thrombi consist of layers of red blood cell masses that are compressed between the seams of fibrin, the leukocytes, and the platelets.

Thrombophlebitis may be secondary to inflammation of the vein wall from chemical and physical trauma or sepsis. It may occur in superficial (subcutaneous) veins or in deep (inter- or intramuscular) veins. Superficial thrombophlebitis is usually self-limiting and rarely leads to pulmonary embolism. Deep-vein thrombophlebitis (or thrombosis) affects small veins, such as the soleal venous sinuses, or large veins, such as the vena cava, and the femoral, iliac, and subclavian veins. In deep-vein thrombosis, the tail of the thrombus can break loose and travel to the lung, resulting in pulmonary embolism, a potentially lethal complication.

In both superficial and deep-vein thrombosis, clinical features vary with the site and extent of involvement. Superficial thrombophlebitis produces visible and palpable signs, such as local heat, pain, redness, and induration along the length of the affected vein. Fever is minimal or absent. Typically, such a lesion is linear, not globular, extends along the course of a subcutaneous vein, and doesn't ulcerate. Deep vein thrombosis may be asymptomatic, or it may produce edema, pain, fever, chills, malaise, cyanosis of the affected arm or leg, and a positive Homans' sign. (Some studies suggest this sign may be unreliable.)

The risk of thrombophlebitis is cumulative whenever venous stasis, local injury to veins, and blood alterations favoring coagulation coexist. These conditions are likely to follow use of oral contraceptives; fractures or other trauma; pregnancy; cesarean section; major surgery; paralysis; prolonged immobilization, sitting, or standing; varicose veins; a familial history of decreased antithrombin III activity; exposure to certain drugs (such as some chemotherapeutic agents); infection; and malignancies.

MEDICAL MANAGEMENT
In all vascular disorders, the goals of treatment are the same: restoring circulation and preventing complications. Because vascular abnormalities are usually chronic, treatment is typically prolonged and difficult—with frequent setbacks. Fortunately, recent advances in diagnostic testing and treatment promise more effective management.

Managing aneurysms
Most arteriosclerotic aneurysms are detected during a routine physical examination as a painless, pulsating abdominal mass, occasionally accompanied by a systolic bruit over the aorta. Several tests (similar for both thoracic and abdominal aneurysms) can confirm a suspected aneurysm.
• *Anteroposterior* and *lateral X-rays* may reveal calcification of the dilated abdominal aorta. A thoracic aneurysm may first be noted on a routine chest X-ray.
• *Ultrasonography* helps determine the size, shape, and location of the aneurysm.
• *Aortography* shows the condition of vessels proximal and distal to the aneurysm and the extent of the aneurysm. This test may underestimate the aneurysm's diameter because it visualizes only the lumen and not the surrounding thrombus.

If rupture is not imminent, elective surgery may be scheduled to allow time for preoperative assessment of the patient's clinical status. What factors influence the scheduling of sur-

gery? The patient's age (physiologic more important than chronologic), the size of the aneurysm, and the risk of surgery weighed against the chance of rupture.

After rupture of an aneurysm, the patient requires immediate surgery. However, if emergency surgery must be delayed, application of medical antishock trousers (MAST suit) helps prevent vascular collapse. In unusual circumstances, a new emergency treatment, balloon tamponade, controls hemorrhage until surgery can be performed. (See *Balloon tamponade for ruptured aneurysm,* page 118.) Usually, surgical repair for abdominal aneurysm requires resection of the aneurysm and replacement of the damaged aortic section with a synthetic graft. Extraanatomic bypass (EAB) and ligation of both the aneurysm and the outflow vessels may be performed on the patient who is a poor risk for major abdominal surgery.

Managing arterial occlusive disease
The following tests can confirm the presence of arterial occlusive disease:
• *Arteriography* shows the location and extent of an occlusion. This test also shows the presence of collateral circulation. It's particularly useful for evaluating candidates for reconstructive surgery.
• *Oculoplethysmography* helps determine the extent of obstruction in the internal carotid artery by comparing the pressures in each eye. A difference greater than 5 mm Hg between the two pressures suggests carotid insufficiency.
• Two noninvasive tests, *plethysmography and Doppler ultrasonography,* show decreased blood flow to the extremity in acute and chronic disease. Measurement of systolic pressures during Doppler ultrasonography helps detect the presence, location, and extent of peripheral arterial occlusive disease.

Treatment of arterial occlusive disease generally depends on the cause, location, and size of the obstruction. In mild chronic disease, treatment aims to modify risk factors— cigarette smoking, hypertension, diabetes, obesity, hyperlipidemia—and to establish an exercise program. In carotid artery occlusion, treatment includes antiplatelet therapy with dipyridamole and aspirin. In patients prone to emboli, it includes anticoagulants. In acute occlusive disease, treatment usually requires surgery to restore circulation to the affected area.
• *Embolectomy* uses a balloon-tipped Fogarty

EMERGENCY MANAGEMENT

Balloon tamponade for ruptured aneurysm

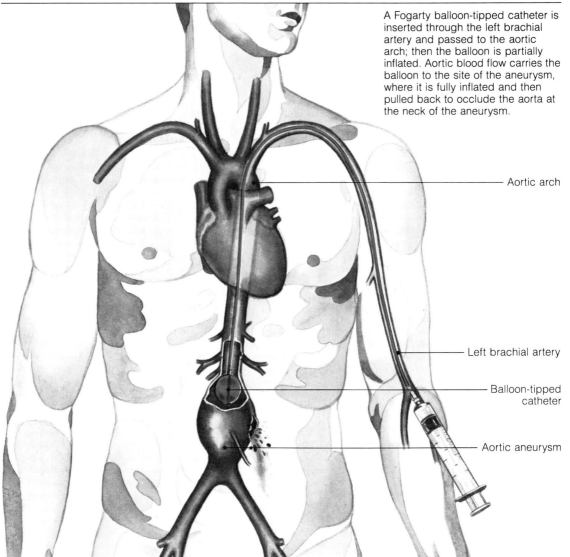

A Fogarty balloon-tipped catheter is inserted through the left brachial artery and passed to the aortic arch; then the balloon is partially inflated. Aortic blood flow carries the balloon to the site of the aneurysm, where it is fully inflated and then pulled back to occlude the aorta at the neck of the aneurysm.

Aortic arch

Left brachial artery

Balloon-tipped catheter

Aortic aneurysm

catheter to remove thrombotic material from the femoral or popliteal artery.

• *Thromboendarterectomy* is the opening of the artery and removal of the obstructing thrombus (atherosclerotic plaque) and the intimal layer of the artery wall. It's usually performed after arteriography, and often used in place of autogenous vein or synthetic bypass surgery. It's most successful in the carotid, aortoiliac, and common femoral arteries.

• *Interposition grafting* is the removal of the thrombosed segment and replacement with an autogenous vein or synthetic graft.

• *Patch grafting* is the removal of the obstructing thrombus and closure of the arteriotomy with an autogenous or synthetic patch to pre-

vent blood vessel narrowing.

• *Bypass grafting* is the diversion of blood flow through an anastomosed autogenous or synthetic graft to bypass the thrombosed arterial segment.

• *Extraanatomic bypass (EAB)* is the diversion of blood flow through an artificial vascular graft from a body area with good arterial flow to a deprived area blocked by disease. It circumvents the traditional, internalized bypass routes. (See *Understanding EAB* on page 120.)

Managing arterial immunity-linked disorders

Confirming the presence of *polyarteritis* requires evaluation of patient history, clinical features, lesion biopsy, and arteriography. Diagnostic tests must rule out other types of vasculitis. Treatment requires vigorous long-term therapy with corticosteroids, usually prednisone, to control symptoms and halt progression. Unfortunately, this disease may progress despite such therapy, and side effects are common. When corticosteroids alone are ineffective, they may be combined successfully with immunosuppressive drugs, such as cyclophosphamide and azathioprine. However, studies of these drugs' effectiveness are still preliminary.

In *Raynaud's disease,* diagnosis must rule out secondary diseases, such as chronic arterial occlusive or connective tissue disease. To control symptoms, the patient should avoid exposure to cold and mechanical injury; and should stop smoking. If symptoms are severe, treatment may include administration of phenoxybenzamine or reserpine. If conservative measures fail to prevent ischemic ulcers, sympathectomy may be helpful.

To confirm *aortic arch syndrome,* aortography of the aortic arch identifies the affected vessels and the extent of damage. Supportive lab results show: elevated white blood cell (WBC) levels and erythrocyte sedimentation rate (ESR); decreased hemoglobin; positive LE cell preparation and complement fixation; and increased alpha and gamma globulins on serum protein electrophoresis. Chest X-rays may reveal cardiomegaly, rib-notching from collateral circulation, and calcification of damaged blood vessels.

Treatment requires surgical repair, with bypass grafting or thromboendarterectomy for symptomatic relief. However, even after surgery, the long-term outlook is poor due to irreversible arterial damage and to the progressive nature of this disease. Treatment with anticoagulants and corticosteroids (prednisone) improves prognosis if it begins before irreversible organ damage has occurred.

Managing varicose veins
The Trendelenburg test and its variations are used to demonstrate blood backflow past incompetent valves to confirm varicose veins. First, the recumbent patient's leg is elevated above the level of the heart to empty the veins; then a tourniquet is applied to occlude the superficial veins. The patient quickly stands up, and the tourniquet is released. If the long saphenous vein is incompetent, blood flows back into the saphenous system; the veins distend, starting at the thigh and ex-

tending down the leg. If two tourniquets are applied and left in place when the patient stands, the filling of the saphenous veins between the tourniquets indicates an incompetent communicating vein. Application of tourniquets at different levels on a leg can precisely locate venous disorders.

Treatment of mild to moderate varicose veins includes application of compression-gradient stockings or elastic bandages to support the veins, improve circulation, and counteract pedal and ankle swelling. Moderate exercise, such as walking, promotes muscular contraction and forces blood through the veins, thereby minimizing venous pooling. Severe varicosities may require stripping and ligation, or, as an alternative to surgery, injection of a sclerosing agent into small venous segments.

Managing thrombophlebitis
Diagnosis of thrombophlebitis must rule out lymphangitis, cellulitis, and myositis. Consequently, laboratory tests include the following:
• *Doppler ultrasonography* identifies impaired venous flow and valve incompetence. A hand-held transducer directs high-frequency sound waves to the vein being tested. Observation of changes in sound-wave frequency during respiration helps detect venous occlusive disease, because venous blood flow normally increases and decreases with respiration.
• *Impedance plethysmography* measures venous blood flow and shows decreased circulation distal to the affected area. This test is more objective than ultrasonography in detecting deep-vein thrombosis. Electrodes from a plethysmograph are applied to the patient's leg and a pressure cuff is applied to his thigh and inflated and deflated. Changes in electrical resistance (impedance) caused by blood volume variations—the result of respiration or venous occlusion—are recorded. Deep-vein thrombosis impedes volume increase and venous outflow.
• *Venography* confirms diagnosis of deep-vein thrombosis, distinguishes blood clot formation from other venous obstruction, and evaluates congenital venous abnormalities. This test is not used for routine screening since it exposes the patient to radiation and can itself cause complications, such as phlebitis, local tissue damage, and, occasionally, deep-vein thrombosis.
• ^{125}I *fibrinogen scan* screens patients at high risk for deep-vein thrombosis, confirms a suspected diagnosis, and detects possible exten-

Understanding EAB

Extraanatomic bypass (EAB) is an artificial vascular graft threaded subcutaneously that carries a limb-preserving blood supply from a body area with good arterial flow to a deprived area. It circumvents the natural channels for blood delivery (blocked by disease), and also skirts the internalized bypass route of the aortofemoral, femoropopliteal, and tibial grafts.

Who's a candidate for EAB?
EAB's a feasible alternative for the patient with vascular disease who needs a bypass but is a poor surgical risk.

EAB may be the surgery of choice for a patient with an existing aortic or femoropopliteal bypass that's become infected or blocked. It may also be used for the patient of advanced age and general debilitation, for the patient with previous abdominal procedures (resulting in excessive scar tissue), or for the patient with limited life expectancy.

And who's not?
EAB, of course, is not for every patient with vascular disease. It isn't the best choice for a younger patient, who can tolerate conventional bypass. Since a traditional aortofemoral graft lasts longer, it would be a more likely surgery for a younger person. Nor is EAB appropriate if diagnostic tests show significant stenosis of the donor artery.

Common bypasses
In the axillofemoral bypass, the axillary artery is exposed via an incision below the clavicle, and the graft is sutured to the donor artery. The tunnel is begun by making an incision in the midaxillary line between the axillary and femoral sites. The groin incision is made, allowing the second segment of the tunnel to be completed. The graft is then pulled through the tunnel and sutured to the recipient femoral artery.

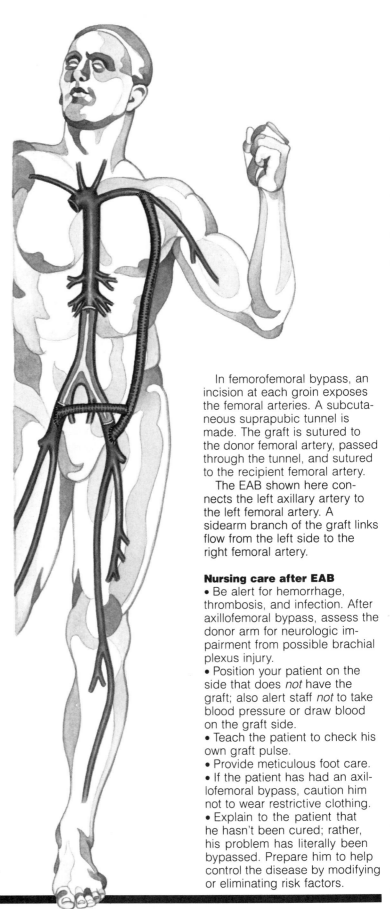

In femorofemoral bypass, an incision at each groin exposes the femoral arteries. A subcutaneous suprapubic tunnel is made. The graft is sutured to the donor femoral artery, passed through the tunnel, and sutured to the recipient femoral artery.

The EAB shown here connects the left axillary artery to the left femoral artery. A sidearm branch of the graft links flow from the left side to the right femoral artery.

Nursing care after EAB
• Be alert for hemorrhage, thrombosis, and infection. After axillofemoral bypass, assess the donor arm for neurologic impairment from possible brachial plexus injury.
• Position your patient on the side that does *not* have the graft; also alert staff *not* to take blood pressure or draw blood on the graft side.
• Teach the patient to check his own graft pulse.
• Provide meticulous foot care.
• If the patient has had an axillofemoral bypass, caution him not to wear restrictive clothing.
• Explain to the patient that he hasn't been cured; rather, his problem has literally been bypassed. Prepare him to help control the disease by modifying or eliminating risk factors.

sion of thrombosis. This test may be used to detect thrombophlebitis in a patient too ill for venography. Labeled fibrinogen injected I.V. collects at sites of active thrombus formation, where an isotope detector measures the increase in surface radioactivity. However, measurements must be made for 2 to 4 days before diagnosis is possible.

Treatment goals are control of thrombus development, prevention of complications, and relief of pain. Superficial thrombophlebitis is self-limiting but severe episodes may require treatment with bed rest, elevation of the affected leg, compression-gradient stockings, and an anti-inflammatory drug, such as phenylbutazone.

Deep-vein thrombosis requires symptomatic treatment with bed rest, elevation of the affected leg (opinions differ on the degree of elevation); warm, moist soaks to the affected area; and analgesics to relieve pain. After an acute episode of deep-vein thrombosis subsides, the patient should wear compression-gradient stockings during hospitalization, and after discharge, as ordered.

Treatment of deep-vein thrombosis requires thrombolytic or anticoagulant therapy. Thrombolytic therapy lyses (destroys) and digests clots already formed; anticoagulant therapy prevents further formation, propagation, and extension. In deep-vein thrombosis, the more acutely ill the patient and the more extensive the thrombosis, the greater the potential benefit from thrombolytic therapy.

Initial treatment of a massive pulmonary embolus or a limb-threatening thrombus begins with administration of a thrombolytic drug, such as streptokinase. (Streptokinase is also used to treat deep-vein thrombosis.) Thrombolytic therapy, followed by anticoagulant therapy, can improve abnormal lung scans, pulmonary arteriograms, and hemodynamic measurements. However, if bleeding occurs, usually due to oozing or excessive bleeding at venipuncture sites, and can't be stopped with application of pressure, thrombolytic therapy is discontinued. Anticoagulant treatment then follows. For example, anticoagulant treatment may begin with heparin sodium because this drug acts immediately to inhibit several steps of the coagulation pathway. Oral anticoagulants, such as warfarin sodium, act more slowly than heparin by interfering with the activation of vitamin K-dependent clotting factors, which are synthesized by the liver. Heparin combines with antithrombin III to potentiate the formation of a thrombin-antithrombin complex to effect coagulation.

Heparin therapy requires careful monitoring—usually with the activated partial thromboplastin time (APTT) test—because individual reponse varies. Heparin therapy for pulmonary embolism and deep-vein thrombosis usually continues for 3 to 5 days before treatment with oral anticoagulants begins. Heparin therapy continues for a total of 7 to 10 days, because warfarin sodium, the commonly used oral anticoagulant, exerts its anticoagulant effect only after 3 to 5 days of therapy. Heparin therapy is discontinued once a therapeutic prothrombin time (PT) is reached. Oral anticoagulant therapy then continues for 3 to 6 months after pulmonary embolism or deep-vein thrombosis.

If anticoagulant therapy fails or is contraindicated, plication of the inferior vena cava is sometimes used to narrow the vessel's lumen and to allow normal blood flow, while trapping the emboli. However, if the patient is a poor risk for abdominal surgery, an intracaval filter may be inserted percutaneously to trap the emboli. Rarely, thrombectomy may be performed, but the formation of new thrombi at the surgical site is a common complication despite the use of heparin.

NURSING MANAGEMENT

If you've ever cared for patients with chronic vascular abnormalities, you know how frustrating and discouraging it can be. And good nursing care means much more than just physical care: Because vascular abnormalities are typically chronic, patients with these conditions are commonly concerned about employment, financial insecurity, or the risk of becoming disabled and dependent on others. Helping these patients challenges all your nursing skills from assessment to evaluation.

Assessing vascular abnormalities

Your assessment of the patient with vascular abnormalities—unless he requires emergency surgery—generally allows you enough time for a carefully detailed nursing history. Here are some priorities to help you get the most information. First, remember that most patients with arterial disorders are elderly, so keep in mind that poor memory could impair some patients' ability to understand and respond to your questions. Examine your patient's attitudes toward his body and his health. Sit close and face your patients, since many may have a hearing and vision loss.

Speak slowly in a low-pitched voice and don't rush the patient's answers. Understand and tolerate the patient's wish to spend more time than you may consider necessary discussing his history, family, and friends.

Ask the patient if he has a history of smoking, GI bleeding, alcohol abuse, hypertension, diabetes, or vascular disease. Determine if your patient's recently recovered from an illness, such as a respiratory infection. Has he experienced general weakness, anorexia, recent weight loss? Does he have a fever? Find out about your patient's current medical regimen and his expectations of treatment.

Ask about any medication he's been taking, since polyarteritis is sometimes precipitated by a drug reaction. Remember to ask about palpitations, angina, shortness of breath, abdominal pain, bloody diarrhea, or blood in the urine. Observe your patient's level of consciousness, noting any episodes of syncope and any sudden changes in mental status that may indicate cerebrovascular insufficiency.

Also, ask about a history of transient paralysis, vision loss, or speech difficulties that resolved spontaneously (evidence of transient ischemic attacks warning of impending stroke). Has your patient suffered any episodes of back and abdominal pain associated with syncope? This may indicate a leaking or expanding aneurysm.

Evaluate leg pain, which can result from arterial or venous insufficiency. Both lead to progressive suffering and disability unless managed promptly and correctly. Remember to ask elderly patients about leg pain even if they don't complain of it, since many consider such pain normal at their age.

If you suspect arterial disorders, ask the patient about pain in the legs related to walking (claudication) or aching pain in the toes that may awaken him at night (rest pain).

If you suspect venous disorders, ask the patient about progressive leg discomfort (unrelated to walking), which worsens by the end of the day or over several days. Elevating the extremities relieves leg discomfort. (Remember, symptoms of arterial disease are aggravated by elevating the extremities.) The patient may also complain of swelling in the extremities from venous insufficiency.

Remember that patients with a history of varicose veins, hypercoagulation, congestive heart failure, or recent major surgery or injury, the obese, the elderly, and women taking oral contraceptives are particularly susceptible to venous disorders in the legs.

Physical examination next

After a detailed history, continue with a head-to-toe review for arterial abnormalities. Check for signs of cerebral ischemia with carotid artery stenosis: Palpate temporal, facial, and carotid pulses. Listen for carotid bruits. Assess for deficits in motor or sensory activity, or diminished or absent reflexes. Check vital signs, noting hypertension or tachycardia. Check for signs of respiratory distress, including dyspnea and paroxysmal cough. (Aneurysm may compress the trachea or bronchus.) Assess for flank and abdominal pain (resulting from decreased mesenteric blood flow or compression of the abdominal organs by aneurysm) and dysphagia (from compression of the esophagus). Remember that 80% of abdominal aortic aneurysms are palpable, even if asymptomatic. If you find evidence of a dissecting or ruptured aneurysm (back and abdominal pain and a tender, pulsating mass), notify the doctor immediately.

Your physical examination should assess the quality of the pulses and note deficits in circulation to the extremities: painful, weak arms or legs; edema. Look for skin changes (integrity, color, temperature, sensation) and postural color changes (blanching and rubor) related to arterial occlusive disease. If appropriate, check for postural color changes: Instruct the patient to elevate his feet for 1 minute and then quickly lower them. Then time the return to normal color. If color fails to return in 15 seconds, arterial insufficiency is moderate; in 30 seconds, marked; and in 60 seconds, extreme. Be sure to include auscultation for bruits. (See *Auscultating for bruits,* page 123.)

During your physical examination for venous disorders, inspect the patient's legs; note symmetry or asymmetry. Also, measure and record calf circumference. Mark the skin at the site of measurement with a felt-tip pen so you can measure precisely the same area again. Look for venous distention, edema, puffiness, palpable venous cords, stretched skin, or induration. Using the back of your fingers, check for increased temperature in the affected leg from inflammation. As you examine your patient's legs, remember that swelling, particularly in loose, connective tissue of the popliteal space, ankle, or suprapubic area, may signal an occluding thrombus. Also, evaluate breath sounds and respiratory patterns to help detect pulmonary emboli.

After you've completed your physical examination, review the results of blood studies,

Auscultating for bruits

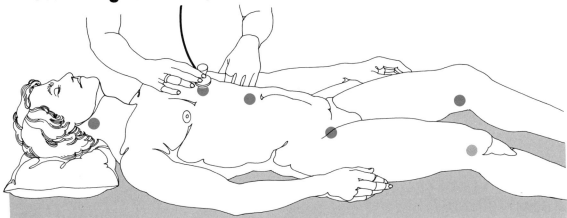

Auscultation of the neck, abdomen, and limbs is essential for complete arterial assessment. Moving from head to toe, auscultate for bruits—swishing sounds caused by turbulent blood flow—in these areas:
• **The neck.** A narrowing or obstruction may cause bruits. A bruit that's loudest close to the jaw is significant since that's where the carotid artery divides; a bruit over the collarbone may have been transmitted up along the arteries from the heart or the aortic root—so listen over the heart, too.
• **The abdomen.** Bruits heard in the abdominal aorta should alert you to assess arterial perfusion in the legs. Absence of pulses indicates decreased blood flow (dissecting aneurysm or arterial embolus is possible).
• **The groin and the inner aspect of the thigh, where the femoral artery runs.** In the lower part of the thigh, slightly above the knee, is the adductor canal, probably the most common site for hardened arteries of the legs to occur.
• **Behind the knee.** Significant narrowing of the popliteal artery can cause bruits.

Preventing problems
Auscultation requires experience, judgment, and finesse. Keep these tips in mind:
• If you press too hard with the stethoscope where arteries are close to the skin, you may compress the artery and create a false bruit. But you do need good contact with the skin.
• It's easy to create a bruit behind the knee. To avoid this, position the patient supinely, put your hand behind the ankle, and lift the leg slightly so the stethoscope can be placed behind the knee without pressure.
• In an overweight person, apply moderate pressure over a big stomach or thigh. Where the vessel is far below the skin, the noise of a bruit may not be very loud, especially when bowel sounds interfere with your hearing. If you hear a bruit, decrease the pressure, but make sure the bruit doesn't disappear.

such as hemoglobin, hematocrit, platelet levels, coagulation studies, triglycerides, blood glucose levels, WBC count, and ESR. Also, check reports from diagnostic tests that evaluate body systems affected by vascular abnormalities: kidney and liver function studies, EKG, radiographs, arteriography, venography, aortography, cardiac catheterization, and ultrasonography. Integrate the findings from these tests with your assessment data.

Planning and implementing care
Now you're ready to develop appropriate nursing diagnoses based on your assessment. (See *Possible nursing diagnoses for vascular abnormalities,* page 124.) These will help you plan nursing goals and interventions for the patient with vascular abnormalities. The following are some typical nursing interventions:

Teach the patient about his disease and provide psychological support. Patients who know little about their disease generally feel anxious about possible complications, surgery, even death. Provide a calm environment and encourage the patient to verbalize his fears. Continually assess the patient's anxiety and plan your teaching accordingly.

Explain the disorder, diagnostic tests, and anticipated surgery. Explain your patient's circulatory problem in simple terms, and discuss his symptoms. Also discuss diagnostic procedures, such as radiographs, EKG, cardiac catheterization with angiography (be alert for complications after this test), and ultrasonography, as appropriate. Explain the anticipated surgery, and show him the synthetic graft for repair of aneurysm, if applicable. Also, prepare him for treatment in the ICU by telling him what sights and sounds to expect. Describe the lines and tubes found in the ICU (central venous pressure, Swan-Ganz catheter, arterial line, indwelling (Foley) catheter, at

Possible nursing diagnoses for vascular abnormalities

Most vascular abnormalities are chronic, with worsening symptoms and progressive deterioration of the patient's condition. Nursing management aims to arrest the disease.

Disorder	Nursing diagnoses	Goals
Aneurysms	• Anxiety due to knowledge deficit related to aneurysms and their complications, and fear of surgery • Potential for postoperative complications of atelectasis, hemorrhage, infection, graft occlusion, and embolization, if aneurysm repair is scheduled • Knowledge deficit related to continuing medical regimen at home	• Reduce anxiety by providing patient teaching • Prevent complications • Provide discharge teaching
Arterial occlusive disease	• Anxiety due to knowledge deficit related to the disease • Impaired circulation to the extremities secondary to occlusion • Pain secondary to ischemia • Potential for injury, infection, and ulcer formation secondary to decreased circulation • Knowledge deficit related to surgery and preoperative procedures • Potential for postoperative complications • Knowledge deficit related to continuing medical regimen at home and steps to prevent progression of the disease	• Reduce anxiety by providing patient teaching • Maintain circulation to the affected part • Relieve pain and promote comfort • Prevent injury, infection, and ulcer formation • Provide preoperative teaching • Prevent postoperative complications • Provide discharge teaching
Polyarteritis	• Anxiety about symptoms and knowledge deficit related to the disorder and its treatment • Potential for complications of corticosteroid therapy	• Reduce anxiety by providing patient teaching • Prevent complications
Raynaud's disease	• Knowledge deficit related to the disease and its treatment • Pain secondary to ischemia	• Provide patient teaching • Relieve pain
Aortic arch syndrome	• Knowledge deficit related to the disease and its treatment • Impairment of peripheral circulation secondary to aortic branch occlusion • Potential for postoperative complications • Depression secondary to poor prognosis	• Provide patient teaching • Maintain circulation to the affected part • Prevent complications • Help patient and family cope with the disease
Varicose veins	• Knowledge deficit related to varicose veins • Impairment of circulation secondary to venous insufficiency • Potential for complications, such as ulcer formation and postoperative infection	• Provide patient teaching • Maintain circulation and promote venous return • Prevent complications
Deep-vein thrombosis	• Knowledge deficit related to deep-vein thrombosis • Potential for pulmonary emboli • Knowledge deficit related to continuing medical regimen at home	• Provide patient teaching • Prevent development of pulmonary emboli • Provide discharge teaching

least one peripheral I.V. line, and a nasogastric tube). Describe the breathing tube that will be in place to ease his breathing and the load on his heart, if its use is anticipated. Teach your patient coughing, deep breathing, pedal or leg exercises, and how to use the incentive spirometer (if appropriate), so he'll be prepared to perform these activities after surgery. Reassure him that a nurse will always be nearby to monitor his condition and provide assistance, as needed.

Explain drug treatment. Give your patient information about any prescribed drugs, their purpose, and possible side effects. For example, treatment of *polyarteritis* may include steroids, which may cause troublesome body changes: moon face, buffalo hump, hirsutism, and purplish striae (Cushing's syndrome).

Provide emotional support if these side effects appear.

The patient who receives drug treatment for *Raynaud's disease* may also develop troublesome side effects: Phenoxybenzamine hydrochloride may cause headache, tachycardia, nasal congestion, and orthostatic hypotension. Cyclandelate may cause headache, nausea, increased perspiration, vertigo, flushing, and tingling. Effects of tolazoline hydrochloride may include GI upset, orthostatic hypotension, chills, tachycardia, and tingling.

The patient with *aortic arch syndrome* needs special psychological support. Encourage him to participate in scheduling procedures, to promote a feeling of some control over this usually fatal disease. Before long-term corticosteroid and anticoagulant therapy begins, explain its purpose, expected results, dosage, and side effects. Stress the need for serial blood studies (prothrombin times) throughout therapy for aortic arch syndrome. Refer the patient to a community agency for rehabilitation or for psychiatric or social services, if necessary.

After effective teaching, the patient is more

Arterial and venous ulcers: A summary comparison

Arterial and venous leg ulcers are not alike. Chronic arterial occlusive disease causes arterial ulcers, which can form whenever a blocked or constricted artery produces ischemia in the distal tissues. As the ischemia worsens, capillary perfusion drops, metabolic exchange decreases, and the skin becomes increasingly fragile and susceptible to trauma. Chronic venous insufficiency causes venous ulcers. Valvular incompetence in the deep veins or the perforating veins causes blood to back up into the superficial veins. As pressure increases from venous hypertension and distension, red blood cells leak through the capillaries into surrounding tissues. Products of red-cell breakdown then infiltrate the subcutaneous tissues and skin of the lower leg. Infiltrated areas become edematous and so fragile that even minor trauma can produce ulceration, which tends to progress, sometimes involving the entire circumference of the leg.

	Arterial ulcers	Venous ulcers
Predisposing factors	• Arteriosclerosis • Advancing age • Diabetes	• History of deep-vein thrombophlebitis • Valvular incompetence in the perforating veins
Associated changes in leg or foot	• Thin, shiny, dry skin • Thickened nails • Absence of hair growth • Temperature variations • Pallor on elevation • Dependent rubor	• Firm ("brawny") edema • Reddish-brown discoloration • Evidence of healed ulcers • Dilated and tortuous superficial veins
Ulcer location	• Between toes or at tip of toes • Over phalangeal heads • On heel • Above lateral malleolus • For diabetic patients: over metatarsal heads, on side or sole of foot	• Anteromedial malleolus • Pretibial area
Ulcer characteristics	• Well-demarcated edges • Black or necrotic tissue • Deep, pale base • Exceedingly painful	• Uneven edges • Ruddy granulation tissue • Superficial • Moderately painful
Nonsurgical treatment	• Wet-to-dry saline solution dressings, loosely bandaged; avoid tape on fragile skin • Bed rest to ensure oxygen and nutrients for healing • Topical antibiotic, if infected • Immobilization, if tendon is exposed, with short-leg fiberglass cast with a window for dressing changes	• Frequent dressing changes with solution, as ordered; tightly bandaged • Limb elevation • Compression bandages to eliminate venous stasis, or Unna's boot, if patient is ambulatory • Systemic antibiotic, if infection or cellulitis is present • Chemical debridement, if necessary, to dissolve necrotic tissue
Surgical intervention	• Vascular reconstruction • Amputation	• Perforating vein ligation • Valvular transposition

PATIENT-TEACHING AID

Caring for your legs and feet

Dear _____

Because of poor circulation in your legs and feet, there's a danger you'll develop leg ulcers. To help prevent these ulcers, follow these guidelines:

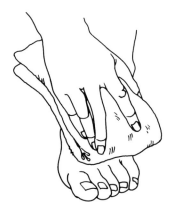

Keep your legs and feet clean, soft, and dry. Wash daily and dry thoroughly by patting with a soft towel, especially between the toes. Apply lanolin or a similar mild cream to keep your skin from cracking. Wear clean, absorbent socks or stockings (preferably cotton or wool).

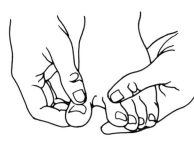

Inspect your legs and feet every day. This is important because you may develop breaks in the skin that you can't feel.

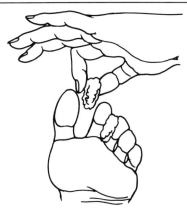

Avoid injury to your legs and feet. Wear shoes that fit correctly, and avoid walking barefoot. Also, put lamb's wool between your toes to prevent rubbing. Lastly, have your doctor or a podiatrist cut your toenails.

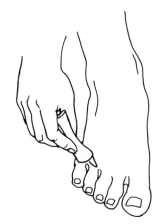

Avoid foot preparations unless the doctor prescribes them. This is important because many foot plasters, corn removers, disinfectants, and ointments are strong enough to injure your feet.

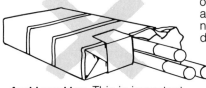

Avoid smoking. This is important because smoking narrows your blood vessels, restricting the blood supply to your skin even more.

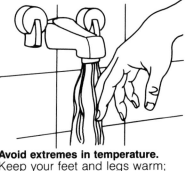

Avoid extremes in temperature. Keep your feet and legs warm; wear cotton or wool socks. Never apply heat (for example, a hot water bottle) to your foot. Test bathwater with your hand (not your foot) before getting into the tub. Also, avoid exposing your legs and feet to the sun, and don't swim in cold water.

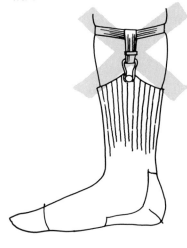

Avoid clothing that restricts your circulation. Don't wear girdles, garters, or socks with tight elastic bands.

Important: Notify your doctor if you get a wound on your leg or foot. Cover the wound with a plain, sterile gauze pad. Do not put ointments (such as hydrocortisone cream) on it.

able to cope with his disease; he seems less anxious and asks appropriate questions about diagnostic procedures and treatment.

Prevent complications. Patients with impaired circulation are susceptible to injury, infection, and leg ulcers; formation of pulmonary emboli (especially in deep-vein thrombosis); complications related to drug therapy; and postoperative complications.

Prevent injury, infection, and leg ulcers. Protect the affected leg with a bed cradle. Provide daily hygiene and observe the skin for scaling and cuts. In immobilized patients, check fragile skin areas frequently for signs of skin breakdown, and treat it aggressively. Warn the patient to avoid injury that might result from decreased sensation in the affected part. Check the patient's pedal pulses; absence of a posterior tibial pulse and dorsalis pedis pulse indicates lower extremity ischemia. Treat ulcers as ordered. (See *Arterial and venous ulcers: A summary comparison,* page 125.)

Prevent pulmonary emboli. Be alert for signs of pulmonary emboli in the patient with thrombophlebitis: sharp chest pain on inspiration, rales, dyspnea, hemoptysis, and hypotension. Position the patient comfortably while maintaining bed rest. Elevate his legs, if ordered (avoid use of pillows). Do not massage or rub the patient's legs. This could break up a clot and release an embolus. Regularly check pulses in all extremities and circulation in the affected leg. If prescribed, apply warm, wet dressings or use a heat cradle.

Prevent complications of drug therapy. Corticosteroids are used to treat polyarteritis and aortic arch syndrome, but they may mask or exacerbate symptoms of intercurrent infections. Watch for fever or other signs of infection. And stress moderate restriction of sodium intake to reduce fluid retention, another side effect of corticosteroid therapy. Also, advise the patient to avoid other drugs that might exacerbate the symptoms of polyarteritis, such as sulfonamides, iodides, penicillins. Help him to develop a drug schedule he can follow at home.

Observe for signs of hemorrhage with thrombolytic and anticoagulant therapy used to treat deep-vein thrombosis. Consider that many drugs can change anticoagulant requirements: antacids, antihistamines, barbiturates, oral contraceptives, vitamin C, and vitamin K (mostly in fresh, leafy vegetables) increase requirements; alcohol, antibiotics, aspirin, cimetidine, diuretics, oral hypoglyce-

mics, phenylbutazone, quinidine, and steroids decrease requirements.

Anticipate and prevent postoperative complications. Know your patient's preoperative status so you'll know what changes and complications may occur. With distal grafting, check distal pulses immediately and report signs of decreased perfusion to the legs. Watch for changes in mental status, which may indicate decreased perfusion to the brain from embolization. Monitor vital signs, distal pulses, and color, temperature, movement, and sensation in the legs every hour for 12 hours and thereafter as ordered. Increased blood flow and changes in lymphatic drainage may cause taut, shiny skin, edema, and generalized redness. Carefully monitor effect of edema on graft and posterior tibial nerve function. Fever may signal respiratory complications, urinary tract infection, or wound contamination.

Maintain hemodynamic stability by assessing pulmonary artery and pulmonary capillary wedge pressures, and report increased drainage on dressings immediately. Also assess for other signs of hemorrhage: tachycardia; hypotension; cool, clammy extremities; and back and abdominal pain after aortic surgery. Encourage coughing and deep breathing. Monitor arterial blood gases and give oxygen, as ordered. Perform chest physiotherapy as ordered, and note character and quantity of secretions.

Check the incision by looking for local inflammation, increased pain, and purulent drainage. Signs of infection include an elevated temperature and changed wound drainage (color, odor). Watch for dehiscence of the suture line. Dressings (adherent or nonadherent) are usually removed by the doctor within 2 or 3 days. However, the incision site is usually left uncovered, except for the groin area, which is usually covered by a 4″ x 4″ cotton gauze dressing to absorb possible drainage.

After an aortic graft, administer intravenous fluids and antibiotics, as ordered. Regularly monitor vital signs for early signs of hemorrhage and assess abdominal girth to check for graft leak or rupture.

After surgery, apply a footboard to prevent footdrop, and a padded bed cradle to keep top covers from pressing on the toes. Help the patient walk as soon as he's able. Early walking dilates collateral vessels, stimulates blood flow and venous return, and improves renal perfusion and respiratory function. Warn the patient against crossing his legs. (See *Exer-*

Exercise—a must

In vascular disorders, exercise is essential to help prevent venous stasis and promote collateral circulation. But individual requirements vary. Elderly patients, for example, are often unable to perform active exercises, and sometimes exercise is not appropriate at all. More often, however, these patients may need your help in performing gentle, passive exercises. So plan your patient's exercise program with his needs in mind.

Unless contraindicated, assist the postoperative patient, while still in the recovery room, to perform passive range-of-motion exercises by flexing and extending his legs. As the patient becomes more alert, tell him to wiggle his toes, rotate his feet at the ankles, and flex and extend his feet alternately.

On the first postoperative day, depending on the patient's condition, begin an active exercise program. Instruct and assist the patient restricted to bed rest to:
• imitate a walking motion for 5 minutes every 2 hours, if lying on his back.
• imitate bicycle pedaling for 5 minutes every 2 hours, if lying on his side. (Do not, however, use this exercise if the patient has a new graft.)
• sit on the side of the bed and support his feet on a stool or a chair.

If the patient is ambulatory, instruct him to walk for 10 minutes every hour and to alternate sitting and lying down. Explain why frequent position changes are necessary, and why he should avoid crossing his legs (compression of blood vessels can restrict blood flow).

If the patient has arterial occlusive disease, encourage walking, swimming, or bicycling. Encourage him to exercise until leg claudication forces him to stop; and then to rest and exercise again. To promote compliance, explore the patient's life-style to help him fit exercise into his daily activities.

Arteriovenous fistulas

An arteriovenous (A-V) fistula is an abnormal connection between an artery and a vein. A-V fistulas may be single or multiple, acquired or congenital. Acquired fistulas, usually single, commonly follow penetrating injuries, blunt trauma, malignancy, infection, and arterial aneurysms. Congenital A-V fistulas, usually multiple, result from defective embryonic development of differentiation into arteries and veins. Congenital fistulas may involve any part of the body. A-V fistulas are also created surgically to provide access for hemodialysis.

In A-V fistulas, arterial blood, following the path of least resistance, flows into the vein, bypassing the corresponding capillary bed. In large fistulas, cardiac output must rise to maintain adequate circulation. Even small fistulas induce increased cardiac output and heart rate, sometimes leading to heart failure. Fistulas may also cause ischemia or venous stasis and varicose veins.

Detecting and treating A-V fistulas

Although initially asymptomatic, an A-V fistula should be suspected in patients with penetrating injuries of the arms or legs. An A-V fistula can be detected as a continuous murmur and palpable vibration over

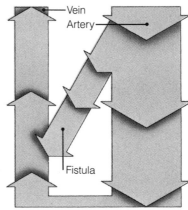

the abnormal communication, which disappears when the feeding artery is compressed. In large fistulas, compression of the feeding artery results in abrupt slowing of the heart rate (Branham's sign). Large fistulas may become infected, and chronic fistulas are distinguished by stasis pigmentation, varicose veins, and cutaneous ulcers. With long-term fistulas, cardiac enlargement is a possibility. Large fistulas between vessels such as the abdominal aorta and the inferior vena cava, where cardiac failure may develop quickly, require immediate surgery. Surgery divides the communication between the artery and vein to reestablish arterial blood flow.

Symptoms of congenital A-V fistulas vary with the location and extent of the abnormal communication. An A-V fistula

should be suspected in the presence of cutaneous hemangioma ("port-wine" type), limb swelling and hypertrophy, visible pulsations, varicose veins in atypical locations, and warmth over the affected part. With arteriovenous fistulas, the deep venous system fails to develop or is obstructed. Treatment varies: It may include support stockings to control venous hypertension and valvular incompetence, excision of a limited fistula (often not feasible), or embolization of the fistula to control blood flow.

Nursing care

Your nursing care of patients with A-V fistulas depends on your skill in physical assessment and nursing diagnosis. A patient with an A-V fistula caused by a penetrating injury or trauma requires supportive, sometimes emergency, care before surgery. This may include maintaining circulation to the affected part, relieving pain, maintaining hemodynamic stability, and providing emotional support. Keep in mind that any abnormal connection between arterial and venous circulation, no matter what the cause, may compromise cardiac output and result in a crisis. Be alert for changes in the patient's vital signs that could indicate hemorrhage and shock. Keep emergency equipment close at hand.

cise—a must on page 127.) Be alert for complications: absence or weakening of pulses, changes in temperature and color, limitation of movement, and paresthesia. Report any of these complications immediately.

You've given effective nursing care for vascular disorders if complications have been prevented or treatment has reduced their severity; if the patient is free of infection and further injury to his legs; if treatment has prevented or minimized ulcers; if the patient is free of postoperative complications, such as atelectasis; if blood pressure, urinary output and acid-base balance are maintained at desirable levels; and if circulation has improved.

Promote adequate circulation. Administer pain medication to the patient with impaired arterial circulation, as ordered, to relieve pain secondary to ischemia. Position the patient comfortably and provide a temperate environment (avoid extremes of cold or heat). Elevate the head of the bed on blocks (avoid the knee gatch), and help him to perform range-of-motion exercises. Assess his circulatory status by checking distal pulses, skin color, and temperature in both legs. Also, note signs of cerebral ischemia and report any sudden changes in mental status that may indicate acute embolization in a patient with aortic arch syndrome.

To promote venous return, obtain compression-gradient stockings, and stress their use, especially if your patient is restricted to bed rest. Administer anticoagulants as ordered, and watch for signs of excessive dosage (bleeding, elevated PT/PTT test).

Evaluate your efforts to maintain circulation. Have the measures you've implemented maintained or improved blood flow to the legs? Is the patient more comfortable? Does he cooperate with procedures you've taught him to maintain circulation?

Teach preventive health. Before the patient is discharged, instruct him about drugs (purpose, route, dosage, timing, frequency, potential side effects); signs and symptoms requiring medical attention; and the importance of follow-up visits. Describe relevant anatomy and review preventive measures that minimize the effects of his disease. Encourage the patient and his family to ask questions. Educate the patient about risk factors. Emphasize the importance of meticulous foot care in preventing infection. Warn the patient to report any lesions on his legs and feet, and any sudden cold or tingling sensations on his feet.

Avoid temperature extremes. Patients with vascular abnormalities are especially vulnerable to tissue damage related to environmental changes in temperature. Tell them that warmth provides or maintains optimal circulation to the extremities and promotes comfort. But warn them against direct or excessive application of heat (hot water bottle or electric pad), which may damage an ischemic area before the patient realizes it. Also, excessive heat raises metabolism, increasing the demand for oxygenated blood beyond what the occluded vessel can provide. Excessive heat injures poorly oxygenated tissues, and gangrene may then follow even slight trauma. Cold injury is similarly damaging, since the resulting vasoconstriction further reduces circulation to an ischemic area.

Instruct the patient with Raynaud's disease to avoid whatever provokes vasoconstriction, including exposure to cold, mechanical or chemical injury, and smoking (nicotine is a vasoconstrictor). Suggest he wear warm clothes in cold weather; turn on the heat in automobiles when traveling; shop in heated stores and avoid unheated buildings; and avoid handling cold items—frozen foods—or defrosting the refrigerator or freezer. Tell him to take extra precautions to avoid injury to fingers and hands from needle pricks and knife

cuts. Explain the effects of stress on vasoconstriction and help the patient develop strategies for avoiding stress.

Maintain an adequate diet. Encourage a balanced and varied diet that maintains desirable weight and provides less fat, more protein, and a good selection of fruits and vegetables. A diet high in protein discourages tissue breakdown. Vitamins, particularly B and C, are also needed. Consult the dietitian for dietary instructions, especially for diabetics and those who may need low cholesterol and low sodium diets. Provide written information for your patient to take home.

Eliminate smoking. Smoking is the single risk factor most strongly associated with arterial disease because it causes vasoconstriction, alters coagulation, and increases carboxyhemoglobin levels and platelet adhesiveness. However, persuading the addicted smoker to stop is difficult.

Establish a continuous program of exercise. For the patient with a venous disorder, regular exercise increases muscle tone and muscle pumping action; walking, for example, promotes muscle contraction and forces blood through the veins, minimizing venous pooling. For the patient with mild arterial occlusive disease, exercise stimulates the development of collateral circulation.

After successful teaching, the patient understands the prescribed treatment: he knows and can demonstrate correct hygiene to prevent complications, and knows and faithfully follows his drug schedule; he wears elastic stockings or bandages during the day, avoids sitting with his legs crossed, and avoids prolonged sitting or standing and wearing restrictive clothing; and he follows an active exercise program.

You've helped the patient with a vascular disorder if he can show adequate understanding of his disease and preventive measures for minimizing its damaging effects, if treatment has maintained or improved circulation, and if complications have been prevented or minimized.

Vascular abnormalities sometimes require emergency care, more often acute care. But most often, they require your perseverance in chronic care. Caring for patients with vascular abnormalities requires your continuous efforts to support, encourage, teach, and motivate the patient in preventive health measures. In managing vascular abnormalities, it's your day-to-day supportive efforts that may count the most.

Points to remember

• Vascular disorders of the arteries, veins, or both at once, affect an increasing segment of the population as more people live longer.
• Abdominal aortic aneurysms (occurring most often in men age 50 to 70) are usually asymptomatic.
• Arterial occlusive disease usually results from atherosclerosis. Diabetes, hypertension, obesity, and smoking are important predisposing factors.
• Treatment to improve circulation and prevent complications may be prolonged, with frequent setbacks. Treatment includes surgical resection for aneurysms; exercise for arterial occlusive disease and certain venous disorders; and thrombolytics and anticoagulants to treat deep-vein thrombosis and to treat or prevent pulmonary embolism.
• Because vascular disorders are typically chronic, patients with these conditions will challenge all your nursing skills from assessment to evaluation.

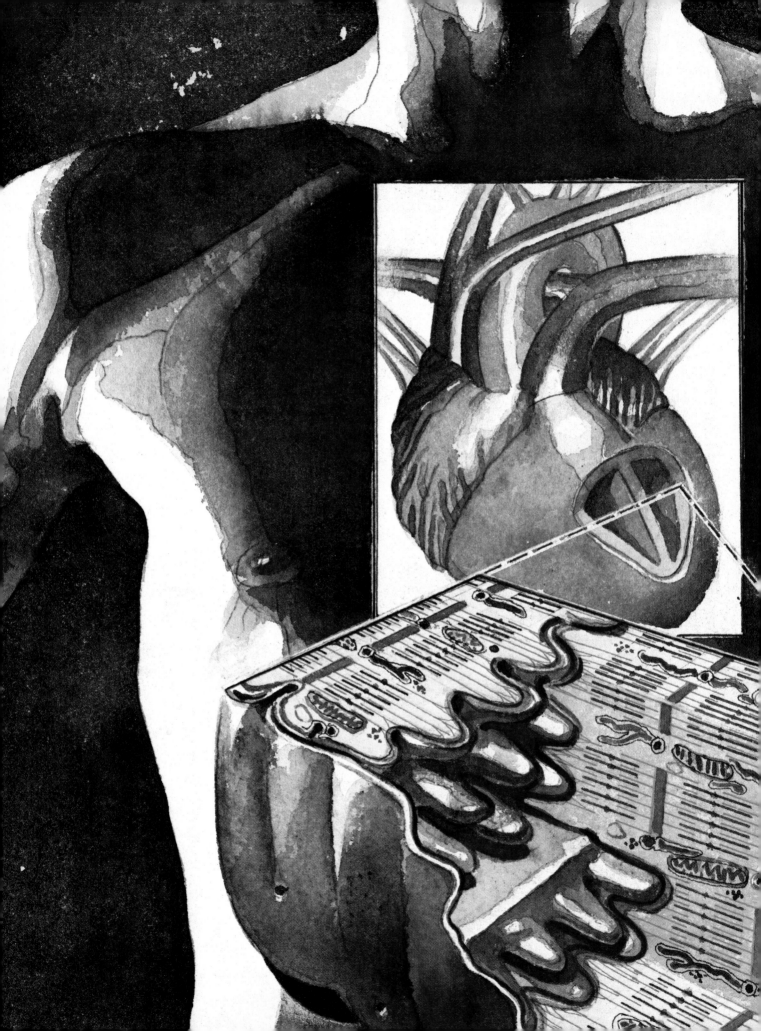

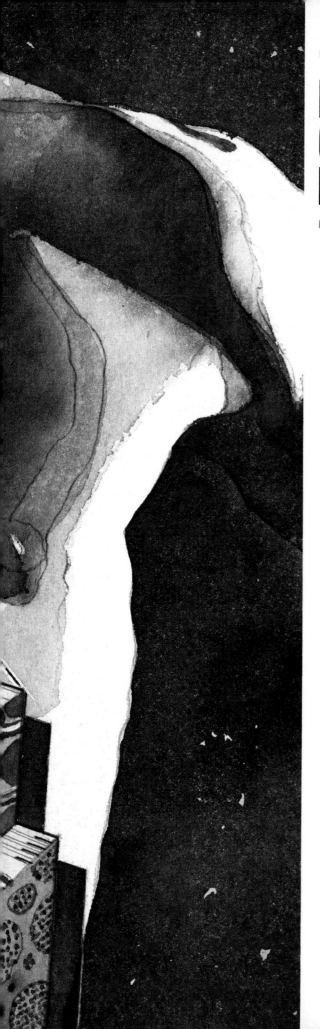

DISORDERS
OF CARDIAC
MUSCULATURE

8 PROVIDING SUPPORT IN CARDIOMYOPATHY

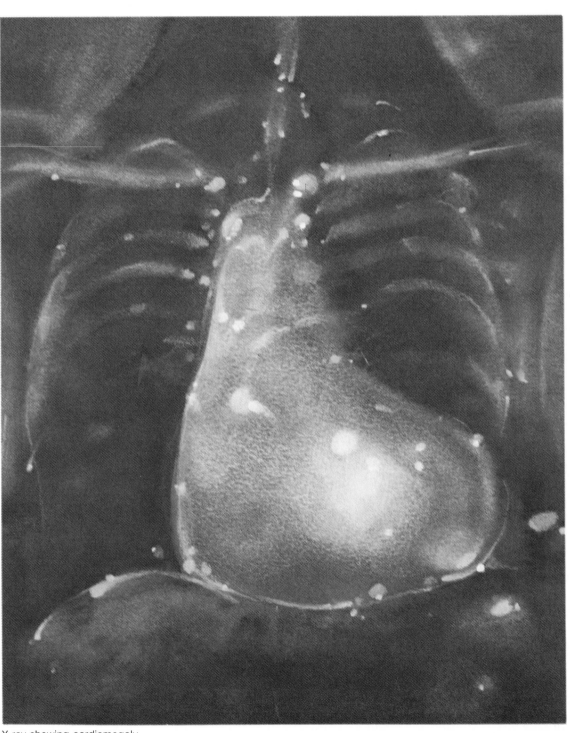

X-ray showing cardiomegaly

Cardiomyopathy. A quick glance at the term tells you it means heart (cardio) muscle (myo) disease (pathy). If you've never had a patient with this disease, the term may convey little more than the dictionary definition. But if you have, you know that cardiomyopathy can be one of the most mystifying cardiovascular diseases. Cardiomyopathy presents many unknowns; its causes are still poorly understood, and curative treatment is rare. To provide effective support for the patient, you must understand that he faces an uncertain, often poor prognosis that may include sudden death, debilitating congestive heart failure, or uncontrollable dysrhythmias. To provide effective care, you must understand the pathophysiology of this disease and become familiar with current treatments.

PATHOPHYSIOLOGY

Reviewing the current classification of cardiomyopathy is a good way to begin discussing the pathophysiology of this mysterious disease. Cardiomyopathy may be broadly classified as primary (idiopathic, or of unknown cause) or secondary (of known cause).

Primary cardiomyopathy, the most common form, carries a poor prognosis. It affects young and old, male and female, and presents a variable clinical picture. It may or may not cause significant symptoms until its advanced stages and often remains undetected until autopsy after sudden death.

Secondary cardiomyopathy carries a somewhat brighter prognosis, its outcome hinging on a timely diagnosis. Early treatment of the underlying systemic cause promises the best chance of recovery or, at least, arrest of cardiac damage. Systemic causes of secondary cardiomyopathy include sarcoidosis; amyloidosis; infectious diseases; neurologic and neuromuscular diseases; chemical, radiation, and drug toxicity; and metabolic, endocrine, and nutritional disorders.

Cardiomyopathy also may be classified as dilated congestive, hypertrophic, restrictive, or obliterative. Of these four, dilated congestive cardiomyopathy is the most common form, restrictive cardiomyopathy is the rarest form, and obliterative cardiomyopathy occurs almost exclusively in tropical areas.

Dilated congestive cardiomyopathy

The term dilated congestive cardiomyopathy conveys two important facts about this form of heart muscle disease—that ventricular dilatation is its hallmark and that symptoms of congestive heart failure are characteristic. Although dilated congestive cardiomyopathy is the most common cardiomyopathy, its etiology is no less obscure than the other cardiomyopathies. Various conditions are associated with dilated congestive cardiomyopathy—among them pregnancy, viral infections, immunologic disorders, and exposure to certain toxic agents. However, the mechanism whereby these conditions induce cardiac damage is unknown; and there's no evidence of a direct cause-and-effect relationship.

One of the most common toxic agents associated with cardiomyopathy is alcohol—the most widely abused substance in the United States. Excessive ingestion of alcohol can produce symptoms of cardiomyopathy that tend to subside with abstinence, but recur with resumption of drinking. However, not everyone who abuses alcohol develops cardiomyopathy. Apparently, some people are simply highly susceptible to alcohol's damaging myocardial effects, a susceptibility that may be aggravated by preexisting heart abnormalities.

Effects of ventricular dilatation

As a result of gross ventricular dilatation, the heart contracts poorly, ejecting only 20% of the blood from the left ventricle (compared with 70% in the normal heart). Because a large volume of blood remains in the ventricle after systole, the ventricular walls become chronically stretched and thinned, thereby inhibiting atrial flow into the ventricle and causing atrial dilatation. Relative stasis of blood in the dilated ventricles predisposes the patient to intracardiac thrombi, which may become the source of pulmonary or systemic emboli.

The signs and symptoms of dilated congestive cardiomyopathy reflect the gradual decline in myocardial contractility and cardiac output. As the heart fails as a pump, stroke volume gradually falls. Initially, the heart attempts to compensate for reduced stroke volume by beating faster. But even with tachycardia, the heart has little reserve to respond well to exercise or stress. (That's why symptoms appear on exertion, even early in disease.) When ventricular dilatation develops from reduced ventricular ejection, the heart's work load and oxygen demands increase. Heart failure ultimately follows, often accompanied by pulmonary congestion and various dysrhythmias.

At first, the patient may report fatigue, palpitations, and mild dyspnea on exertion—signs of left ventricular failure. Paroxysmal nocturnal dyspnea and a dry, irritating cough at night are also characteristic. Dependent edema, liver engorgement, and jugular vein distention—signs of right ventricular failure—may then quickly follow.

When tachycardia is present, the first heart sound may be distant and muffled at the mitral and tricuspid areas, and heart sounds may mimic embryocardia. In embryocardia, as in fetal life, the first and second heart sounds are difficult, if not impossible, to distinguish. Muffling of the first heart sound associated with tachycardia strongly suggests cardiomyopathy, because most other conditions that produce tachycardia intensify the first sound. The third heart sound, or ventricular gallop, commonly occurs—the result of rapid filling of the dilated, flabby left ventricle.

Usually, blood pressure remains normal or decreases, and pulse pressure decreases from poor cardiac output. Initially, the chest X-ray shows cardiomegaly, especially a prominent left ventricle. As the disease progresses, the chest X-ray typically shows gross cardiomegaly and, perhaps, pleural effusion and evidence of pulmonary emboli.

Histologic findings in dilated congestive cardiomyopathy are nonspecific, shedding little light on the cause of ventricular dilatation. Interstitial fibrosis is usually present, and myofibrils appear long and attenuated. However, actual necrosis and inflammatory exudate between myocardial cells are rarely present.

Hypertrophic cardiomyopathy

Decidedly different from dilated congestive cardiomyopathy is the hypertrophic form of heart muscle disease. Its hallmark is a bizarre hypertrophy that affects all heart muscles, but is most prominent in the left ventricular septal wall. In fact, the septum may be large enough to bulge into the right ventricular chamber.

This septal enlargement greatly reduces the left ventricular outflow tract within the heart. Obstruction of the outflow tract may result if the hypertrophied septum abuts the anterior mitral valve leaflet during systole. Thickening of the mitral valve leaflets, the result of increased contact and friction in the small ventricular chamber, also contributes to this obstruction. In severe obstruction, the outflow tract may become a mere slit. The bulging ventricular septum also distorts the papillary

muscles, resulting in mitral regurgitation.

Unlike dilated congestive cardiomyopathy, hypertrophic cardiomyopathy doesn't enlarge the ventricular chambers; their size remains normal or decreases. However, the increased muscle mass stiffens the ventricles, increasing resistance to blood flow from the left atrium. Impaired atrial emptying often causes atrial dilatation.

Bizarre, focal disorganization of myofibrils is a characteristic histologic finding in hypertrophic cardiomyopathy. Normally, myofibrils are arranged in a parallel fashion. But in hypertrophic cardiomyopathy, focal areas of hypertrophied myofibrils, arranged in whorls or at random, are interspersed with larger areas of parallel hypertrophied myofibrils. This irregular alignment of myofibrils interferes with effective contraction and relaxation. Some myofibrils contract at abnormal angles to each other, thereby creating abnormal tensions; some myofibrils also contract while others relax.

Idiopathic hypertrophic subaortic stenosis

Hypertrophic cardiomyopathy with obstruction is known as idiopathic hypertrophic subaortic stenosis (IHSS). This rather unwieldy term accurately describes the disorder. *Idiopathic* describes the obscure pathogenesis of IHSS, although it's known to be inherited through a non-sex-linked autosomal dominant gene. One hypothesis suggests that the myofibril disarray in the septum results from an *in utero* response to altered catecholamine metabolism—an alteration caused by a hereditary neural crest abnormality. Support for this hypothesis comes from the unusually high incidence of other coexisting conditions associated with catecholamine dysfunction, such as pheochromocytoma and Friedreich's ataxia.

Hypertrophic, of course, describes the enlargement of the ventricular septum; and *subaortic,* the location of septal hypertrophy. *Stenosis* describes the narrowing or obstruction of the left ventricular outflow tract.

The severity of outflow tract obstruction in IHSS is not constant. It can vary from examination to examination and even from heartbeat to heartbeat. The obstruction may worsen on its own over the course of time, or it may not. Most important, it can be influenced by the heart's contractility and the size of the left ventricular cavity during systole. Contraction of the left ventricle triggers the outflow tract obstruction. Consequently, any factor

Pathologic changes in cardiomyopathy

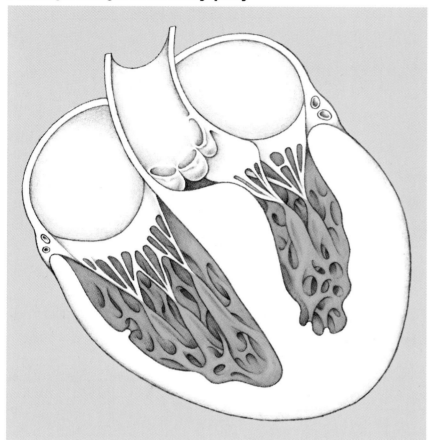

Heart with IHSS
Asymmetric septal enlargement, narrowing of the left ventricular outflow tract, and thickening and displacement of the mitral valve characterize this cardiomyopathy. Outflow tract obstruction may result if the hypertrophied septum abuts the anterior mitral valve leaflet during systole.

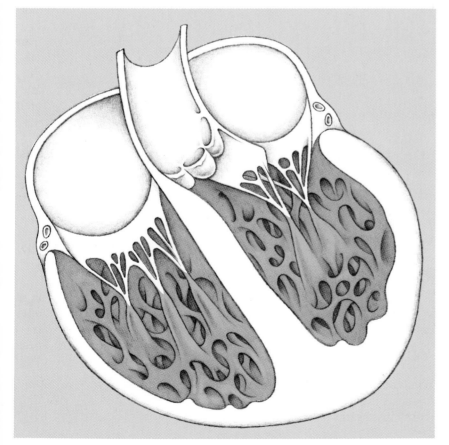

Heart with dilated congestive cardiomyopathy
Gross dilatation is the hallmark of this cardiomyopathy, and causes the heart to assume a globular shape. Because of ineffective ventricular contraction, a large volume of blood collects in the heart, and the ventricular walls become chronically stretched and thinned.

Factors affecting the obstruction in IHSS

Increased obstruction
Agents that increase the force of cardiac contraction:
Digitalis
Isoproterenol

Agents that decrease left ventricular volume:
Diuretics
Blood loss
Nitrates
Exercise
Tachycardia
Sudden assumption of upright position
Valsalva's maneuver
Nonsinus rhythms

Decreased obstruction
Agents that decrease the force of cardiac contraction:
Beta-adrenergic blockers, such as propranolol
Methoxamine
Phenylephrine
Verapamil
Supine or squatting position
Expansion of blood volume

that affects the rate or force of contraction can influence the obstruction. Exercise, for example, stimulates the release of catecholamines, which increases contractility and intensifies the obstruction.

The size of the ventricular cavity during systole influences the degree of contact between the hypertrophied septum and the anterior mitral valve leaflet. Consequently, any factor that affects ventricular size can influence the obstruction.

Sudden death: The ultimate threat

Unfortunately, IHSS carries a significant risk of sudden death, even in totally asymptomatic children and young adults. Typically, sudden death resulting from IHSS follows physical exertion.

Although the exact mechanism of sudden death in IHSS is unknown, ventricular dysrhythmias are highly suspect. Certain atrial dysrhythmias also may be implicated as a primary cause. In atrial dysrhythmias, absence of atrial systolic contraction can cause a sudden, fatal decrease in left ventricular volume and outflow. Atrial dysrhythmias also may degenerate into ventricular fibrillation, resulting in syncope and, if untreated, death.

Fortunately, IHSS does present a few diagnostic signs besides sudden death. Practically pathognomonic of this disorder is a low-pitched, apical systolic ejection murmur, heard best at the lower left sternal border and at the apex. This characteristic murmur results from turbulent blood flow through the narrowed or obstructed outflow tract. It's intensified during Valsalva's manuever or when the patient sits upright or stands suddenly; it disappears if he squats. If congestive heart failure develops, this murmur diminishes or disappears.

Angina may also occur in the patient with IHSS. Outflow tract obstruction increases oxygen demand by increasing the left ventricular work load; the resultant disproportion between oxygen supply and demand causes angina. Because the degree of obstruction may vary without provocation or in response to changes in position or to drugs, angina may occur at rest. Syncope also may occur at rest or during exercise.

In a patient with mild to moderate symptoms, the course of IHSS may vary, with intervals of spontaneous improvement. But if the outflow tract obstruction is severe, congestive heart failure may gradually claim the patient's life.

MEDICAL MANAGEMENT

Diagnosis of cardiomyopathy—and the identification of its particular form—often requires extensive diagnostic testing. Accurate diagnosis is critical for selecting effective treatment.

Diagnosis by exclusion

Because cardiomyopathy may mimic several common cardiovascular diseases, its diagnosis challenges the most skilled clinician. Typically, this diagnosis results from systematic exclusion of other diseases. In dilated congestive cardiomyopathy, diagnosis must rule out other causes of congestive heart failure; in hypertrophic cardiomyopathy, other causes of mitral regurgitation.

The following diagnostic tests make differential diagnosis possible.

Electrocardiography (EKG). Typically, this noninvasive test shows nonspecific ST segment and T wave changes; left atrial and ventricular enlargement, especially in dilated congestive cardiomyopathy; and right ventricular enlargement in advanced disease. In IHSS, pronounced Q waves often are mistaken for evidence of an old posterolateral myocardial infarction, but they actually result from marked septal hypertrophy. Two or more components of Wolff-Parkinson-White syndrome—a short PR interval, a delta wave, and a prolonged QRS complex—also appear in 25% of patients.

In dilated congestive cardiomyopathy, the EKG commonly shows atrial fibrillation, but it also may show atrial flutter, A-V junctional rhythm, supraventricular tachycardia, and ventricular tachycardia. The EKG also reveals left bundle branch block in about 10% of patients.

Chest X-ray. Even in the early stages of dilated congestive cardiomyopathy, this test demonstrates cardiomegaly. As the disease progresses, the chest X-ray may show dilatation of the main pulmonary arteries and pulmonary infarction. In advanced stages, it characteristically shows a grossly enlarged cardiac silhouette, caused by dilatation of all four heart chambers and pericardial effusion. In IHSS, it may show an enlarged cardiac silhouette, sometimes with a bulge in the left ventricle. Since the severity of enlargement doesn't correspond to the severity of outflow tract obstruction, the chest X-ray isn't useful for monitoring the progression of IHSS. However, it can exclude aortic stenosis by failing to show aortic dilatation and aortic valve calcification.

Cardiomegaly: A characteristic X-ray sign

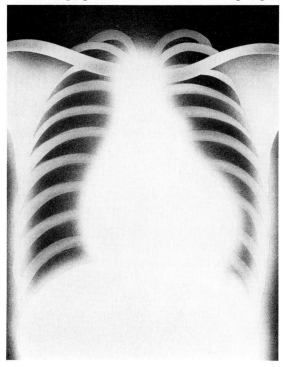

Cardiomegaly typically appears at all stages of dilated congestive cardiomyopathy. In this simulated postero-anterior X-ray of a patient with end-stage disease, the heart assumes a greatly dilated "water bottle" shape.

Echocardiography. In dilated congestive cardiomyopathy, this noninvasive test outlines ventricular dilatation, poor movement of a thin posterior left ventricular wall, and para-doxical motion of a thin septum. In IHSS, echocardiography determines the relative thickness of the enlarged septum and records abnormal motion of the anterior mitral valve leaflet. In fact, it has become the primary test for detecting IHSS and for screening members of the patient's family for this disease.

Blood tests. Typically, these tests are unremarkable. Measurement of complement and rheumatoid factor, detection of parasites, and evaluation of other immunologic changes may help pinpoint secondary disease involving the heart. Measurement of cardiac enzymes—creatine phosphokinase (CPK), lactic dehydrogenase (LDH), and serum glutamic-oxalo-acetic transaminase (SGOT)—may help detect myocardial damage. However, elevated levels of these enzymes also accompany skeletal muscle damage.

Radionuclide tests. Gated cardiac blood pool imaging and thallium stress imaging are the most commonly used radionuclide tests. Gated cardiac blood pool imaging helps monitor the course of the disease and the patient's

response to therapy by assessing cardiac chamber size, regional wall motion, and the ejection fraction. It also may demonstrate asymmetric septal enlargement, cavity obliteration, and a filling defect near the outflow tract in IHSS. Thallium stress imaging aids differential diagnosis by detecting ischemic areas that are characteristic of coronary artery disease.

Cardiac catheterization. This invasive procedure may include coronary angiography, contrast ventriculography, and hemodynamic monitoring. Coronary angiography can definitively rule out coronary artery disease by failing to show arterial constriction. In dilated congestive cardiomyopathy, contrast ventriculography reveals a diffusely enlarged, hypokinetic left ventricle. Hemodynamic monitoring confirms pump failure, but it provides no specific diagnostic information.

In IHSS, contrast ventriculography demonstrates marked thickening of the ventricular wall with a small, irregular cavity that's often obliterated during systole. Hemodynamic monitoring provides specific—and often diagnostic—information. For example, arterial pulse pressure demonstrates a characteristic spike-and-dome pattern: pressure rises rapidly, falls in mid-systole, then rises again. Measurement of the pressure gradient between the left ventricular cavity and the outflow tract confirms subaortic obstruction and helps evaluate its severity.

Treating dilated congestive cardiomyopathy

When dilated congestive cardiomyopathy results from a specific condition or a known systemic disease, the obvious first step is to treat the underlying cause. The second is to improve pump performance and relieve the symptoms of heart failure by interrupting the cycle of compensatory mechanisms. Triggered by reduced cardiac output, these compensatory mechanisms—increased sympathetic activity, ventricular dilatation, and hypertrophy—act to increase cardiac output. However, they do so by increasing ventricular work load and can eventually cause further deterioration of the patient's condition.

The goal of treatment is, in part, the same as that of the compensatory mechanisms: to increase cardiac output. However, it also must improve pump performance and reduce work load. Typically, treatment may include these measures:

• digitalis to strengthen myocardial contractil-

ity and diuretics to reduce circulating blood volume and circulatory congestion
• vasodilators to increase cardiac output by reducing resistance to ventricular outflow and improving myocardial perfusion (In acute congestive failure, treatment may require intravenous infusion of nitroprusside until the patient's condition stabilizes. Oral vasodilators can be used thereafter.)
• anticoagulants to prevent systemic and pulmonary emboli
• antiarrhythmics to minimize the frequency of ventricular dysrhythmias with myocardial ischemia
• oxygen to decrease respiratory effort and enhance myocardial oxygenation
• supportive measures—prolonged bedrest or restricted activity; a nutritious, low-sodium diet to curb fluid overload; and vitamin supplements
• abstinence from alcohol.

Treating IHSS
Effective treatment involves relaxing the stiffened left ventricle and relieving the outflow tract obstruction by surgical or nonsurgical measures. Because exercise stimulates the release of catecholamines, which intensify outflow tract obstruction, restricting physical activity is a vital part of nonsurgical treatment. Weight reduction, another nonsurgical treatment, helps reduce the heart's work load in an obese patient.

Drug therapy usually includes propranolol, a beta-adrenergic blocking agent. By blocking the sympathetic receptors that stimulate heart rate, propranolol allows more time for ventricular filling. By decreasing the force of contraction, it reduces outflow tract obstruction.

Verapamil and certain vasoconstrictors also can influence contractility and often relieve symptoms of IHSS in patients who fail to respond to other measures. Verapamil decreases contractility by impeding the entry of calcium into the myocardial cells. Intravenous administration of vasoconstrictors, such as methoxamine and phenylephrine, decreases heart rate and contractility by increasing impedance to left ventricular outflow.

Notice the critical difference in drug therapy. While vasodilators help to correct dilated congestive cardiomyopathy, their effects—reduced venous return to the heart and increased heart rate and contractility—would *worsen* outflow tract obstruction in IHSS. Consequently, the administration of nitrates to relieve chest pain in IHSS may lead to syn-

Understanding compensatory mechanisms
In dilated congestive cardiomyopathy, chronic ventricular dilatation is responsible for heart failure and reduced cardiac output. Reduced cardiac output triggers increased sympathetic activity, which causes further dilatation and hypertrophy of the diseased heart. These three compensatory mechanisms improve cardiac output at the expense of increased ventricular work.

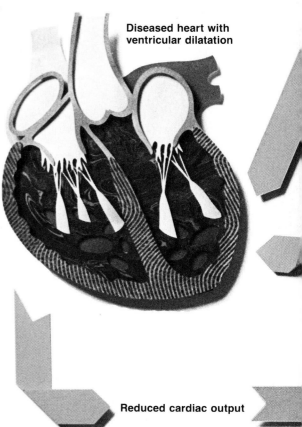

Diseased heart with ventricular dilatation

Reduced cardiac output

cope or, at worst, sudden death.

In some patients with IHSS, activity restrictions, weight reduction, and drug therapy fail to relieve severe symptoms of outflow tract obstruction. For these patients, septal myotomy-myectomy may become the next treatment step. This surgical procedure widens the outflow tract through dissection and removal of a portion of the hypertrophied septum. This procedure can significantly improve IHSS, but it does carry an 8% mortality rate.

NURSING MANAGEMENT
When caring for the patient with cardiomyopathy, knowledge of pathophysiology and medical treatment is certainly a must. But recognizing the emotional strain that cardiomyopathy's uncertain prognosis places on the patient and his family is equally important. Your ability to identify and deal effectively with the patient's diverse problems can do much to-

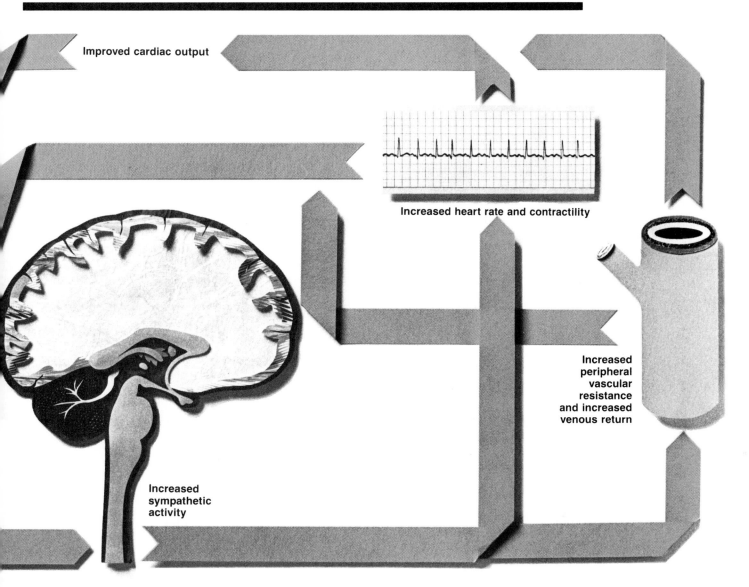

Improved cardiac output

Increased heart rate and contractility

Increased peripheral vascular resistance and increased venous return

Increased sympathetic activity

ward helping him understand, accept, and cope with this disease.

Begin assessment with the history
When taking the patient's history, be sure to include the following steps:

Review the patient's medical history. Find out when cardiomyopathy was first detected and the details of subsequent care. Also identify any pathologic changes in the pulmonary, renal, or neurologic system that have resulted from compromised cardiac function and may influence your care plan.

Ask the patient to describe his symptoms. Obtain answers to these questions: Do you tire easily? When did you first notice the feeling of weakness and fatigue? Is it getting worse? Have you experienced any chest pain? If you have, does the pain radiate? How often does it occur? Do you get breathless during exertion? Is your breathlessness related to the onset of chest pain? Have you fainted or felt lightheaded recently? Does your weight fluctuate? Are your ankles or feet frequently swollen?

Evaluate the patient's understanding and acceptance of cardiomyopathy. Keep in mind that many patients experience profound anxiety and depression, so be especially supportive. Encourage the patient to express his concerns. Is he preoccupied with death? Is he worried about meeting occupational, community, or family responsibilities? Remember, the better the patient understands and accepts his disease, the more likely he is to follow the prescribed treatment regimen.

Determine patient adherence to prescribed treatment. Find out if the patient has observed dietary and exercise restrictions. Ask the names and dosages of any prescription and over-the-counter drugs he's taking. Also ask about consumption of beer, wine, or other forms of alcohol: how often, how much, and for how long?

How nitrates intensify outflow tract obstruction in IHSS

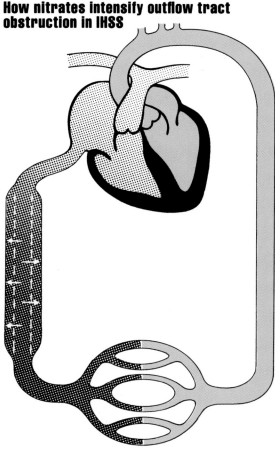

Vasodilating drugs, such as nitrates, permit venous pooling in the periphery, which reduces venous return to the heart. This, in turn, reduces preload, resulting in a smaller left ventricular chamber.

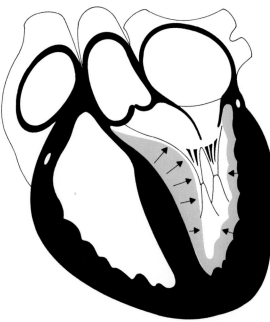

A smaller ventricular chamber brings the hypertrophied septum and anterior mitral valve leaflet closer together, increasing the extent of contact during systole. Increasing the extent of contact intensifies outflow tract obstruction and can result in syncope or, at worst, sudden death.

After you complete the patient's history, you're ready to conduct the physical examination, using the techniques of inspection, palpation, and auscultation.

Perform the physical examination

Begin the physical examination with inspection. Observe for signs of congestive heart failure, such as cyanosis and edema. Also inspect the patient's neck for jugular venous distention and visible carotid artery pulsations.

Then, palpate the carotid artery for rapid pulsations with a biphasic upstroke. Next, palpate the peripheral pulses for rapid, irregular beats or beats of small volume with a characteristic double impulse *(pulsus bisferiens)*. Check for pulse deficit—a characteristic sign of atrial fibrillation. Also palpate the extremities for edema and the right epigastrium for hepatic engorgement and tenderness.

Now, auscultate the heart for diffuse apical impulses, a pansystolic murmur, mitral or tricuspid regurgitation, and S_3 and S_4 gallop rhythms. Auscultate over the left sternal border and at the apex for a low-pitched apical systolic ejection murmur. Typically, this murmur is intensified during Valsalva's maneuver or when the patient sits upright; it disappears if he squats. Also auscultate for rales that accompany congestive heart failure.

If the patient is connected to a cardiac monitor, check for dysrhythmias, such as sinus tachycardia or atrial fibrillation.

Shape data into nursing diagnoses

With the data collected from the patient's history and the physical examination, you're ready to formulate nursing diagnoses and establish related goals and interventions. Nursing diagnoses define the patient's actual or potential problems that you're qualified to treat. In cardiomyopathy, your nursing diagnoses typically address physical, emotional, and cognitive problems.

Reduced cardiac output. After formulating this nursing diagnosis, your goals are to achieve adequate cardiac output, to maintain hemodynamic stability, to prevent complications, and to reduce patient anxiety.

When planning nursing interventions to meet your goals, recognize that reduced cardiac output occurs most often in patients with dilated congestive cardiomyopathy. When the heart fails as a pump, drug therapy is the most effective means of restoring adequate cardiac output. In acute heart failure, I.V. infusion of sodium nitroprusside causes rapid arterial and venous dilatation, decreasing afterload and preload and increasing cardiac output. Because sodium nitroprusside acts so powerfully and quickly, use an infusion pump to control the flow rate precisely. In chronic heart failure, oral and sublingual vasodilators help maintain cardiac output.

Other drugs that improve cardiac output include digitalis, which strengthens myocardial contractility, and diuretics, which reduce total blood volume and circulatory congestion. A low-sodium diet also helps curb fluid overload. Remember, these drugs improve cardiac output in dilated congestive cardiomyopathy, *not* in IHSS.

An especially critical nursing intervention that goes hand in hand with sodium nitroprusside therapy is hemodynamic monitoring after insertion of a balloon-tipped pulmonary artery catheter. Hemodynamic monitoring helps to evaluate the patient's response to therapy and to prevent further complications. For example, pulmonary capillary wedge pressure (PCWP) accurately reflects left ventricular end-diastolic pressure. Consequently, elevated readings indicate left ventricular failure or cardiac insufficiency. When monitoring the patient's hemodynamic status, keep these target values in mind: cardiac output > 4 liters/minute, systolic blood pressure > 90 mm Hg, PCWP > 13 to 22 mm Hg.

Also monitor intake and output. In acute heart failure, measure urine output hourly. Weigh the patient daily to assess fluid retention and check for peripheral edema.

Because reduced cardiac output increases susceptibility to venous stasis and thrombus formation, apply antiembolism stockings. Perform passive range-of-motion exercises or, if the patient's condition permits, encourage active range-of-motion exercises. Watch for calf pain and tenderness.

Remember that the patient with acute heart failure is typically dyspneic, which causes extreme anxiety. Offer support and reassurance to help relieve anxiety. After successful treatment of the acute stage, increase the patient's activity level gradually, and monitor him for dysrhythmias.

Ineffective ventilation related to fluid accumulation in the lungs. After formulating this nursing diagnosis, your goals are to provide adequate oxygenation, to prevent complications, and to comfort the patient and reduce his anxiety.

When planning nursing interventions to

Using palpation

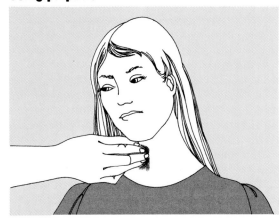

Check the carotid artery for rapid pulsations with a palpable biphasic upstroke.

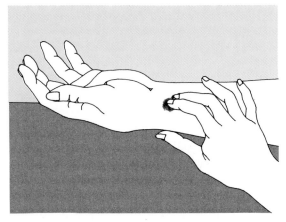

Palpate the peripheral pulses for rapid, irregular beats or beats of small volume with a characteristic double impulse (*pulsus bisferiens*).

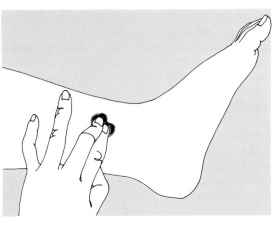

Palpate the ankles and other extremities for edema.

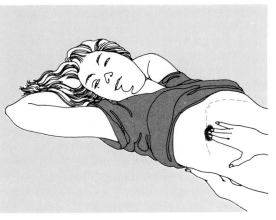

Palpate the right epigastrium for liver engorgement.

Detecting complications of septal myotomy-myectomy

After septal myotomy-myectomy, observe the patient carefully for cardiovascular, respiratory, and renal complications. Anticipating these complications promotes prompt treatment and improves the patient's prospects for recovery.

Dysrhythmias
Monitor the patient's heart rate and rhythm continuously. Watch especially for heart block and atrial fibrillation. (Abnormal conduction often follows surgery near the AV conduction network. Left bundle branch block may develop, or existing conduction defects may progress to complete heart block).

Record all rhythm disturbances. Note any associated changes in the patient's condition or activities, such as movement in bed or sudden onset of diuresis. Notify the doctor if dysrhythmia continues or is life-threatening.

If necessary, prepare the patient with heart block for pacemaker insertion. Administer antiarrhythmic drugs (digoxin, quinidine, propranolol), as ordered, for atrial fibrillation. Recognize that cardioversion may be necessary for persistent atrial fibrillation; defibrillation, for ventricular fibrillation.

Low cardiac output
Monitor the patient's vital signs frequently and evaluate fluid balance. Watch for cold, clammy, mottled skin; narrowing pulse pressure; thready peripheral pulses; decreased urinary output; rales; and elevated central venous and/or pulmonary capillary wedge pressure. Notify the doctor of significant changes in the patient's clinical status.

Administer blood and/or colloid solutions, vasopressors, or diuretics, as ordered.

Cardiac tamponade
Watch for rapid decrease in blood pressure, narrowing pulse pressure, elevated central venous and pulmonary capillary wedge pressures, paradoxical pulse, and distant or muffled heart sounds. Notify the doctor if any of these signs occur. If necessary, prepare the patient for pericardiocentesis.

Respiratory failure
Continuously monitor breath sounds, arterial blood gases, and other measures of respiratory function, especially if the patient is connected to a ventilator.

Maintain airway patency with adequate humidification of inspired air to loosen secretions and suctioning. Administer medication, as ordered, to prevent pain during coughing and deep breathing or to promote maximal ventilator functioning for the intubated patient. Perform chest physiotherapy to help mobilize and eliminate secretions. Encourage use of incentive spirometry and/or other breathing exercises to promote maximal ventilation as well as early ambulation.

Renal failure
Measure and record the patient's urine output and specific gravity hourly. Notify the doctor if output is less than 20 ml/hr or as specified.

Watch for persistent low urinary output; elevated blood urea nitrogen, creatinine, and serum potassium levels; elevated urine sodium and decreased urine potassium levels; and persistent proteinuria and hematuria.

Administer fluid challenges or vasopressors, as ordered. Prepare the patient for dialysis.

---

meet your goals, recognize that therapy to restore adequate cardiac output also decreases associated pulmonary congestion. But this alone doesn't ensure adequate oxygenation; the remaining functional alveoli must be supplied with oxygen to achieve optimal gas exchange. Administer oxygen through a nasal cannula or a mask. Determine the flow rate by assessing the oxygen saturation of the patient's arterial blood. Be sure to insert an arterial line beforehand to eliminate repeated punctures and minimize discomfort. Offer emotional support because dyspnea causes extreme agitation.

Chest pain resulting from decreased myocardial perfusion. After formulating this nursing diagnosis, your goals are to relieve discomfort and to prevent complications.

Remember that septal hypertrophy in IHSS decreases myocardial perfusion by obstructing left ventricular outflow. Effective drug therapy reduces this obstruction and, consequently, relieves chest pain caused by decreased myocardial perfusion. Propranolol, a beta-adrenergic blocking agent, and verapamil, a calcium antagonist, reduce outflow tract obstruction by decreasing contractility.

Nitroglycerin, however, increases outflow tract obstruction and is therefore contraindicated in IHSS.

Potential for complications related to septal myotomy-myectomy. When the patient's scheduled for septal myotomy-myectomy, study the goals and related nursing interventions outlined above.

Syncope related to decreased cerebral blood flow from left ventricular outflow tract obstruction. After formulating this nursing diagnosis, your goals are to reduce outflow tract obstruction and to prevent patient injury.

Administer the prescribed drugs to reduce outflow tract obstruction. Also, accompany the hospitalized patient when he's out of bed and take other appropriate measures to prevent falls.

Fatigue related to inadequate cardiac output and/or heart failure. After formulating this nursing diagnosis, your goals are to promote rest and patient comfort. To achieve these goals, schedule your care with the patient's need for rest in mind. Allow short rest periods between care procedures and before and after meals. Gradually increase the patient's activity level, as tolerated.

Anxiety. This may be related to breathlessness or to fear of disability or death. To relieve such anxiety, you'll need to reassure the patient frequently and stay with him during acute episodes of dyspnea. Allow the patient time and encourage him to express his feelings about death and about cardiomyopathy's effect on his life. Answer any questions about the disease or about impending diagnostic or therapeutic procedures. If necessary, obtain an order for a sedative to help relieve acute anxiety.

Altered body image. Your goals are to promote acceptance of cardiomyopathy and effective coping mechanisms. Encourage the patient to share his feelings about cardiomyopathy with you, his family, and his close friends to help relieve anxiety. He's likely to have many repressed feelings—disbelief, anger, and a sense of helplessness are but a few. Encourage him to express these feelings, and be flexible with visiting hours. Of course, balance your willingness to listen with a respect for the patient's privacy. If you believe the patient isn't coping effectively, don't hesitate to refer him for psychosocial counseling.

Encourage the patient's independence to ease acceptance of cardiomyopathy. Independence helps restore the patient's sense of control over his life and supports his self-image. To promote this sense of control, encourage his participation in treatment decisions whenever possible.

Knowledge deficit. This diagnosis addresses the patient's lack of knowledge about the cause, effects, and treatment of his disease. Typically, your goals are to increase the patient's understanding of cardiomyopathy and to promote compliance with the prescribed treatment. Emphasize the importance of taking prescribed drugs, as ordered. Teach the patient about cardiomyopathy, its symptoms, and measures to control them. Be sure to warn the patient against:
• straining during defecation or other actions that elicit Valsalva's maneuver. Advise the patient to use a stool softener to prevent constipation.
• sitting bolt upright or standing up too quickly. This aggravates outflow tract obstruction in IHSS.
• emotional and physical stress. Suggest regular rest periods during the day. Warn the patient with IHSS against strenuous physical activity, which may cause syncope or sudden death.
• obesity. Help the obese patient undertake a weight-loss program to decrease the heart's work load.

Finally, stress the permanent need for regular cardiac checkups. Although the patient's disease may remain stable for years, never showing severe symptoms or causing him problems, its course is unpredictable. Be sure the patient knows that he should call the doctor immediately if symptoms of cardiomyopathy worsen.

Once you've defined the patient's problems and taken steps to treat them, what's next? More than likely, a new set of problems. As the patient's condition changes, so will his problems. Continuing assessment is mandatory to keep up with the patient's changing clinical status and to update your care plan.

Evaluate your care plan
You'll know that your care plan was successful when the patient:
• maintains hemodynamic stability, adequate cardiac output, and adequate oxygenation.
• obtains relief of chest pain.
• openly expresses his feelings about cardiomyopathy and its effect on his life-style.
• can describe cardiomyopathy's effect on the heart, its symptoms, and measures to control them.
• understands and follows the prescribed treatment regimen.
• demonstrates no evidence of therapy- or disease-related complications.

A final word
Cardiomyopathy hands the patient a difficult prognosis and requires drastic changes in life-style. Like many cardiovascular diseases, it's certain to test the patient's coping ability. Your sympathetic understanding of the patient's problems can do much toward helping him understand and live with this mysterious disease.

Points to remember

• The etiology of cardiomyopathy usually remains obscure, and treatment is largely palliative rather than curative.
• Signs and symptoms of heart failure are characteristic in dilated congestive cardiomyopathy.
• Left ventricular outflow tract obstruction in IHSS can be influenced by various drugs and physiologic maneuvers. Nitroglycerin intensifies this obstruction and should never be given to relieve chest pain.
• Although the exact mechanism of sudden death in IHSS is unknown, the proper use of drugs and avoidance of strenuous exercise help reduce the risk.

9 DEALING WITH INFLAMMATORY CONDITIONS

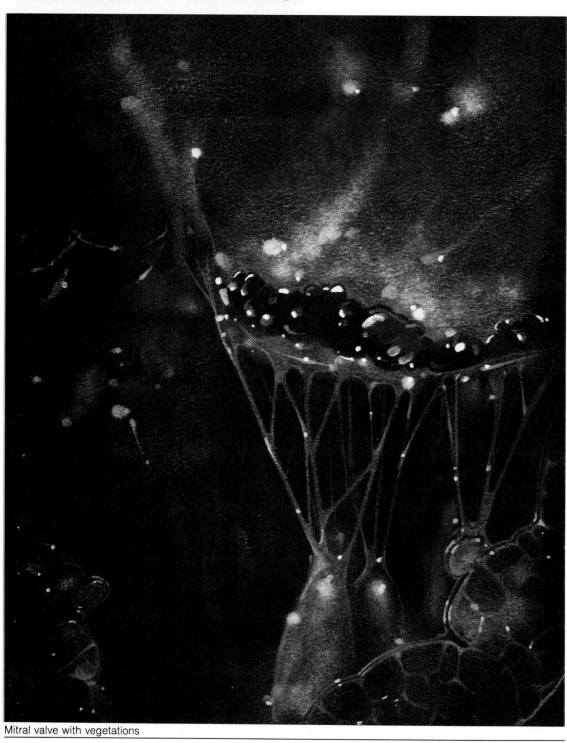

Mitral valve with vegetations

When infection and inflammation develop in the heart, their characteristic signs—unmistakable at external sites—have no diagnostic value. To make diagnosis more difficult, the signs of cardiac inflammation that *are* externally perceptible often mimic those of other cardiovascular disorders. Consider infective endocarditis, for example. This condition commonly produces fever and heart murmurs. However, these characteristic signs may be associated with sharp chest pains and distended jugular veins, which could obscure and delay accurate diagnosis and allow the onset of complications.

Because cardiac inflammation has potentially devastating effects, learning to identify its often elusive signs is critical. It requires thorough understanding of inflammation, its specific effects in cardiac disorders, and keen assessment skills.

How inflammation develops

Inflammation develops in four phases: release of histamines and other substances from injured tissue; vasodilation, with increased blood flow and congestion in the affected area; infiltration of leukocytes (monocytes, neutrophils) into the area to phagocytize the pathogens; and tissue repair, involving clotting and scar formation. These cellular changes produce characteristic effects. Vasodilation causes redness, increased blood flow causes heat, and fluid exudates cause swelling and pain.

PATHOPHYSIOLOGY OF CARDIAC INFLAMMATION

Although inflammation is normally a protective mechanism, its effects on the heart are potentially devastating. For example, in myocarditis, pericarditis, endocarditis, and rheumatic fever, scar formation and other healing processes cause debilitating structural damage, especially in the valves. Myocarditis causes degeneration and necrosis of poorly oxygenated myocardial cells. Pericarditis may cause restricted cardiac filling when a fibrinous exudate causes adjacent structures to adhere to each other. Rheumatic fever and endocarditis commonly cause valvular damage. Endocarditis also promotes formation of blood clots on roughened valvular surfaces; these clots may embolize and cause widespread infarctions in the lungs, brain, spleen, or kidneys.

Myocarditis

Myocarditis, a focal or diffuse inflammation of the myocardium, produces multiple and severe clinical effects. Typically, its signs and symptoms include heart murmurs caused by dysfunctional valves, and chest pain. It may result in cardiac dilatation, mural thrombi, infiltration of circulating blood cells around coronary vessels and between myocardial fibers, and degeneration of the myocardium. Aschoff bodies, characteristic nodular lesions of rheumatic myocarditis, may form within the heart's interstitial tissues.

Pericarditis

Mild inflammation of the visceral and parietal pericardium typically produces no external signs and may go unrecognized. However, if inflammation leads to a large accumulation of fluid in the pericardial sac, the heart will fail to expand and fill with blood, resulting in reduced cardiac output and, possibly, cardiac tamponade and death. In constrictive pericarditis, fibrous tissue resulting from a previous inflammation tends to contract, restricting the heart's ability to distend during diastole and impairing cardiac filling. As a result, venous pressure rises.

Endocarditis

Endocarditis—the inflammation of the cardiac endothelium—usually results from bacterial infection of normal or damaged heart valves. However, it may also result from abnormal growths on the closure lines of previously damaged or, occasionally, normal valves. These growths—swollen collagen fibers stabilized by fibrin—may separate from the valve and embolize, causing widespread infarction in the myocardium, kidney, brain, and other organs.

In infective endocarditis, circulating pathogens become trapped and form vegetative growths on inflamed areas. These vegetations have three layers: a thick inner layer composed of platelets, fibrin, white blood cells, and collagen; a middle layer composed mostly of bacteria; and an outer layer of fibrin and additional bacteria. As healing progresses, fibrinous tissue covers the outer layer; leukocytes invade and engulf the middle layer; and hyalinization and calcification occur in the necrotic inner layer.

Endocarditis most commonly affects the mitral and aortic valves. Vegetations on these valves may perforate the valve leaflets, obstruct the valve orifices, and spread to the chordae tendineae, causing necrosis, or to the

Causes of inflammatory heart conditions

Myocarditis
Viral infection, especially Coxsackie A and B strains
Bacterial and parasitic infection
Rheumatic fever
Toxins

Pericarditis
Viral, bacterial, or fungal infection
Rheumatic fever
Postcardiac injury
Uremia
Toxins

Endocarditis
Nonbacterial growths because of rheumatic fever, systemic lupus erythematosus, and other collagen diseases
Bacterial (streptococcal and staphylococcal) or fungal (*Candida, Aspergillus, Histoplasma*) infections
Infections related to I.V. drug abuse
Congenital heart disease
Prosthetic valve surgery

Rheumatic fever
Group A beta-hemolytic streptococcal infection, usually of throat or middle ear

Effects of rheumatic fever on heart wall layers

Rheumatic fever can affect one or more layers of the heart wall. If it affects all three layers, the condition is called rheumatic pancarditis.

Rheumatic myocarditis
Aschoff nodules usually form in the connective tissue surrounding small arteries in the myocardium. These nodules result from accumulation of leukocytes in inflamed tissues. The nodules eventually heal and become fibrotic.
Rheumatic myocarditis may cause temporary loss of myocardial contractility, but rarely causes permanent damage.

Rheumatic pericarditis
Lesions result from diffuse, nonspecific fibrinous inflammation. They may cause pericardial friction rub, but usually cause no serious, long-term effects.

Rheumatic endocarditis
Tiny, beadlike excrescences form along the edges of valve leaflets and can cause permanent, severe valvular dysfunction.

papillary muscles, causing dysfunction and, rarely, rupture.

Fever and heart murmur are the most common signs of endocarditis. Other signs include petechiae of the skin and the buccal, pharyngeal, or conjunctival mucosa, and splinter hemorrhages in the nail beds.

Rheumatic fever

This disorder is thought to reflect hypersensitivity to group A beta-hemolytic streptococcal infections of the throat or middle ear. Antibodies that combat these infections produce inflammatory lesions in other tissues, especially the joints and heart valves. Early stage valvular lesions, composed of cellular infiltrate, injure the tissues and cause scar formation. Eventually, scarring distorts the valve and may lead to stenosis or regurgitation.

Classic signs and symptoms of rheumatic fever include migratory joint pain, fever secondary to streptococcal infections, and, occasionally, skin lesions. In up to 50% of patients, carditis develops and affects the myocardium, pericardium, endocardium, or the heart valves. In severe carditis, congestive heart failure may develop.

MEDICAL MANAGEMENT

Inflammatory heart conditions are notoriously difficult to diagnose. The two major reasons for this are the characteristically long latent period between the initial infection and overt cardiac damage, and the nonspecificity of associated symptoms. Typically, cardiac damage resulting from infection and inflammation evolves slowly and produces recognizable symptoms only after many years—usually after illness, pregnancy, or advancing age overstresses the weakened heart. Because cardiac function deteriorates so gradually, it produces subtle and nonspecific symptoms, such as gradually worsening weakness.

Thus, detecting and identifying cardiac inflammation accurately is possible only with a thorough and reliable history, complete physical examination, and special laboratory tests. Except in late stages, when cardiac complications are obvious, the most useful tests are certain blood tests that confirm infection.

Blood tests detect infection

In inflammatory heart conditions, the erythrocyte sedimentation rate (ESR) usually increases, and the complete blood count reveals leukocytosis, a classic sign of infec-

tion. Serum glutamic-oxaloacetic transaminase (SGOT) and total lactic dehydrogenase (LDH) levels increase, and LDH_1 levels may exceed LDH_2 levels. In acute rheumatic fever, the antistreptolysin-O titer (ASO) increases in more than 75% of patients.

Cultures detect causative organisms

Blood and throat cultures can help detect the cause of infective endocarditis and rheumatic fever. In infective endocarditis, three or more blood cultures during a 24- to 48-hour period identify the causative organism in up to 90% of patients. However, negative blood cultures may occur during antibiotic therapy or in patients with vegetative growths on the tricuspid or pulmonic valve.

A throat culture that's positive for group A streptococci can indicate acute rheumatic fever, but can also indicate a carrier state. However, a negative culture doesn't rule out rheumatic fever, since streptococci may have disappeared from the throat or be difficult to detect once signs and symptoms of rheumatic fever appear.

Special tests detect cardiac complications

Chest X-rays may reveal enlargement of one or more heart chambers, and *angiography* may reveal the degree of valvular stenosis or regurgitation. In acute pericarditis, chest X-rays may appear normal. However, cardiac blood pool imaging may detect fluid accumulation or pericardial thickening. *Computerized axial tomography* also detects pericardial thickening and tumors. *Echocardiography* allows diagnosis of pericardial effusion, valvular stenosis, and left atrial and ventricular dilatation in rheumatic heart disease. *Electrocardiography* can detect conductive disturbances and dysrhythmias resulting from cardiac inflammation and valvular dysfunction. *Cardiac catheterization* allows study of chamber pressures and blood gas levels to evaluate valvular damage.

Treatment: Drugs, support, and surgery

After identifying the cause of an inflammatory heart condition, treatment can include drug therapy, supportive measures, or surgery to repair or replace diseased valves.

Drug therapy. Myocarditis caused by bacterial infection requires antibiotics; associated congestive heart failure requires diuretics to reduce fluid retention, and digitalis to strengthen myocardial contractility. However, digitalis must be given cautiously, since some patients show a paradoxical sensitivity to even small doses. Dysrhythmias require cautious administration of antiarrhythmics, such as quinidine or procainamide, since these drugs depress myocardial contractility.

In pericarditis, salicylates and indomethacin usually relieve pain and reduce inflammation. If they don't, corticosteroids may be used; however, if steroid therapy is discontinued, symptoms may recur. In cardiac tamponade, drug therapy aims to correct its cause: bacterial infections require specific antibiotics; tuberculosis requires ethambutol, rifampin, and isoniazid; and idiopathic pericarditis requires corticosteroids.

In infective endocarditis, drug therapy varies, depending on the pathogen and the presence of complications. Generally, penicillin and an aminoglycoside (gentamicin or streptomycin) are given for 4 to 6 weeks to eliminate the pathogen.

In fungal endocarditis, treatment includes amphotericin B, but its therapeutic serum levels may cause toxic side effects. Because of this toxicity and the complications of continuing infections, which may cause large emboli, early valve resection is almost always required.

In rheumatic fever, antibiotics are administered to eliminate group A beta-hemolytic streptococci and prevent contagion. Although antibiotics help prevent subsequent streptococcal infections and recurrence of rheumatic fever, they can't modify the course of an acute rheumatic episode or prevent carditis. However, antibiotic prophylaxis does reduce the risk of cardiac damage, which rises with each acute episode of rheumatic fever. If carditis is absent, antibiotic prophylaxis should continue for at least 5 years; if it's present, prophylaxis may continue for life.

Anti-inflammatory drugs suppress many signs and symptoms of rheumatic fever, and may obscure diagnosis in mild or questionable cases. In mild or absent carditis, salicylates effectively decrease fever and joint inflammation. In severe carditis with congestive heart failure, corticosteroids may replace salicylates.

Supportive treatment. Bed rest helps prevent complications and minimizes the heart's work load, promoting healing. Pericarditis requires bed rest as long as pain and fever persist; myocarditis and endocarditis require only partial bed rest. Rheumatic fever requires bed rest during the first 3 weeks of illness, when carditis usually appears. Thereafter, physical activity can increase progres-

sively, depending on clinical findings and the patient's response to treatment. If cardiac function has deteriorated to congestive failure, treatment should include activity restrictions to minimize myocardial oxygen demand, supplemental oxygen therapy, sodium restriction, and diuretics and digitalis.

If pericarditis leads to cardiac tamponade, the doctor may perform pericardiocentesis—the aspiration of fluid from the pericardial sac. Blood pressure and cardiac output may improve dramatically with removal of as little as 25 ml of fluid. Recurrent pericarditis may require partial pericardectomy, to create a window that allows fluid to drain into the pleural space. Constrictive pericarditis may require total pericardectomy to permit adequate filling and contraction of the heart.

Surgery. Long-term management of patients with inflammatory heart conditions varies with the degree of cardiac involvement. For example, most patients with aortic regurgitation, who are relatively asymptomatic in childhood, show progressive disability as adults. Severe aortic regurgitation may eventually require valve replacement.

In endocarditis, prosthetic valve replacement should be postponed until the patient completes drug therapy. Valve replacement should be considered for patients with recurrent emboli despite adequate drug therapy. Immediate valve replacement is necessary in life-threatening congestive heart failure resulting from valvular regurgitation.

NURSING MANAGEMENT
Inflammatory heart conditions involve long-term treatment and possible serious complications. As a result, you'll need to continually monitor your patient, modifying your care plan according to his changing clinical status.

Take a careful patient history
In the initial interview, ask the patient to describe his chief complaint. Explore his reasons for seeking treatment, including the onset and duration of symptoms, the use of drugs and other treatments and their effectiveness, and any aggravating or alleviating factors. Symptoms of inflammatory heart conditions may resemble those of the common cold, and the patient may not seek treatment until they become severe (chest pain or syncope) or persist for several weeks.

If the patient reports chest pain, ask him to describe the pain. Is it sharp? Does it burn? Where is it? Remember that substernal chest pain, sharp and knife-like or dull and oppressive, may indicate acute pericarditis. Also, ask if he's had palpitations or a history of murmurs.

Ask the patient if he's had rheumatic, congenital, or syphilitic heart disease, which may lead to valvular disease. Ask also if he's had prosthetic valve replacement surgery.

Check for recent infection, dental treatment, surgery, or endoscopic procedure involving the upper respiratory, genitourinary, or lower gastrointestinal tract. Ask about frequent self-injections (insulin, narcotics), which may lead to bacterial endocarditis.

Perform the physical exam
The physical examination provides a valuable baseline that helps you identify subsequent changes in the patient's condition. Check vital signs first to detect such abnormalities as fever or tachycardia. Then, auscultate for heart murmurs (such as a systolic murmur related to mitral insufficiency) and for pericardial friction rub (a grating sound as the heart moves in its protective sac). Pericardial friction rub, a classic sign of pericarditis, may have up to three audible components, corresponding to atrial systole, ventricular systole, and the rapid-filling phase of ventricular diastole.

Using an ophthalmoscope, examine the patient's retina for Roth's spots—hemorrhages with pale, white centers, located near the optic fundus, that may be an early sign of bacterial endocarditis. Next, observe for petechiae on the mucous membranes of the mouth, and on the conjunctiva, neck, wrists, and ankles. Check the nail beds for splinter hemorrhages; the pads of the fingers and toes for Osler's nodes (tender, raised, subcutaneous nodules); and the palms and soles for Janeway lesions (slightly raised, hemorrhagic spots).

Palpate for splenomegaly, another common sign of endocarditis. Also, note any uncoordinated spastic movements—a sign of Sydenham's chorea. Check the trunk and extremities for erythema marginatum, a transient, migratory rash of reddish lesions with clear centers that blanch upon pressure. Both are signs of rheumatic fever.

Observe for complications. Be alert for signs of pericardial effusion, a major complication of acute pericarditis. In this condition, fluid accumulation in the pericardial space prevents adequate filling of the cardiac chambers. Blood backs up into the venous system, even-

tually leading to jugular venous distention. Dyspnea, varying levels of consciousness, and a paradoxical pulse (a difference of more than 8 to 10 mm Hg in systolic pressures taken at expiration and at inspiration) also indicate pericardial effusion. In a large pericardial effusion, percussion of the lower half of the sternum reveals increased cardiac dullness because of fluid accumulation. In chronic constrictive pericarditis, observe for peripheral edema as well.

Be especially alert for cardiac tamponade, the most perilous complication of pericarditis. The accumulation of fluid in the pericardium initially limits diastolic filling, causing diminished cardiac output and a decline in arterial pressure and coronary artery filling. This sequence of events further compromises cardiac function and eventually results in ischemia, which further decreases cardiac function. In a patient with cardiac tamponade, your assessment will reveal continuously declining blood pressure, paradoxical pulse, neck vein distention, and muffled heart sounds. If you detect tamponade, notify the doctor immediately.

Formulate nursing diagnoses
After collecting subjective data from the patient history and objective data from the physical examination, you're ready to formulate the nursing diagnoses, set goals, and plan interventions. Typically, four nursing diagnoses relate to inflammatory heart conditions.

Potential for pericardial effusion and cardiac tamponade from pericarditis. Your goal is to prevent or resolve pericardial effusion or cardiac tamponade. To achieve this goal, you'll need to monitor the patient's hemodynamic status, observe for signs of cardiac tamponade, and, if necessary, assist with pericardiocentesis. Be sure to explain all procedures to the patient and his family to help relieve their anxiety.

Monitor hemodynamic status. First, check for signs and symptoms of increased central venous pressure, such as jugular vein distention, dyspnea, and fullness in the chest. Also, observe for decreased blood pressure, paradoxical pulse, narrowing pulse pressure, sinus tachycardia (indicating reduced stroke volume), and weak or absent peripheral pulses (indicating reduced circulating blood volume). Watch for signs of impaired cerebral perfusion, and record serial EKGs to detect decreased QRS complexes. Make sure a pericardiocentesis set is readily available.

Pathways of infective endocarditis

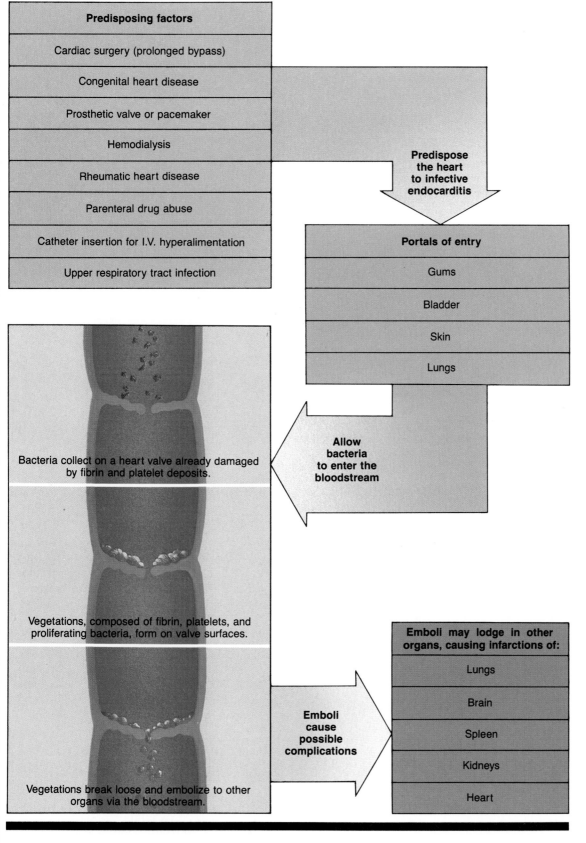

Predisposing factors
Cardiac surgery (prolonged bypass)
Congenital heart disease
Prosthetic valve or pacemaker
Hemodialysis
Rheumatic heart disease
Parenteral drug abuse
Catheter insertion for I.V. hyperalimentation
Upper respiratory tract infection

Predispose the heart to infective endocarditis

Portals of entry
Gums
Bladder
Skin
Lungs

Allow bacteria to enter the bloodstream

Bacteria collect on a heart valve already damaged by fibrin and platelet deposits.

Vegetations, composed of fibrin, platelets, and proliferating bacteria, form on valve surfaces.

Vegetations break loose and embolize to other organs via the bloodstream.

Emboli cause possible complications

Emboli may lodge in other organs, causing infarctions of:
Lungs
Brain
Spleen
Kidneys
Heart

In infective endocarditis, bacteria enter the blood-stream and become trapped and form vegetative growths on damaged heart valves. These growths may perforate the valve leaflets and obstruct the valve orifices. Sometimes, they spread to the chordae tendineae and the adjacent endocardium. The vegetative growths may also break loose from the valve surface and embolize, causing widespread infarction.

Pericarditis: The inflammatory response

Pericarditis, an inflammation of the protective sac that encloses the heart, produces an exudate that may compress the ventricles and impair heart function if not surgically corrected. Usually, it results from pneumonia, tuberculosis, or myocardial infarction, but may also follow nonbacterial inflammation, penetrating or blunt chest wounds, or connective tissue diseases. This generalized sequence shows the course of bacterial inflammation of the pericardium, illustrating the body's defenses at work.

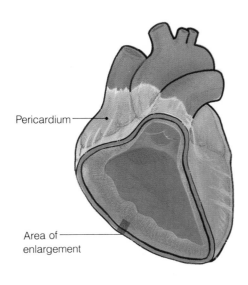

Pericardium

Area of enlargement

1. Pericardial tissue damaged by bacteria releases chemical mediators of inflammation (such as prostaglandins, histamines, bradykinins, and serotonins) into surrounding tissue.

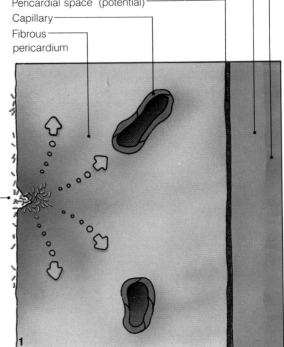

Myocardium
Serous pericardium (visceral layer)
Pericardial space (potential)
Capillary
Fibrous pericardium

Bacteria

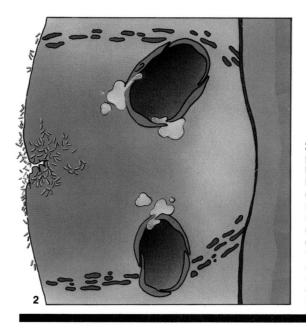

2. Vessels dilate and increase in permeability due to the action of histamines and other mediators. Local blood flow to the area (hyperemia) increases. Venule and capillary walls leak fluids and proteins (including fibrinogen) into tissues, causing extracellular edema. Clots of fibrinogen and tissue exudate form a wall, blocking tissue spaces and lymph vessels in the injured area. This wall hampers the spread of bacteria and toxins to adjoining healthy tissues.

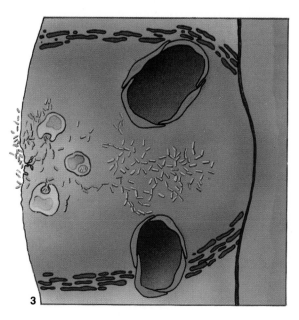

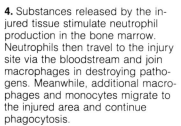

3. The macrophages already present in the tissues begin to phagocytize the invading bacteria, but usually fail to stop the infection.

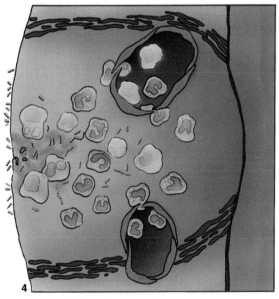

4. Substances released by the injured tissue stimulate neutrophil production in the bone marrow. Neutrophils then travel to the injury site via the bloodstream and join macrophages in destroying pathogens. Meanwhile, additional macrophages and monocytes migrate to the injured area and continue phagocytosis.

5. After several days, the infected area becomes filled with an exudate (pus) consisting of necrotic tissue and dead and dying bacteria, neutrophils, and macrophages. Pus formation continues until all infection ceases, forming a cavity that remains until after tissue destruction stops. The contents of the pus cavity autolyze and are gradually reabsorbed into healthy tissue.

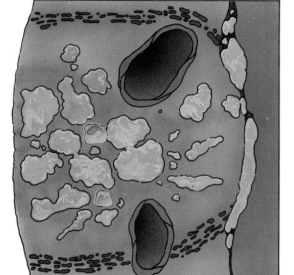

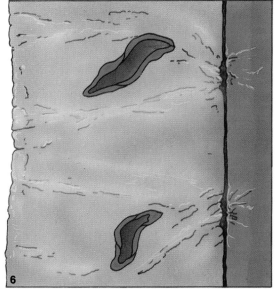

6. As the end products of the infection slowly disappear, fibrosis and scar tissue formation take place. Scarring may be extensive and may ultimately cause heart failure.

Effects of rheumatic fever on valvular function

Acute rheumatic fever causes gross changes in the mitral and aortic valves—edema, erosion of the valve leaflets along the closure line, and formation of beadlike vegetations along the inflamed leaflet edges. In many patients, the vegetations occur simultaneously on adjacent leaflets, which become scarred and partially fused together during healing.

The three detailed views at right show a mitral valve in a possible progression from rheumatic inflammation to stenosis and regurgitation.

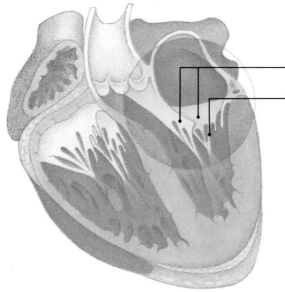

— Mitral valve leaflets

— Chordae tendineae

Vegetations on valve leaflets

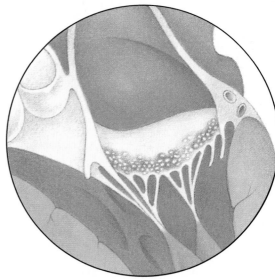

In this view, the mitral valve leaflets have become inflamed, and a thin line of rheumatic vegetations has formed along the delicate leaflet edges. These vegetations form when fibrin and platelets accumulate on the damaged surface of the valve.

Mitral stenosis

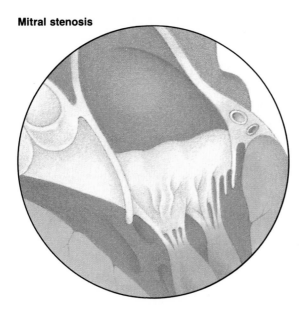

In mitral stenosis, the most common valvular defect associated with recurrent episodes of rheumatic fever, inflammation causes shrinkage of the chordae tendineae. The left atrium attempts to force blood through the narrow valve opening into the left ventricle, eventually causing left atrial enlargement, pulmonary congestion, and right ventricular hypertrophy and failure. Unfortunately, symptoms of mitral stenosis don't usually appear until the valve opening has been reduced by 50%.

Mitral regurgitation

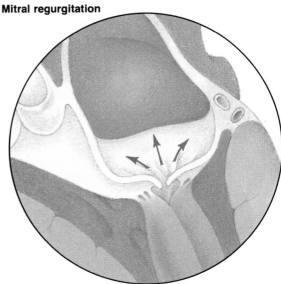

Some degree of regurgitation (backflow) of blood into the atrium may coexist with stenosis, because the dysfunctional valve cannot close tightly.

Be alert for cardiac tamponade. If tamponade develops, place the patient in the low Fowler position, and administer oxygen as ordered. Keep cardiopulmonary resuscitation equipment and drugs close by for immediate use. Frequently monitor central venous pressure, blood pressure, and pulse rate, as ordered; monitor peripheral pulses for perfusion and changes in degree of paradoxical pulse. Also, monitor the EKG for signs of tachycardia. Watch for changes in the patient's mental status and for Kussmaul's sign—absence of a normal decline in blood pressure during inspiration, because of restricted diastolic filling.

Prepare the patient for pericardiocentesis if pericardial effusion develops, if hemodynamic status worsens, or if you suspect pus in the pericardial sac. Maintain a patent I.V. line.

Assist with pericardiocentesis to relieve tamponade. During pericardiocentesis, monitor the EKG for premature ventricular contractions and elevated ST segments, which may indicate that the needle has touched the ventricle; for an elevated PR segment, which may indicate that the needle has touched the atrium; and for large, erratic QRS complexes, which may indicate penetration of the myocardium. Monitor vital signs every 5 to 15 minutes. Observe for clots in the aspirate, indicating puncture of a heart chamber. If puncture occurs, notify the doctor immediately. Otherwise, simply label all specimens properly and send them to the laboratory for analysis.

Evaluate your interventions. Consider them effective if the patient's hemodynamic status stabilizes (or if pericardiocentesis relieves cardiac tamponade) and if the patient and his family have understood all procedures and report less anxiety.

Potential for development and migration of emboli. This is most acute if the patient has endocarditis. Your goal is to promote bed rest to help prevent formation or migration of emboli. Discuss the potential for embolization, as well as its causes and treatment, with the patient to reduce anxiety.

If an echocardiogram is available, check its results for vegetations on heart valves, which increase the risk of embolization. Watch for signs and symptoms of embolization, and report them immediately.

Evaluate your interventions. Is the patient comfortable? Has an embolus formed? If so, has it migrated and caused injury to other organs?

Potential for valvular regurgitation from vegetative growths on valve leaflets. Your goal is to help prevent or correct valvular regurgitation. After reviewing the patient's chart, assess the precordium for signs and symptoms of mitral, aortic, or tricuspid regurgitation. These valves are rarely affected simultaneously. (See pages 154 and 155.)

Report any signs of valvular regurgitation to the doctor. Continue or initiate prescribed treatment for endocarditis or congestive heart failure. If the patient is scheduled for prosthetic valve surgery, explain the procedure as well as preoperative and postoperative care. To ease the patient's anxiety, provide reassurance, listen sympathetically to his fears, and encourage his questions.

Consider your interventions effective if valvular regurgitation has been prevented or resolved, if perivalvular leaks have been avoided postoperatively, and if the patient reports decreased anxiety.

Knowledge deficit about inflammation, treatment, and preventive care. Begin by explaining the inflammatory response and its effects on the heart. Also, explain the use of monitors and the purpose of diagnostic tests. Teach the patient the purpose, dosage, schedule, route of administration, and potential side effects of prescribed drugs. If appropriate, tell him that drug therapy must continue until cultures are negative for the causative organism. Emphasize that prophylactic antibiotic therapy is needed to prevent further valvular damage that might result from infections caused by dental treatment, childbirth, surgery, or endoscopic studies, intubation, or catheterization of the respiratory, GI, or genitourinary tracts. Be sure the patient knows reportable signs and symptoms, especially of infection. Warn him to avoid exposure to infection and to maintain good health through proper diet, exercise, and rest.

Does the patient ask appropriate questions about his condition and its treatment? The patient who understands his condition is more likely to comply with treatment and less likely to suffer relapse than the patient who fails to understand it.

A final word

The uncertainties of inflammatory heart conditions will challenge all your nursing skills. Understanding the inflammatory response and its effects on the heart helps remove some of these uncertainties and promotes careful, competent patient care.

Signs and symptoms of embolization

Brain
Altered mental status, paralysis, aphasia, ptosis, incontinence, seizures, nausea, vomiting, elevated blood pressure

Circulatory system
Coronary arteries: signs and symptoms of MI, abscess, pericarditis
Peripheral arteries: positive Homans' sign, tenderness, pain, swelling, erythema, gangrenous fingers or toes, and coolness, blanching, and decreased or absent pulse in an extremity

Lungs
Dyspnea, tachypnea, pleuritic pain, tachycardia, pallor, cyanosis

Kidneys
Lower back or flank pain, hematuria, oliguria

Spleen
Pain in upper left quadrant that radiates to left shoulder, local tenderness, abdominal rigidity, friction rub

Valvular heart diseases

Disease	Description and causes	Signs and symptoms
Aortic stenosis	• Stiffened valve leaflets fail to open properly, resulting in impaired blood flow from the left ventricle. • Usually caused by rheumatic fever (ages 30 to 70) or calcification of aortic valve (after age 70).	• Angina pectoris, syncope upon exertion. • Left ventricular failure, indicated by signs of pulmonary congestion: dyspnea, orthopnea, paroxysmal nocturnal dyspnea.
Aortic regurgitation	• Diseased aortic valve fails to close properly, causing blood backflow into left ventricle during diastole. • Usually caused by valve damage from rheumatic fever, syphilis, or endocarditis. Sometimes associated with Marfan's syndrome and rheumatoid arthritis.	• Rapidly rising and falling pulses, dysrhythmias, wide pulse pressure in severe regurgitation. Dyspnea progressing to paroxysmal nocturnal dyspnea and orthopnea, which indicates pulmonary congestion. • Severe blood backflow may cause pulmonary edema.
Mitral stenosis	• Stiffened valve leaflets cannot open properly, impairing blood flow from left atrium to left ventricle. • Most commonly caused by rheumatic fever. Sometimes associated with congenital anomalies, such as tetralogy of Fallot.	• Dyspnea on exertion; fatigue; rapid, irregular pulse; palpitations; increased left atrial pressure; pulmonary hypertension; right ventricular hypertrophy and failure. • Loud S_1 or opening snap, with rumbling diastolic murmur at apex.
Mitral regurgitation	• Diseased valve cannot close tightly, causing blood backflow from left ventricle to left atrium during systole. • May be caused by rheumatic fever, prolapsed valve, left ventricular dilation, papillary muscle dysfunction and, in acute regurgitation, by ruptured chordae tendineae.	• Dyspnea and fatigue commonly develop late in chronic regurgitation; symptoms of pulmonary edema in acute regurgitation. Palpitations and chest pain suggest nonrheumatic disease origin. • Holosystolic murmur at apex, possible split S_2, and S_3.
Mitral prolapse	• Enlarged valve leaflets bulge backward into left atrium during ventricular systole. • Usually idiopathic and benign. Commonly inherited.	• Sharp chest pain unrelated to exercise, fatigue, palpitations, lightheadedness, syncope, dyspnea. • Mild or late systolic click followed by a late, high-pitched and musical systolic murmur at apex.
Tricuspid stenosis	• Stiffened tricuspid valve leaflets cannot open properly, impairing blood flow from the right atrium to the right ventricle during diastole. • Most commonly caused by rheumatic fever; often associated with mitral stenosis; sometimes congenital.	• Increased right atrial pressure causes chamber dilatation and hypertrophy, increased pressure in the vena cava, and eventual right ventricular failure. • Blowing diastolic murmur along left sternal border. Changes on inspiration are diagnostic.
Tricuspid regurgitation	• Diseased valve fails to close properly, causing blood backflow from right ventricle into right atrium during systole. • Usually occurs in right ventricular failure, and, at times, in left ventricular failure and pulmonary hypertension.	• Increased right atrial pressure causes signs of right ventricular failure: distended neck veins, peripheral edema, ascites, hepatomegaly, hydrothorax, nausea, and vomiting. • Blowing holosystolic murmur at lower left sternal border, augments during inspiration.
Pulmonic stenosis	• Stiffened pulmonic valve leaflets impair blood flow from the right ventricle. • Rare disorder, often caused by congenital heart defect.	• Right ventricular hypertrophy, right ventricular failure. • Systolic ejection murmur over the pulmonic area, with a widely split second sound and systolic ejection click.
Pulmonic regurgitation	• Diseased pulmonary valve cannot close properly, causing blood backflow into the right ventricle during diastole. • Generally caused by congenital heart disease. Often associated with other valvular or heart defects.	• Fluid overload in right ventricle leads to hypertrophy and eventual failure of ventricle. Fatigue, dyspnea, and syncope may indicate severe pulmonary hypertension. • Diastolic murmur at left sternal border increases with inspiration.
Papillary muscle dysfunction and rupture	• Dysfunction: may affect mitral or tricuspid valve. Ineffective closure causes regurgitation or prolapse into atria during systole. Usually results from ischemic disease. • Rupture: usually results from infarction of the muscle in coronary artery disease.	• Dysfunction: signs of underlying heart disease. • Rupture: severe dyspnea, chest pain, syncope, hemoptysis, pulmonary edema, hyperdynamic apical pulse, tachycardia, hypotension, and signs of hypoperfusion.

Treatments	Nursing interventions
• Drug therapy includes nitrates, digitalis, diuretics, rheumatic prophylaxis. • Valve replacement is often preferred, since symptoms generally occur late in the disease.	• Monitor vital signs (including apical pulse), lung and heart sounds, ABGs, hemodynamic status, chest X-rays, intake/output, weight. Watch for signs of drug side effects, pulmonary edema, ventricular failure. • After surgery, be alert for dysrhythmias, thrombi, hypotension, and pulmonary emboli.
• Prompt, vigorous treatment of infections and dysrhythmias. Drug therapy includes digitalis glycosides, diuretics, nitroglycerin and, for the patient with syphilitic aortitis, penicillin. • Patients symptomatic with exertion despite drug therapy require surgery.	• Monitor vital signs (including apical pulse), lung and heart sounds, ABGs, hemodynamic status, chest X-rays, intake/output, and weight. Watch for signs of ventricular failure, pulmonary edema, and drug side effects. • After surgery, be alert for dysrhythmias, thrombi, hypotension, and pulmonary emboli.
• Prophylaxis for endocarditis may be required; digitalis, quinidine, diuretics, vasodilators, sodium restriction, and activity limitation for atrial fibrillation or CHF. • Valve replacement or commissurotomy.	• Monitor vital signs (including apical pulse), lung and heart sounds, ABGs, hemodynamic status, chest X-rays, intake/output, and weight. Watch for signs of pulmonary edema, right ventricular failure, eventual left ventricular failure, and drug side effects. • After surgery, be alert for hypotension, dysrhythmias, thrombi and pulmonary emboli.
• Prophylaxis for endocarditis may be required; digitalis, quinidine, diuretics, vasodilators, sodium restriction, and limited activity for atrial fibrillation or CHF; and hydralazine for reducing preload and afterload. • Valve replacement or reconstruction.	• Monitor vital signs (including apical pulse) frequently, avoid overhydration, and assess lung and heart sounds. Check for signs of decompensation, pulmonary edema, right ventricular failure, eventual left ventricular failure, and drug side effects. • After surgery, be alert for hypotension, dysrhythmias, thrombi and pulmonary emboli.
• Nitroglycerin may relieve chest pain. Propranolol increases ventricular volume and corrects dysrhythmias. Prophylaxis for endocarditis may be required. • Valve replacement in severe symptoms.	• Reassure patient to control anxiety. Explain his condition, its treatment, and possible complications. • Watch for drug side effects; reinforce prophylactic drug therapy.
• Pulmonary and systemic congestion are treated with digitalis, diuretics, and sodium restriction. Prophylaxis for endocarditis may be required. • Valve replacement or ring annuloplasty in moderate to severe stenosis.	• Monitor vital signs (including apical pulse), ABGs, hemodynamic status, chest X-rays, intake/output, and weight. Watch for signs of ventricular failure, pulmonary edema, and drug side effects. • After surgery, be alert for hypotension, dysrhythmias, thrombi, and pulmonary emboli.
• Treatment is usually symptomatic: prophylaxis for endocarditis, digitalis, diuretics, sodium restriction, and activity limitation. • Surgery for isolated tricuspid regurgitation is seldom necessary. Valve replacement or annuloplasty may be done concurrently with mitral valve surgery.	• Monitor vital signs (including apical pulse), ABGs, hemodynamic status, chest X-rays, intake/output, and weight. Watch for signs of ventricular failure, pulmonary edema, and drug side effects. • After surgery, be alert for hypotension, dysrhythmias, thrombi, and pulmonary emboli.
• Treatment aims to correct symptoms of systemic congestion. Anticoagulants may be used if pulmonary emboli develop. • Valvotomy in severe or progressive symptoms.	• Watch for signs of ventricular failure and drug side effects. • After surgery, be alert for hypotension, dysrhythmias, thrombi, and pulmonary emboli.
• Without underlying disease, pulmonic regurgitation is generally well tolerated, and treatment consists of prophylactic antibiotics and continuous observation. • When pulmonic regurgitation results from other diseases, treatment is symptomatic.	• Monitor vital signs (including apical pulse), lung and heart sounds, ABGs, hemodynamic status, chest X-rays, intake/output, and weight. • Watch for signs of ventricular failure and drug side effects. • After surgery, be alert for hypotension, dysrhythmias, thrombi, and pulmonary emboli.
• Dysfunction: symptomatic (may include propranolol, nitroglycerin, digitalis, diuretics, and vasodilators). Severe mitral regurgitation and refractory heart failure may require mitral valve replacement. • Rupture: mitral valve replacement is treatment of choice. Preoperative therapy may include I.V. diuretics.	• Watch for signs of heart failure or reduced cardiac output. Auscultate for systolic murmur or S_4. • Reinforce the patient's coping mechanisms; encourage coughing and deep breathing. • After surgery, be alert for hypotension, dysrhythmias, thrombi, and pulmonary emboli.

• Although inflammation is normally a protective mechanism, when it affects the heart it may cause myocardial, endocardial, pericardial, and valvular diseases.
• Rheumatic fever commonly occurs after a streptococcal infection of the throat or middle ear, most often in persons between ages 5 and 15.
• Signs of pericardial effusion include jugular vein distention, dyspnea, paradoxical pulse, and varying levels of consciousness.
• Paradoxical pulse is a difference of more than 8 to 10 mm Hg in systolic pressures taken at inspiration and at expiration.
• Cardiac tamponade, a life-threatening complication of pericarditis, requires immediate treatment.
• Myocarditis requires careful monitoring to prevent digitalis toxicity.

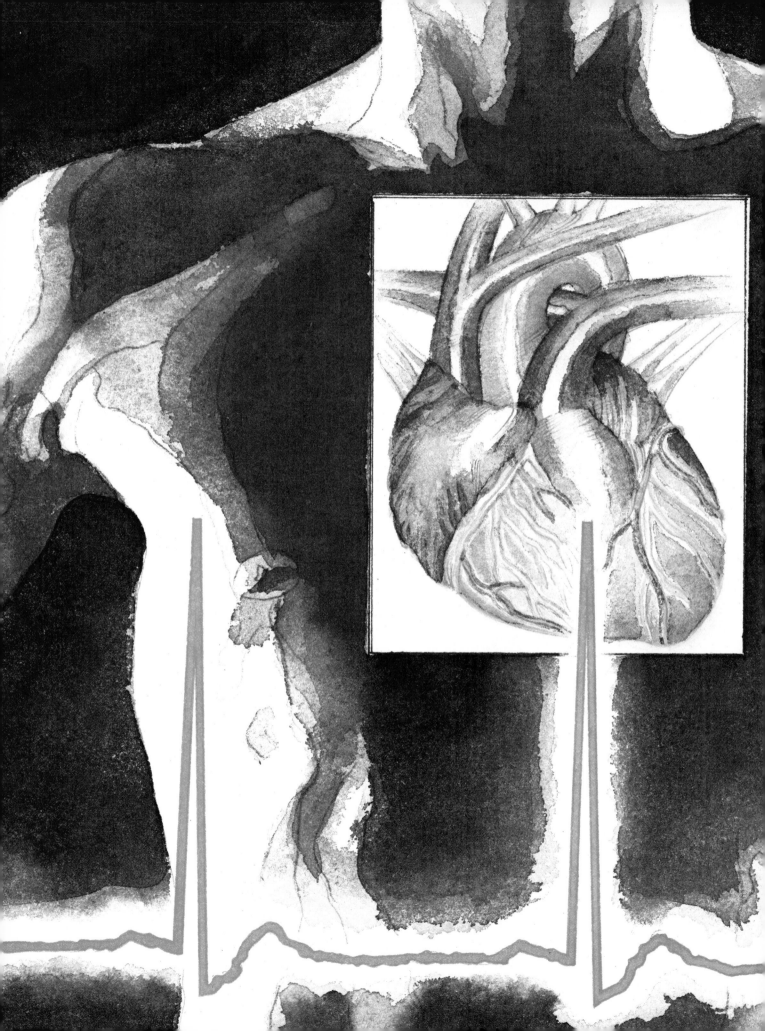

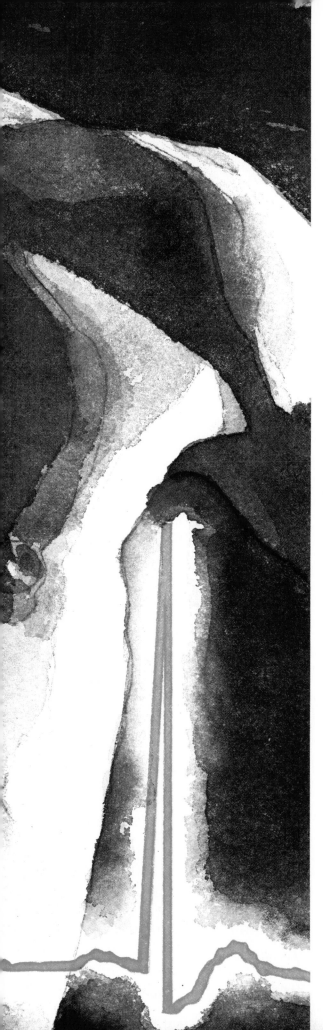

DISORDERS OF ELECTROCONDUCTION

10 RECOGNIZING DYSRHYTHMIAS

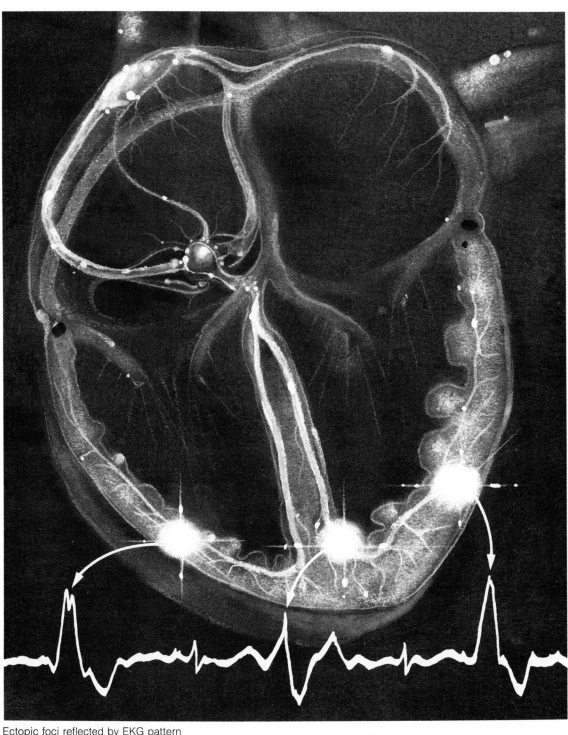

Ectopic foci reflected by EKG pattern

Even if you never expect to work in a coronary-care unit (CCU), you should know how to recognize dysrhythmias and know what to do about them. And there's much to know. Dysrhythmia may be one of many abnormal variations of cardiac rhythm and rate (also called arrhythmias) or of impaired conduction, such as heart block. It may be a single, continuing abnormality, such as persistently rapid heart rate; or multiple, intermittently recurring abnormalities, such as premature ventricular contractions (PVCs). Dysrhythmia may be mild, asymptomatic, and clinically insignificant, like respiratory sinus arrhythmia (in which the heart rate changes with respiration and which requires no treatment); or, like ventricular fibrillation, it may be catastrophic, requiring immediate resuscitation.

The clinical significance of dysrhythmia depends largely on its site of origin and also on the patient's cardiac status and hemodynamic reaction: a typically major dysrhythmia, such as PVCs, may require no hospital treatment, yet a relatively minor one, such as atrial fibrillation, may need treatment in the CCU if the patient has symptoms. To deal with dysrhythmia correctly, you must unerringly distinguish the benign from the catastrophic.

PATHOPHYSIOLOGY

The physiologic effects of dysrhythmia vary significantly according to the cause and to cardiac and vascular capacity to compensate. The normal heart adapts quickly to changes in heart rate and rhythm by compensating with coronary vasodilation, which provides sufficient oxygen to meet the demands of an increased work load. However, a diseased heart is less likely to adapt effectively. For example, the presence of coronary artery obstruction prevents adequate oxygenation; thus, dysrhythmia that increases oxygen demand can lead to progressive myocardial ischemia and, as compensatory mechanisms fail, heart failure. In this situation, dysrhythmia may precipitate or aggravate angina or congestive heart failure. Also consider that dysrhythmias that impair AV synchrony (such as AV dissociation) also reduce cardiac output.

No matter what the cause, reduced cardiac output causes forward heart failure, requiring vasoconstriction of the renal, mesenteric, cerebral, and musculoskeletal circulations to maintain blood pressure. Thus, the symptoms associated with dysrhythmia are the classic ones related to impaired cardiac output—

pallor, cold and clammy extremities, reduced urine output, weakness, chest pain, dizziness, and (if cerebral circulation is severely impaired) syncope.

In a patient with a normal heart, dysrhythmia typically produces few symptoms. But even in a normal heart, persistently rapid or very irregular rhythms can strain the myocardium and meaningfully impair cardiac output. For example, ventricular tachycardia can lead to ventricular fibrillation and sudden death.

Dysrhythmias are generally classified according to their site of origin, as supraventricular or ventricular. Site of origin partially influences their effect on cardiac output and blood pressure and determines their clinical significance. Ventricular dysrhythmias, through their inherent effect on cardiac output, are potentially more life-threatening than supraventricular dysrhythmias.

Supraventricular dysrhythmias

The supraventricular dysrhythmias include those that originate at the sinoatrial node, the atria, and the junctional (AV) node.

Sinoatrial (SA) node dysrhythmias. These dysrhythmias usually spring from autonomic hyperactivity, and rarely from disorders of the SA node itself. Such hyperactivity may be sympathetic or parasympathetic and may result from stress, metabolic changes, drugs, cardiac disease, or noncardiac diseases, such as anemia or thyrotoxicosis.

Any of these autonomic influences may cause the SA node to produce impulses too quickly, causing sinus tachycardia; to produce them too slowly, causing sinus bradycardia; or to prevent their transmission entirely, causing sinus arrest or sinus block. Autonomic influences may also change cardiac rhythm in synchronization with the patient's respiratory cycle (sinus arrhythmia).

In SA node dysrhythmias, heart rate may vary from below 60 to 160 beats/minute. The EKG configuration and rhythm are normal, except in sinus arrest and SA block. Since these impulses originate in the SA node, the P wave is normal. And because SA node disturbances do not affect ventricular depolarization, the QRS configuration is normal.

A severe form of sinus dysrhythmia, often associated with decreased cerebral perfusion, is sick sinus syndrome (SSS). This syndrome generally describes a broad category of rhythm disturbances that includes sinus bradycardia, tachy-brady syndrome, or sinus block

How to calculate heart rate

To calculate heart rate, you must know EKG graph paper measurements. EKG graph paper is divided into millimeter (mm) squares that measure time on the horizontal axis and wave amplitude on the vertical axis. When paper speed is 25 mm/sec, each mm square equals 0.04 second; each 5 mm square equals 0.20 second. You can calculate heart rate with the following methods:

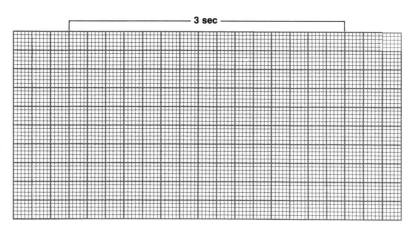

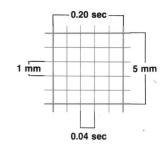

1. If the heart rate is regular, count the number of large (0.20 second) boxes between two consecutive QRS complexes and divide the constant (300) by this number to derive the heart rate in beats/minute.

In this example, the heart rate is 300 ÷ 3 = 100 beats/minute.

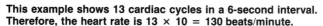

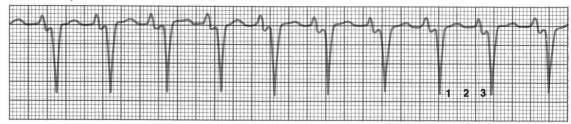

2. If the heart rate is irregular, count the number of cardiac cycles (the intervals between two consecutive R waves) that are recorded within 6 seconds. Multiply this number by 10.

This example shows 13 cardiac cycles in a 6-second interval. Therefore, the heart rate is 13 × 10 = 130 beats/minute.

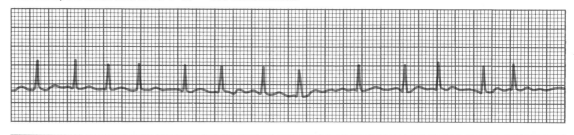

with intermittent episodes of rapid supraventricular arrhythmias. Strictly defined, true SSS is marked by profound bradycardia, long periods of cardiac arrest, supraventricular tachycardia, and shortened SA recovery time after cardioversion. Syncopal episodes related to SSS or tachy-brady syndrome are called Stokes-Adams attacks.

Atrial dysrhythmias. These dysrhythmias result when an atrial pacemaker usurps the role of the SA node pacemaker. Atrial dysrhythmias are classified as supraventricular because the atrial pacemaker originates at a site above the AV node. If the pacemaker "wanders" through the atria from the SA node, it is called a "wandering pacer."

How does an atrial pacemaker usurp control in atrial dysrhythmias? The atrial pacemaker may produce a premature atrial contraction, which occurs before normal release of the impulse at the SA node, or extremely rapid impulses. Such rapid impulses occur in atrial tachycardia (160 to 250 beats/minute), atrial flutter (250 to 400 beats/minute), and atrial fibrillation (>400 beats/minute). At these dangerously rapid rates, the ventricular myocardium cannot contract efficiently nor recover adequately between contractions. Inefficient myocardial contractions reduce coronary blood flow and lead to angina and congestive heart failure.

Rapid atrial rhythms may be accompanied by varying degrees of second-degree AV block. This block, which is physiologic, protects the ventricular mechanism from the effects of rapid impulse formation. This is a protective mechanism and doesn't reflect pathology.

In atrial dysrhythmias, the EKG shows P waves induced by atria rather than SA node, with normal QRS complexes (atrial dysrhythmias don't affect the ventricular complex).

Junctional (nodal) dysrhythmias. These dysrhythmias result from disturbances in which the AV node functions as the heart's pacemaker, or in which the AV node blocks impulses from the AV node to the ventricles. In the first case, impulses travel retrograde and antegrade from the AV node. Such dysrhythmias include junctional rhythm, junctional tachycardia, premature junctional contractions, and junctional escape complexes. They produce characteristic EKG configurations. Depending on the sequence of atrial activation, a P wave may be observed before or after the QRS complex or may be buried within the complex. The P wave appears inverted in leads II, III, and aVF. The PR interval will be short if it precedes the QRS complex. Since ventricular activation occurs normally, the QRS will be normal.

In the second case, ischemia, electrolyte abnormalities, or drug toxicity delays or blocks impulses at the AV node for abnormally long intervals. Normally, impulses coming from the SA node delay at the AV node for 0.20 seconds or less before passing to the bundle of His. These dysrhythmias include first-, second-, and third-degree heart block.

Preexcitation syndromes. Wolff-Parkinson-White and Lown-Ganong-Levine syndromes occur when an atrial impulse prematurely activates the ventricular muscle. Premature activation usually results from an accessory pathway that conducts impulses faster, but recovers more slowly than the AV pathway. This difference in refractiveness allows a phenomenon called circuit reentry. If the impulse is delayed long enough in a pathway of slow conduction or speeded up in an area of fast conduction, it may still be active when the surrounding myocardium repolarizes. Thus, the impulse can then reenter the surrounding tissue or circuit and produce an ectopic beat.

Preexcitation syndrome often results in debilitating reentrant tachycardia and/or atrial fibrillation. (If atrial fibrillation coincides with antegrade conduction in the accessory pathway, ventricular fibrillation—and sudden death—may result.) In preexcitation syndromes, the EKG shows a shortened PR interval, and a normal or widened QRS complex.

Ashman phenomenon

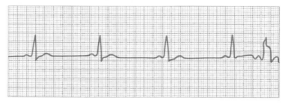

This phenomenon reflects the relationship between the length of the cardiac cycle and refractoriness of cardiac tissue. Theoretically, an aberration of conduction will occur when a short cycle follows a long one, because the refractory period varies with the length of the cycle. Any impulse that ends a short cycle that is preceded by a long one is more likely to encounter refractory tissue. For example, in sinus bradycardia complicated by premature atrial contraction (PAC), the cycle of sinus bradycardia is long; but because PAC shortens the cardiac cycle, the PAC will be conducted aberrantly, usually in an RBB pattern. (See rhythm strip above.)

In the past, the Ashman phenomenon was associated with atrial fibrillation. However, because so much concealed conduction occurs in atrial fibrillation, it's not possible to tell exactly when bundle branch activation, one of the mechanisms of aberrant conduction, occurs.

Ventricular dysrhythmias

Ventricular dysrhythmias can result from ventricular irritability or from conduction disturbances resulting from injury, ischemia, edema, or toxicity in either bundle branch. Ventricular irritability may result from myocardial ischemia secondary to coronary artery disease or congestive heart failure, or follow physical stimulation during cardiac catheterization or invasive monitoring. Often, the irritable focus results from an ischemic area of tissue next to scar tissue from an MI. If a ventricular aneurysm is present, the focus is often part of the weakened, ischemic myocardium.

Ventricular irritability may progress from occasional PVCs, bigeminy, trigeminy, and couplets to ventricular tachycardia and to ventricular fibrillation. Other ventricular dysrhythmias include: "Torsades de Pointes," Romano-Ward syndrome, and ventricular standstill (asystole). In all ventricular dysrhythmias, impulses arise below the AV node.

Ventricular conduction disorders. Intraventricular conduction defect (block) may reflect right bundle branch block (RBBB), left bundle branch block (LBBB), hemiblock, or a delayed conduction in any fascicle of the bundle branches. (The left bundle branches into two fascicles or small bundles. The right bundle branch consists of one main fascicle.)

Since LBBB usually accompanies left ventricular disease, its prognosis is worse than RBBB. In both left and right bundle branch block, the QRS complex is widened because of

Axis deviation

Quadrants of
axis deviation

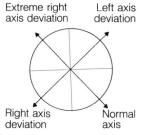

Extreme right   Left axis
axis deviation   deviation

Right axis   Normal
deviation   axis

Normal axis

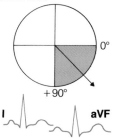

I   aVF

Left axis deviation

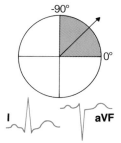

I   aVF

Right axis deviation

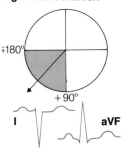

I   aVF

Extreme right axis deviation

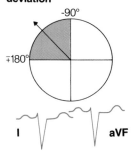

I   aVF

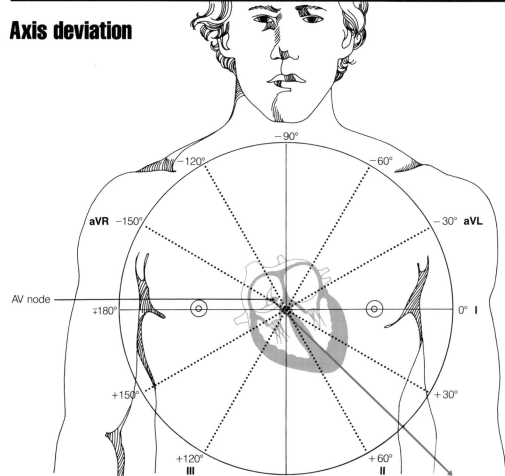

AV node

Mean QRS vector

Vectors represent the magnitude and direction of the heart's electrical forces. The mean QRS vector, the sum of the heart's small vectors, represents the axis or general direction of ventricular depolarization. The exact direction of the mean QRS vector is determined by plotting frontal plane leads in degrees on a hexaxial figure drawn over the patient's chest.

Normally, the mean QRS vector points downward and to the patient's left side. An abnormality in the heart causes the vector to shift or deviate, but the AV node is always the tail of the vector. For example, in hypertrophy of one ventricle, increased electrical activity on one side displaces the vector to that side. In MI, the vector usually points away from the infarcted area since this area shows no electrical activity.

The mean QRS vector points to only one of four possible quadrants. Several methods precisely calculate the electrical axis of the heart. The easiest way to *estimate* the axial quadrant is to determine direction of QRS deflections in leads I and aVF. Positive deflections in leads I and aVF reflect a normal axis. Positive deflections in lead I and negative in aVF reflect left axis deviation; negative deflections in lead I and positive in aVF reflect right axis deviation; negative deflections in leads I and aVF reflect extreme right axis deviation.

abnormal ventricular conduction. Instead, hemiblock results in axis deviation.

MEDICAL MANAGEMENT
Diagnosis of dysrhythmia is always based on patient history and symptoms (tachycardia, palpitations, anginal pain, extreme dyspnea, edema, faintness) and detailed cardiovascular examination that includes a 12-lead EKG.

Effective medical treatment of dysrhythmia should return pacer function to the sinus node; increase or decrease ventricular rate to normal; regain AV synchrony; and maintain NSR. Such treatment corrects abnormal rhythms through therapy with antiarrhythmic drugs; electrical conversion with precordial shock (defibrillation and cardioversion); physical maneuvers (carotid and vagal [Valsalva maneuver]); temporary or permanent placement of a pacemaker to maintain heart rate; and surgical removal or cryotherapy of an irritable ectopic focus to prevent recurring dysrhythmias. Dysrhythmias often respond to treatment of the underlying disorder, such as correction of hypoxia. However, dysrhythmia associated with heart disease often requires continuing and complex treatment.

Conversion with antiarrhythmic drugs
Drug therapy is often the initial treatment for converting a dysrhythmia to NSR. Depending on the dysrhythmia, treatment for a life-threatening dysrhythmia, such as ventricular tachycardia, may begin with an I.V. lidocaine bolus, followed by continuous infusion of lidocaine. If lidocaine is ineffective, bretylium or procainamide may be infused instead. After cardiac rhythm stabilizes, treatment may continue with oral procainamide, disopyramide, verapamil, or another drug—while I.V. infusions taper off. Some centers report more effective results with other oral drugs— mexilitene, tocainide, or aprindine.

When drug therapy fails to provide adequate control of symptoms resulting from dysrhythmia, electrophysiological studies (EPS) may help determine the most effective drug and its dosage. EPS provides much information about the heart's conduction mechanisms, and new insights into the causes and treatment of dysrhythmias. For instance, EPS has led to the development of a new surgical procedure, endocardial stripping, for removal of an irritable focus.

In some centers, EPS is used to induce dysrhythmia in a patient with an incapacitating or potentially life-threatening dysrhythmia (such as Wolff-Parkinson-White syndrome or recurrent ventricular tachycardia) to verify effective drug dosage in a closely controlled situation with minimal risk to the patient.

Conversion with precordial shock
Defibrillation and cardioversion are the two common uses of precordial shock for correction of tachycardia or other life-threatening dysrhythmias. Precordial shock delivers a controlled electrical current to the heart through paddles placed externally on the chest wall or electrodes placed directly on the myocardium during surgery. The brief electric current completely depolarizes the myocardium, usually terminating ventricular fibrillation and other dysrhythmias, and allows the SA node to regain control of cardiac pacing. Defibrillation is the application of an electrical current to convert ventricular fibrillation to NSR. Synchronized cardioversion is the application of an electric current to convert refractory atrial, junctional, and ventricular tachydysrhythmias. In cardioversion, the electrical discharge is synchronous with QRS waves; in defibrillation, the discharge is asynchronous (see *How to defibrillate*, page 164).

Another application of precordial shock—an implantable automatic defibrillator—is currently being tested for patients with refractory tachydysrhythmias. This device automatically delivers a 25-joule defibrillatory discharge when it senses potentially lethal ventricular dysrhythmias, such as ventricular fibrillation. If the initial discharge fails to convert the rhythm, the device automatically recycles three more times with the third and fourth discharges each delivering 30 joules.

Conversion with carotid massage and Valsalva maneuver
Carotid massage is the application of manual pressure to the left or right carotid sinus to decrease the heart rate. This procedure requires continuous EKG monitoring as pressure is applied, first to one carotid sinus, then to the other, each time for no longer than 5 seconds. Pressure is released when any sign of rhythm change appears on the EKG monitor. Pressure should never be applied simultaneously to both sinuses, because this may cause complete asystole and significantly impair cerebral blood flow. EKG monitoring is particularly important if the patient has atrial flutter or supraventricular tachycardia with AV block: slowing the heart rate by carotid massage may worsen AV block and induce junctional or ventricular escape rhythms.

Valsalva maneuver, which increases intrathoracic pressure by forcible exhalation against a closed airway, may also be used to increase vagal tone and convert a dysrhythmia to NSR. Intrathoracic pressure is created by having the patient inhale deeply, hold his breath and strain hard for at least 10 seconds. Coughing, gagging, or self-induced vomiting may occasionally produce a similar effect. The Valsalva maneuver is contraindicated if the patient has severe coronary artery disease, acute MI, or moderate to severe hypovolemia.

Pacemakers: Permanent or temporary
A pacemaker is driven by a lithium-powered pulse generator. Its electrical impulses are transmitted to and from the heart through an electrode lead wire, which runs from the battery pack to the heart. The electrode may be *unipolar*, with a positive electrode (cathode) inside the heart and a negative (anode) outside the heart in subcutaneous tissue; or *bipolar*, with both electrodes lying against the

Dysrhythmias and sudden death
Most cases of sudden death occur before the victim reaches the hospital. In 75% of the victims of sudden death (defined as death within 1 hour of onset of symptoms), the EKGs recorded by rescue workers within minutes of collapse show ventricular fibrillation. In the remaining 25%, sudden death results from asystole, idioventricular rhythm, sinus bradycardia, and acute heart block with Stokes-Adams attacks.

These fatal dysrhythmias have multiple causes.
Cardiovascular causes (80% to 90%):
• coronary artery spasm, especially with unstable angina
• small-vessel coronary disease
• valvular aortic stenosis
• idiopathic hypertrophic subaortic stenosis
• cardiomyopathy
• pulmonary hypertension
• dissecting aortic aneurysm
• ruptured aortic aneurysm.
Noncardiovascular causes:
• massive intracerebral and subarachnoid hemorrhage
• massive gastrointestinal hemorrhage
• aspiration of a food bolus.

How to defibrillate

Before defibrillation, check the manufacturer's specifications for the difference between the stored energy and the charge delivered through the paddles. Then, set the dial to the level needed for defibrillation. (Note: Some EKG machines and temporary pacemakers are not defibrillator-shielded. Disconnect such units before defibrillation.)

• *Lubricate the paddles to facilitate conduction and prevent burns.* You can use cream, paste, a gel pad, or saline-soaked gauze sponges. If you're using cream or paste, squeeze a ring of lubricant around the disk, and then rub the disks together to spread the lubricant over the entire disk surface. Or use one gel pad or four sponges per paddle to lubricate each disk.

• *Wipe any lubricant off your hands before discharging the paddles* to prevent arcing, which can cause a shock or burn.

• *To start the charging cycle, activate the charge control button.* The meter needle will move gradually to the selected energy level; when it stops, the machine is charged. (Some machines have a digital readout; others sound an alarm when fully charged.)

• *Position the paddles.* To position standard paddles on a man, put one paddle beneath his clavicle, to the right of the upper end of his sternum; put the other paddle on the left lateral chest wall, to the left of the cardiac apex. To position paddles on a woman, place them at the mid- or anterior-axillary level, not over the breasts. (Note: When positioning paddles, keep your fingers off the discharge buttons, so that you don't discharge them accidentally.)

To position A/P paddles, put the flat paddle under the patient's body, behind the heart and just below the left scapula. Put the other paddle over the

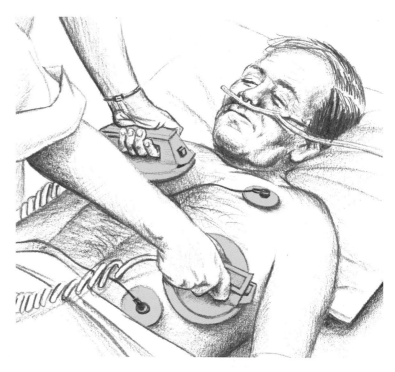

left precordium, directly over the heart. With A/P paddles, the discharge button is located on the anterior paddle only. *Never use standard paddles for A/P placement.*

• *Before discharging the standard paddles,* look around to be sure no one's touching the patient or the bed (be sure you're standing clear, too) and say loudly, "Stand clear." Give other members of the code team time to step away.

• *Discharge the paddles by pressing both buttons simultaneously* with at least 20 to 25 pounds of forearm pressure per paddle. (A discharging control is usually on both handles, but may be on only one.) Be sure to use arm pressure rather than shoulder pressure so that the paddles won't slip out of position.

Defibrillate adults at 200 watt-seconds (or joules), as ordered. If unsuccessful, defibrillate again at the same setting.

• *After defibrillation, check the patient's pulse, and check for any changes on the monitor.* He may need sodium bicarbonate or epinephrine. If the patient

requires a third shock, increase the energy level to 360 watt-seconds.

• *If the paddles have been recharged but not used, clear the charge by turning off the machine or by pressing the "bleed" button, if applicable.* Don't discharge paddles into each other or into the air.

• *Clean the lubricant off the patient's skin and the paddle disks with soap and water.* Residual lubricant can corrode the metal paddles and can cause arcing of the electrical current.

• *Document the procedure and any changes in the patient's heart rhythm.* Record the date, time, lead, and watt-seconds (or joules) on the recording strip or code form. Treat any burns as ordered; document their size, appearance, and your care.

• *Prepare the defibrillator unit for reuse, and restock necessary supplies.* Someone should check the defibrillator unit at the beginning of every shift to be sure it's working. The hospital's engineering department should regularly check it and the EKG machine and make needed repairs.

myocardium. In a bipolar system, two insulated conductors connect electrodes to the generator. The unipolar electrode produces tall EKG pacing spikes because of the distance between the two poles. The bipolar electrode produces short spikes.

Temporary pacemakers are commonly used in temporary situations (drug intoxication, acute MI with transient heart block), prophylactic situations (acute VT and new BBB), and in patients scheduled for implantation of a permanent pacemaker. In such patients, they support cardiovascular function until spontaneous pacing is restored or permanent pacing is possible. They can also be used independently to correct conduction disturbance, to slow or accelerate impulse formation, and to usurp control of tachydysrhythmias and ectopic activity. Such control is particularly important in patients with acute MI complicated by complete heart block, with digitalis toxicity, and with heart block following recent cardiac surgery. Temporary pacing is also used in complete heart block with intermittent asystole; episodes of ventricular tachycardia or fibrillation; heart block that shifts between the second and third degrees; sinus bradycardia; cardiac arrest; and permanent pulse generator replacement. When diagnostic tests confirm irreversible cardiac damage with complete conduction block, the patient needs a permanent pacemaker to maintain heart rate.

The newest of the standard pacemakers is the programmable pacemaker, which combines the advantages of standard pulse generator pacemakers—rate stability and automatically programmed pulse width increase—with noninvasive, push-button rate programming. A pacemaker rate controller permits changes in the pacing rate on a permanent programmable pacemaker without surgery.

Electrophysiologic mapping

If electrophysiologic studies determine that drug therapy cannot control dysrhythmias satisfactorily, other procedures may be used to suppress the irritable focus: cryotherapy, aneurysmectomy, internal defibrillation, and a new procedure, endocardial stripping (also called "The Pennsylvania Peel"). Endocardial stripping—excision of an irritable focus (or foci) during open heart surgery—is an alternative treatment for recurrent ventricular tachycardia and sudden death syndrome.

These special procedures require preliminary electrophysiologic studies (called mapping) of the area to be removed. The electrophysiologist divides the ventricle into numbered sections and electrically stimulates each section, in turn, to locate the most irritable tissue. If the patient's condition is unstable or requires defibrillation to terminate the dysrhythmia, mapping may have to be done while the patient is on coronary bypass. After mapping, the irritable focus (or foci) is "scraped" or "peeled" from the myocardium. If mapping reveals a ventricular aneurysm with a focus inside it, aneurysmectomy is necessary. However, if some foci are in inoperable areas, antiarrhythmic drug therapy may still be necessary postoperatively.

NURSING MANAGEMENT

To identify and manage dysrhythmia correctly, you must determine the patient's cardiac, electrolyte, and overall clinical status, noting the effect on cardiac output and whether the dysrhythmia is life-threatening. Careful nursing assessment makes this possible.

First, a detailed history

If the patient's dysrhythmia is benign or not immediately life-threatening, you'll have time to take a careful history. Find out if the patient has any preexisting dysrhythmia; when and how often current dysrhythmia is most likely to occur; what provokes it; what symptoms accompany it (especially syncope); how long it lasts; and what treatment is effective. Record the patient's complaints or symptoms in his own words.

Also ask about current health problems, particularly heart disorders. Ask if the patient is receiving any drugs or other treatment. Check laboratory test results for noncardiac causes—potassium or calcium imbalance, hypovolemia, anemia, hypoglycemia, diabetes, hypothyroidism, hyperthyroidism, or impaired liver or renal function. Ask about smoking and use of caffeine.

Physical examination next

Look for hemodynamic consequences of dysrhythmia. Your first priority, especially in an emergency or if you detect dysrhythmia on a monitor, is to determine how the patient tolerates the abnormal rhythm. Assess for signs of inadequate cerebral perfusion (confusion, loss of consciousness, fainting, decreased urine output). If the patient is unconscious, check airway, breathing and circulation and, if necessary, begin CPR. Also assess for signs of decreased myocardial perfusion (chest pain,

Pacemaker placement

Temporary

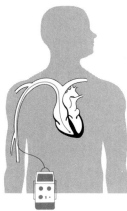

Temporary pacemakers are inserted via the subclavian, jugular, antecubital, or femoral vein. Under fluoroscopic guidance, the doctor threads the catheter through a vein to the right ventricle.

Permanent

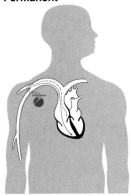

Permanent pacemakers are inserted transvenously via the cephalic or subclavian vein into the right atrium or the apex of the right ventricle. The newest pacemaker modes allow for both atrial and ventricular pacing. The internal pulse generator is usually implanted in a pocket the doctor forms in the anterior chest.

shortness of breath) and signs of inadequate peripheral vascular perfusion (pale, dusky, gray, cool, clammy, or dry skin). Then, check for an apical-radial pulse deficit, and make sure his pulse is palpable. Watch for blood pressure changes, such as a significant drop from previously recorded pressures or the presence of only a palpable pressure.

Next, try to identify the dysrhythmia. If a 12-lead EKG is available, systematically inspect QRS complexes, P waves, and a clear pacemaker spike, if present. What is the site of origin? Is the dysrhythmia junctional, ventricular, or supraventricular?

Try to identify a cause. Was there a precipitating event, such as exercise, stress, or vagal stimuli (such as straining with a bowel movement)? Was the patient having chest pain when the rhythm changed? Was he due for administration of an antiarrhythmic drug?

Nursing diagnosis

When you have a clear idea of the severity and type of dysrhythmia and some idea of the cause or precipitating factors, you're ready to develop nursing diagnoses, establish treatment goals, and plan care accordingly. In patients with dysrhythmia, your nursing diagnoses and planned care will be similar to the following:

Anxiety related to knowledge deficit regarding diagnosis, possible therapy, and prognosis. To reduce the patient's anxiety, encourage him and his family to verbalize their fears. Encourage him to tell you about any symptoms, such as palpitations, dyspnea, or sensations of irregular beat. Also, maintain a quiet, calm environment and help the patient understand dysrhythmia and its implications. Explain all scheduled tests and procedures (including pacemaker insertion and surgery). If dysrhythmia requires emergency treatment, offer the conscious patient calm, reassuring, emotional support. If severe anxiety persists, administer a sedative, as ordered.

Potential for recurring dysrhythmia related to electrical instability. Your goal is to prevent the recurrence of dysrhythmia. Administer antiarrhythmic drug treatment, as ordered. If you're giving these very potent drugs intravenously, use an infusion pump or microdrip administration. Check every 15 minutes to ensure delivery of the correct dosage. Since antiarrhythmics are potentially lethal and dosage may need adjustment, watch carefully for symptoms of toxicity.

If the patient is receiving digitalis or has received it within the last 48 hours, also watch for digitalis toxicity (nausea, vomiting, diarrhea, increased ectopy, heart block), particularly if the patient needs cardioversion. If you suspect or recognize digitalis toxicity, inform the doctor. He'll postpone cardioversion. Meanwhile, make sure an I.V. line is in place and patent, and keep emergency equipment, antiarrhythmic drugs, and a pacemaker readily available. If the patient is alert, explain cardioversion to him. Continue to monitor cardiac rhythm, noting increased ectopy. Notify the doctor, as ordered.

Potential for decreased tissue perfusion related to decreased cardiac output. Your goal is to prevent ischemic complications by maintaining adequate cardiac output. Check blood pressure every 2 hours for decreased systolic pressure and narrowed pulse pressure showing reduced effective volume. If systolic pressure falls below 100 mm Hg or the limit set by the doctor, report it immediately, check blood pressure frequently, and try to identify the cause of the hypotension. Consider these possible causes: drug therapy, MI, and hypovolemia.

Watch for and immediately report any signs and symptoms of inadequate cerebral perfusion: yawning, mental confusion, dizziness, Stokes-Adams syndrome, convulsions, Cheynes-Stokes respirations. Then try to rule out other causes, such as use of antiarrhythmics or sensory deprivation. Be alert for signs and symptoms of inadequate myocardial perfusion: angina, MI, left heart failure with pulmonary edema, and increased ectopy.

Inadequate renal perfusion. Check urine output every 8 hours; every 1 to 2 hours if oliguria develops; every hour if anuria develops. If indicated or ordered, weigh the patient daily and monitor results of laboratory tests: blood urea nitrogen (BUN), creatinine clearance, electrolyte balance (particularly, potassium), and acid-base balance. Watch for changes in mental status (lethargy, confusion, anorexia, nausea, vomiting) that may indicate fluid imbalance. Know if the drug you're administering is excreted in the urine. If it is, report altered urine output promptly.

Inadequate peripheral perfusion. Check all pulses for equality and quality. Assess for pallor, cooling of extremities, and clamines from peripheral arterial constriction. Report any of these signs immediately.

If necessary, assist with insertion of intraarterial lines and/or pulmonary artery line

Types of pacemakers

A three-letter identification code for implantable cardiac pacemakers helps you to sort out their complex characteristics. The first letter identifies the paced chamber: V stands for ventricle, A for atrium, and D for double (atrium and ventricle). The second letter identifies the sensed chamber: A or V. The third letter identifies the response mode: I for inhibited and T for triggered. The letter O means no specific comment is applicable. Possible pacemaker combinations include: VOO, AOO, DOO, VVI, VVT, AAI, AAT, VAT, and DVI.

Pacemakers are commonly grouped by pacing mode:
• **Fixed rate pacemakers** (AOO, VOO, DOO) keep a steady rate (usually 70 beats/minute) regardless of the patient's own cardiac impulses. Because such pacing interferes with normal cardiac activity, it may become dangerous when threshold for ventricular fibrillation is low (for example, after MI). Fixed rate pacemakers are rarely used.
• **QRS-inhibited pacemaker** (VVI), a demand pacemaker with an inhibited response mode, prevents firing of an impulse when the pacemaker senses an R wave.
• **QRS-triggered pacemaker** (VVT) fires in the absolute refractory period when it senses the R wave. Thus, when natural cardiac rhythm is adequate, this pacemaker fires but causes no cardiac response. However, if cardiac rate falls below the pacemaker's preset rate, the artificial discharge stimulates the myocardium.
• **Atrial synchronized pacemaker** (VAT) uses an atrial electrode to sense normal atrial depolarization. After an appropriate delay to permit atrial transport, it triggers a ventricular electrode to pace the ventricle. If the atrial rate exceeds 130 beats/minute, the pacemaker transmits every other impulse to the ventricle. If the rate falls below 60, it initiates fixed pacing at 60 beats/minute.
• **Atrioventricular sequential pacing** (DVI) imitates the normal sequence of electrical activity in the heart, maintaining cardiac output 22% higher than conventional pacemakers. It uses two separate electrodes to pace the atrium and ventricle in sequence. However, it's inhibited by ventricular activity.

Pacemakers can also be grouped according to their use:
• **Ventricular pacemakers** (QRS-inhibited, QRS-triggered, and some temporary pacemakers) are primarily (95%) used to treat sinus bradycardia. They may be permanent or temporary.
• **Atrial pacemakers** (AAI, AAT, and some temporary pacemakers) are used when AV conduction is intact, especially for symptomatic bradycardia and sick sinus syndrome, with or without congestive heart failure and low cardiac output. Rapid atrial pacing is helpful to end intractable supraventricular and ventricular tachydysrhythmias. Atrial pacemakers are hemodynamically superior to ventricular pacemakers because they maintain ventricular filling. However, maintaining electrode contact with atrial tissue can be difficult. Reliable lead fixation can remedy this problem.
• **Atrial synchronous** (VAT and some temporary pacemakers) are commonly used when complete heart block prevents use of an atrial pacemaker or when another condition prevents ventricular pacing because the patient needs atrial contraction to maintain cardiac output.

(Swan-Ganz) so drugs can be given, as ordered, to improve peripheral perfusion. Also, position the patient to avoid compromising circulation.

Potential for embolism formation related to pooling of blood from irregular myocardial contraction. To help prevent embolization, find out if the patient has a previous history of thromboembolic disease. If he does, or if his condition requires prolonged bed rest, apply antiembolism stockings and encourage range-of-motion exercises. Encourage ambulation as soon as possible. If he has chronic atrial fibrillation, a condition at higher risk for emboli, and requires cardioversion, make sure he receives anticoagulant therapy first. In any patient at high risk for emboli, watch for sudden onset of chest pain; signs and symptoms of respiratory distress; altered mental status; unexplained restlessness or anxiety; and decreased temperature, sensation, or pulses in extremities.

Potential for cardiac arrest related to extreme cardiac instability. Be prepared to perform lifesaving resuscitation correctly. Keep emergency equipment and drugs readily available. Keep up to date on CPR techniques (see *The ABCs of CPR,* pages 168 and 169). Make sure you are familiar with and know how to draw up and administer emergency drugs. Check the defibrillator, and be prepared to defibrillate if necessary (see *How to defibrillate,* page 164).

Self-care deficit related to lack of knowledge about pacemaker insertion. Provide individualized teaching. Explain how the pacemaker functions, and how it will correct the patient's condition. Provide written information when-

EMERGENCY MANAGEMENT

The ABCs of CPR

Once you've determined that the victim actually has suffered respiratory and cardiac arrest, recall the ABCs of cardiopulmonary resuscitation (CPR): open the Airway, restore Breathing, and restore Circulation. Administer CPR until one of the following occurs:

• The victim responds with spontaneous breathing and circulation.
• Another qualified person takes over life-support efforts.
• The victim has been transferred to an emergency medical facility, where qualified personnel take over.

• You're too exhausted to continue giving CPR.
  To give CPR effectively you should complete a course taught by a certified CPR instructor. The drawings below review the CPR techniques currently recommended by the American Heart Association.

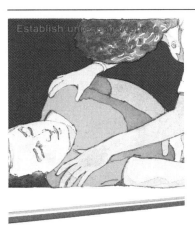

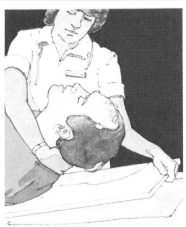

Establish unresponsiveness
• When you first discover the victim, look at him closely. Shake him gently by the shoulders and loudly call out "Are you okay?" This shaking and shouting will establish whether or not he's unconscious. If he's unconscious and you're alone, call for help. (See illustration at far left.) Begin the CPR procedure until help arrives.
• If the victim isn't lying on a hard surface, place a cardiac arrest board (or the headboard of the bed, if detachable, or some other flat, rigid support) under his back to ensure that subsequent compression steps will be effective. (See illustration at left.)

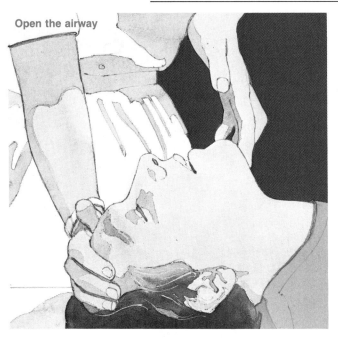

Open the airway

Open the airway
• Open the victim's airway. The most common cause of airway obstruction in an unconscious person is his tongue, which has relaxed and fallen into the airway. Because the tongue is attached to the lower jaw, moving the lower jaw forward will lift the tongue away from the back of the throat, thereby opening the airway.

You can use three methods to open the victim's airway: the head-tilt/chin-lift (the method recommended by the National Conference on Cardiopulmonary Emergency Cardiac Care), the head-tilt/neck-lift (the most commonly used method), or the jaw-thrust without head-tilt.
• To use the head-tilt/chin-lift method, place your hand that's closer to the victim's head on his forehead, and tilt his head slightly. Then, place the fingertips of your opposite hand under his lower jaw on the bony part near the chin. Next, gently lift the victim's chin up, taking care not to close his mouth.
• To use the head-tilt/neck-lift method, place the palm of your hand that's closer to the victim's shoulders under his neck. Place the hand lifting his neck close to the back of his head to minimize

cervical-spine extension. Then gently press back on the victim's forehead while lifting up and supporting his neck. (See illustration at left.)
• Use the jaw-thrust without head-tilt method if you suspect the victim has a neck or spine injury. Kneel at the victim's head, facing his feet. Place your thumbs on his mandible near the corners of his mouth, pointing your thumbs toward his feet. Then, position the tops of your index fingers at the angles of his jaw.

Now, push your thumbs down as you lift up with the tips of your index fingers. This action should open the victim's airway.
• After opening the airway, see if this action has restored breathing. Put your ear over the victim's mouth and nose while you look toward his chest and abdomen. Then, listen for air movement and observe if his chest or abdomen is moving up and down. Next, feel with your cheek for any flow of air. If the victim has started to breathe, maintain his airway until help arrives.

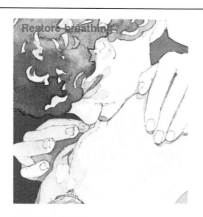

Restore breathing

• If the victim hasn't started to breathe, close his nostrils with the thumb and index finger of your hand on his forehead.
• Open your mouth wide and place it over the victim's mouth, sealing it tightly so no air can escape. (See illustration at left.)
• When using the head-tilt/neck-lift method, remember to support his neck with one hand while you pinch his nares.
• Deliver four quick full breaths, but do not allow the victim to exhale between these breaths. These four breaths maintain positive pressure in the airway. Even if the victim has stopped breathing for only a short time, some of the lungs' alveoli may have already collapsed. Positive pressure helps reinflate them. When you see the victim's chest rise, and then fall after your fourth breath, you have verified that air is entering and escaping from his lungs.

If the victim wears dentures, keeping them in place will usually make ventilation easier. However, if his dentures start to slip, be sure to remove them.

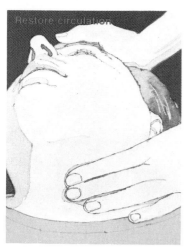

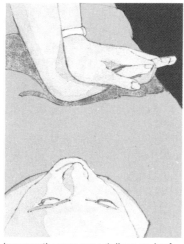

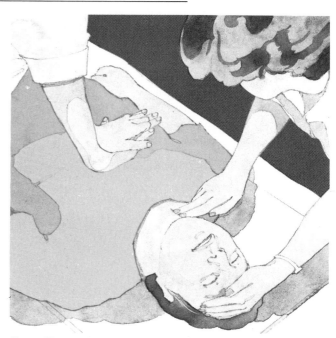

Restore circulation

• Keep your hand on the victim's forehead to maintain the head-tilt position. Use your other hand to find the carotid artery on the side closest to you, in the groove beside the larynx. Use your index and middle fingers to palpate the artery gently for 5 to 10 seconds. (See illustration above.)

If you find a pulse, don't give cardiac compressions, but do ventilate the patient at the rate of 1 breath every 5 seconds (12 breaths per minute). Continue to check his pulse after every 12 breaths.

If you find no pulse, prepare to begin cardiac compression. Position yourself close to the victim's side, with your knees apart. This position gives you a broad base of support.
• Use the fingers of your hand that's closer to the victim's feet to find the correct hand position. Locate the lower margin of his rib cage and trace it to the notch where his ribs meet his sternum. Place your middle finger on the notch.
• Place your index finger of the same hand next to your middle finger. Then place the heel of your other hand next to your index finger on the long axis of the victim's sternum, as shown. This is the correct position for cardiac compression. If your hands are placed incorrectly, you may deliver an ineffective compression that could lacerate the victim's liver, fracture a rib, or break off the xiphoid process.
• Place the hand you used to locate the notch over the heel of your other hand. Interlock or extend your fingers to keep them off the victim's ribs and to maintain vertical pressure through the heel of the hand touching his sternum. Align your shoulders over your hands, keeping your elbows straight. Keeping your fingers off the victim's ribs and your shoulders aligned ensures that you'll compress downward, not laterally. Lateral compressions won't deliver sufficient pressure.

Using the weight of your upper body, compress downward about 1½ to 2 inches (3 to 5 cm), concentrating the pressure through the heels of your hands. (See illustrations above and at right.) Don't deliver bouncing compressions, because they're less effective and could injure the victim. Then, relax the pressure completely to let the heart fill with blood, but don't remove your hands from his chest or you'll lose your hand position.
• If you're the only rescuer, time your compressions at a rate of 80 per minute. Count: "One and two and three and..." up to the count of fifteen. Then deliver two quick breaths without allowing the victim to exhale between them. (Actually, you'll be delivering 60 compressions per minute, because of the delay needed to ventilate the victim.) Perform CPR for 1 minute, and check pulse for 5 seconds. If it's absent, resume CPR with two ventilations to ensure that oxygen is in the lungs before beginning compressions.

If another person trained in CPR arrives while you can still continue, one of you can perform compressions while the other ventilates the victim and checks his carotid pulse to monitor effectiveness of compressions. The person doing ventilations also instructs the person doing compressions to stop them, checks for spontaneous pulse and respirations, describes the patient's status, and gives one breath. The compressor then resumes compressions. Apply five compressions to one ventilation. Perform at least two cycles before rescuer and compressor switch positions.

Caring for pacemaker patients

If your patient has a temporary or permanent pacemaker, you'll need to provide special nursing care and comprehensive patient teaching.

Temporary pacemaker care
If a patient has a temporary pacemaker, record on his chart the date and method of insertion, the location (atrial or ventricular) of the pacemaker, and its type, rate, threshold (MA) settings, times turned on or off, and frequency of use.

To maintain pacemaker function, continuously monitor the EKG for frequency of pacing need, maintenance of preset rate, capture, sensing, and paced QRS or P configuration. After insertion of a temporary pacemaker and every 8 hours thereafter, check the connections, battery, pulse at the insertion site, and consistency between the pacemaker setting and the actual rate and stimulation and sensitivity thresholds when the pacemaker is on and off. Every 24 hours or as indicated, check the threshold; every 4 hours or as indicated, check vital signs and the sense/pace needle. (See *Troubleshooting pacemaker problems*, page 171.)

To maintain equipment, place a plastic cover over the dials to keep the box and wires dry. Clean the box with water or alcohol; or gas-sterilize it, but never autoclave it. Clean nondisposable catheters in bactericidal solution, and then gas-

sterilize them. Before defibrillation, find out if the doctor wants the pacemaker disconnected.

To prevent infection at the insertion site, cleanse the skin with antiseptic solution, apply antibiotic ointment and dry, sterile dressings daily. To prevent ulceration of underlying tissue, pad the area beneath the wires. Inspect the site every 4 hours for tenderness, redness, swelling, and discoloration. When you remove the catheter, culture the tip if it has been in place for over 1 week, if signs of infection are present, or if insertion was traumatic.

To prevent microshock, insulate the external metallic parts of the pacing catheter. When you handle these parts, wear dry rubber or plastic gloves. Protect these parts of newer models by imbedding them in the insulated pacemaker terminals or by covering them with clear tape or a dry, surgical rubber glove. Make sure all equipment is properly grounded, using a three-prong plug; don't use adapters. Don't use extension cords or equipment that has frayed wires or other signs of disrepair. If you're not sure equipment is in good condition, check with the hospital electrician. Prevent the patient from contacting metal. Warn him not to touch a television set. Don't touch the patient or his bed while touching electrical equipment. Avoid using electrical beds that are not specifically approved; unplug lamps attached to metal beds; and

make sure electrical equipment, such as a respirator, doesn't touch the bed. Place a "microshock precaution" sign over the bed, and explain the sign to the patient and his family.

To maintain the patient's comfort, give medication for pain, as ordered. If the patient has pain or discomfort in his legs or arms, check pulse and perfusion distal to the cutdown every 8 hours. Position the affected extremity comfortably; and to avoid stiffness, help the patient gently exercise it regularly.

Permanent pacemaker care
If a patient has a permanent pacemaker, record on his chart the date and location of the insertion, the manufacturer's model and serial numbers for the generator and leads, the set rate, EKG tracings with and without a magnet held over the generator, amplitude of pacemaker artifact, and threshold measurements at insertion.

To maintain pacemaker function, continuously monitor the patient's EKG for the first 24 hours; then analyze the EKG every 4 hours for maintenance of the preset rate, capture, paced QRS configuration, amplitude of pacemaker artifact, sensing, competition, and ventricular dysrhythmias. Check consistency against baseline values.

Every 4 hours, check blood pressure, respiration, and temperature; and count apical and radial pulses for 1 minute. Every 2 hours, quickly check these pulses. Report any rates below

ever possible. Offer explanations in terms the patient understands.

Anxiety related to knowledge deficit of endocardial stripping. Give adequate preoperative teaching. Begin by explaining the procedure. Tell the patient that, after surgery, two temporary pacer wires will protrude through an incision and will be covered with a sterile dressing. These electrodes are available for emergency pacing, to terminate a dysrhythmia. They are removed after his con-

dition has been stable for a few days.

Self-care deficit related to lack of knowledge about home medical regimen. Provide adequate discharge teaching. Help the patient and his family understand maintenance treatment of dysrhythmia. Explain normal heart function, dysrhythmias and the symptoms they cause, factors that might provoke them, what to do about them, and everything the patient needs to know about drug therapy (purpose, dosage, timing, side effects). If the patient has the pacing rate or an apical-radial pulse deficit.

Watch for signs of pacemaker failure (decreased blood pressure, decreased urinary output, Stokes-Adams syndrome, palpitations, chest pains, dyspnea and fatigue, lightheadedness). Also, watch for signs of pacing catheter displacement (intermittent or complete pacing failure, abnormal pacemaker stimulation).

To avoid such displacement, make sure the patient doesn't raise his arms above the shoulder until the doctor orders range-of-motion (ROM) exercises, usually around the third postoperative day. Enforce bedrest for 24 hours and reduced activity for another 48 hours.

To make sure that equipment (batteries, pacing catheter) is working well, watch for ventricular premature beats, frequency, and coupling interval; and check for sensing or competition.

To avoid infection, inspect the insertion site at regular intervals and whenever the patient reports discomfort. Check for signs of infection, skin break- down, or hematoma. Check temperature every 4 hours. If a closed-wound drain is in use, empty it every 8 hours or as needed. When you remove the pressure dressing, replace it with a sterile dressing. Change the sterile dressing daily. Give antibiotics for 5 to 7 days after implantation, as ordered.

To promote comfort, assist and encourage the patient to begin ROM exercises for the affected shoulder, as ordered, usually 5 to 7 days after pacemaker insertion. Administer an analgesic, as needed.

Troubleshooting pacemaker problems

Problem	Signs	Possible causes	Possible solutions
Failure to capture (pacemaker transmits impulses to heart but fails to stimulate it)	• Apical rate below pacemaker setting • Pacemaker spike not followed by QRS complex on EKG • Continuous sense/pace dial movement	• Dislodged catheter • Pacemaker end-of-life or battery depletion • Fractured lead wire • Change in output threshold (stimulation threshold)	• Turn patient on left side to aid catheter contact with myocardium. • Replace the battery. • Lead wire replaced by doctor. • Notify doctor and monitor patient closely. Doctor may increase output threshold or reposition catheter. (*Note:* In some institutions, nurse may increase stimulation threshold before calling doctor.)
Failure to sense (pacemaker fails to detect ventricular depolarization and functions independent of heart rate)	• Apical rate higher than pacemaker setting and irregular • Pacemaker beats follow normal beats at a rate higher than pacemaker setting • Continuous sense/pacer dial movement	• Mode dial accidentally set at *fixed* mode • Dislodged catheter • Competition between pacemaker's rhythm and patient's rhythm, possibly resulting in ventricular fibrillation	• Turn the dial to *demand* mode. • See "Failure to capture." • Turn the pacemaker off. Call the doctor to reposition the catheter. Monitor the patient closely to make sure his heart rate can maintain adequate cardiac output.
Firing loss (combined failure to sense/capture caused by mechanical failure of the unit)	• No pacing seen • No sense/pace dial movement	• Dislodged catheter • Pacemaker accidentally turned off • Battery failure • Loose catheter terminals • Pacemaker generator worn out • Broken catheter wires	• See "Failure to capture." • Turn the pacemaker on. • Replace the battery. • Tighten terminals; wear rubber gloves to avoid microshock. • Replace generator. Monitor apical rate and blood pressure until pacemaker functions correctly. • Catheter wires replaced by the doctor. Monitor the patient closely.

a pacemaker, explain how it works and how to care for it. Teach him when and how to take his pulse for 1 minute and when to notify his doctor of changes.

Evaluate your care
You know you've given good nursing care for dysrhythmia if your patient understands his dysrhythmia, its treatment, and the prescribed regimen for maintenance; is free of complications upon discharge; or has survived an emergency situation in which you acted quickly and skillfully.

Practice makes perfect
If you work in an area without continuous monitoring equipment, you can still practice recognizing dysrhythmias by reading charts and analyzing the EKGs placed in them. In time, and with much practice, you should be able to recognize dysrhythmias quickly and accurately and know how to treat them.

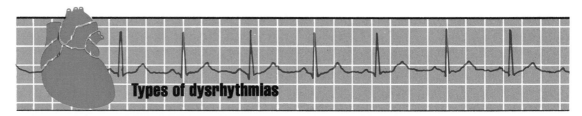

Types of dysrhythmias

Sinoatrial dysrhythmias

Sinus bradycardia

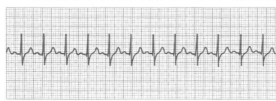

Causes
- Increased intracranial pressure; increased vagal tone due to straining at stool, vomiting, intubation, mechanical ventilation; sick sinus syndrome or hypothyroidism
- Treatment with beta blockers and sympatholytic drugs (Normal sinus rates return when drugs are stopped.)
- May be normal in athletes or young adults

Description
- Rate < 60 beats/minute.
- QRS complex follows each P wave.
- Normal AV conduction occurs (1:1 AV response with a normal PR interval).
- Marked sinus bradycardia may severely decrease cardiac output.
- Marked sinus bradycardia may be associated with prolonged PR interval.

Sinus tachycardia

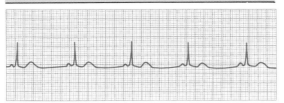

Causes
- In acute MI, sinus tachycardia may be one of the first signs of CHF, cardiogenic shock, pulmonary embolism or infarct extension.
- Normal cardiac response to demand for increased blood flow during exercise, stress, pain, fever, hypo- or hyperthyroidism
- Treatment with adrenergics, anticholinergics, and some antiarrhythmics

Description
- Rate is 100 to 160 beats/minute. (Tracing shows 130 beats/minute.)
- Impulse formation and conduction are normal.
- Prolonged sinus tachycardia may lead to ischemia and myocardial damage by raising oxygen requirements.

Sick sinus syndrome

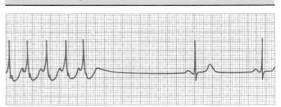

Causes
- Ischemic, rheumatic, or inflammatory disease, sinus node involvement by pericarditis; cardiomyopathy, especially amyloidosis; Friedreich's ataxia, progressive muscular dystrophy; collagen disease or metastasis. Possibly idiopathic.
- Surgical injury

Description
- Tachycardia and bradycardia may alternate and be interrupted by long sinus pauses, resulting in Stokes-Adams syndrome (decreased cerebral perfusion resulting in loss of consciousness).

Sinus arrhythmia

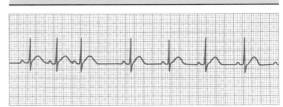

Causes
- Vagal effect of respiration on the heart rate increases with inspiration and decreases with expiration.
- From medication, as in digitalis toxicity

Description
- Difference between shortest and longest PP interval > 0.12 sec. (Difference shown in waveform 0.26 sec)
- P waves are identical.
- Rhythm varies.
- Impulse formation and conduction are normal.

Sinus arrest

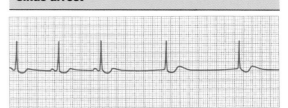

Causes
- Vagal stimulation, digitalis, acetylcholine, potassium, or quinidine toxicity
- Acute inferior wall myocardial infarction
- Often a sign of sick sinus syndrome
- Acute myocarditis

Description
- PP interval is not a multiple of the sinus cycle.
- Sinus node fails to generate impulse.
- Junctional escape beats occur frequently.

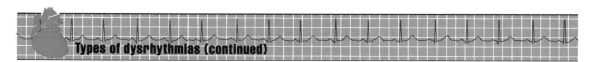

Types of dysrhythmias (continued)

Sinus exit block

Causes
• Vagal stimulation, digitalis, acetylcholine, potassium, or quinidine toxicity
• Acute inferior wall myocardial infarction
• Often a sign of sick sinus syndrome
• Acute myocarditis

Description
• Block occurs between actual discharge of the SA node and arrival of the impulse in atrial tissue.
• Block may be 1°, 2°, or 3°.
• 1° is concealed and may be indistinguishable from normal sinus rhythm.
• 2° may be Type I or Type II (see below).
• 3° is clinically indistinguishable from sinus arrest.

Second-degree sinoatrial exit block, Type I (Wenckebach)

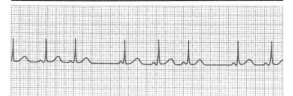

Causes
• Acute inferior wall myocardial infarction
• Often a sign of sick sinus syndrome
• Acute myocarditis

Description
• PP intervals progressively shorten until there is a pause in atrial activity.
• Duration of the pause is less than twice the shortest PP interval.
• Identical PR intervals occur as long as AV conduction is intact.

Second-degree sinoatrial block, Type II

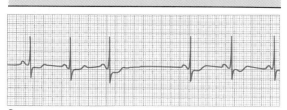

Causes
• Acute inferior wall myocardial infarction
• Often a sign of sick sinus syndrome
• Acute myocarditis

Description
• Blockage of the sinus impulse, unlike Type I, occurs without any preceding increase in conduction time.
• PP interval is twice the length of the basic sinus rhythm.

Wandering pacemaker

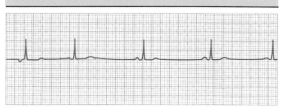

Causes
• May occur in normal heart
• Seen in rheumatic pancarditis as a result of inflammation involving the SA node, digitalis toxicity, sick sinus syndrome

Description
• Irregular P interval with changing P-wave configuration and PR intervals.
• Unchanged configuration of QRS complexes.
• Pacemaker travels downward from the SA node through the atrium, toward or into the AV junction. If pacemaker wanders to AV junction, P waves usually become inverted in leads II and III, and the PR < 0.12 sec.
• Rate varies.

Atrial dysrhythmias

Premature atrial contraction (PAC)

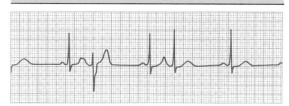

Causes
• Congestive heart failure, ischemic heart disease, acute respiratory failure, or COPD
• May result from treatment with digitalis, aminophylline, or adrenergic drugs; or from anxiety and excessive use of caffeine
• Occasional PAC may be normal

Description
• Premature, occasionally abnormal-looking P waves occur.
• QRS complexes follow, except in very early or blocked PACs.
• P wave is often buried in the preceding T wave and can often be identified in the preceding T wave.
• Premature beat may be conducted aberrantly, as shown.

continued

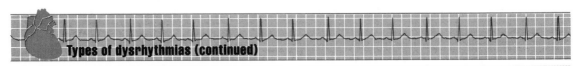

Types of dysrhythmias (continued)

Paroxysmal supraventricular tachycardia (PSVT) or paroxysmal atrial tachycardia

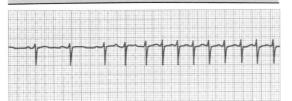

Causes
• May occur in otherwise normal, healthy persons with physical or psychologic stress, hypoxia, hypokalemia; may be associated with excessive use of caffeine or other stimulants, with use of marijuana, and with digitalis toxicity
• Intrinsic abnormality of AV conduction system; can be forerunner of more serious ventricular arrhythmia
• Congenital accessory atrial conduction pathway

Description
• Heart rate > 140 beats/minute; rarely exceeds 250 beats/minute.
• P waves are regular but aberrant; difficult to differentiate from preceding T wave.
• Onset and termination of dysrhythmia occur suddenly but may be prevented by tachycardia. Such tachycardia often begins during sleep and awakens the patient.
• PSVT may cause palpitations, light-headedness, and exhaustion.
• When atrial rate is exactly twice the ventricular rate, patient is said to have PSVT with 2:1 block (common in digitalis toxicity).

Atrial flutter

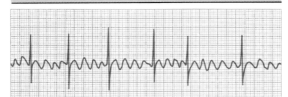

Causes
• Heart failure, valvular heart disease, pulmonary embolism, digitalis toxicity, postoperative coronary revascularization; atrial flutter is rare in the absence of organic heart disease.

Description
• Impulse arises from atrial ectopic foci.
• Ventricular rate (usually 60 to 100 beats/minute) depends on degree of AV block and is usually regular. Irregular ventricular rhythm may mean patient is ready to convert to atrial fibrillation (a favorable sign: atrial fibrillation is more responsive to drug therapy than atrial flutter).
• Atrial rate is 250 to 400 beats/minute and usually regular.
• QRS complexes are uniform in shape, can be regular or irregular depending on the degree of AV block.
• Flutter waves have sawtooth configuration.
• It may be difficult to distinguish between atrial flutter and coarse atrial fibrillation.

Atrial fibrillation

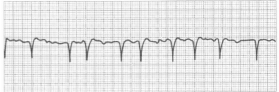

Causes
• Congestive heart failure, COPD, hyperthyroidism, hypertension, sepsis, pulmonary embolus, mitral valve disease, digitalis toxicity (rarely), atrial irritation, postcoronary bypass, or valve replacement surgery
• Cause often unknown

Description
• Impulse forms in atrial ectopic areas.
• Atrial rate > 400 beats/minute.
• Ventricular rate varies, and ventricular rhythm is grossly irregular.
• QRS complexes are uniform in shape, but the rhythm is irregular.
• No P waves; or P waves appear as erratic, irregular baseline f waves.

Junctional (nodal) dysrhythmias

Accelerated idiojunctional rhythm

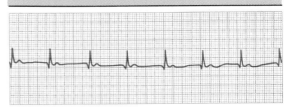

Causes
• Enhanced automaticity, usually from digitalis toxicity
• Inferior wall myocardial infarction or ischemia, hypoxia, vagal stimulation
• Acute rheumatic fever
• Valve replacement surgery

Description
• Rate: 60 to 100 beats/minute.
• Junctional dysrhythmias begin insidiously with few isolated PJCs.
• As junctional pacemaker begins to take over sinoatrial pacemaker, AV dissociation may occur—junctional focus paces the ventricles while the sinus node paces the atria.
• P waves may precede, be hidden within (absent), or follow QRS.

Junctional tachycardia

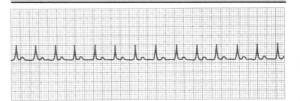

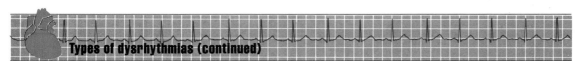

Types of dysrhythmias (continued)

Causes
• Digitalis toxicity, myocarditis, cardiomyopathy, myocardial ischemia, or infarct

Description
• Ventricular rate is 100 to 180 beats/minute (tracing shows 135 beats/minute).
• Onset of rhythm is often sudden, occurring in bursts.

Premature junctional contractions or complexes (PJC or PNC)

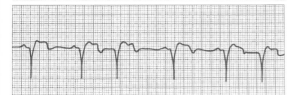

Causes
• Myocardial infarction or ischemia, excessive caffeine ingestion, and most commonly digitalis toxicity (from enhanced automaticity)

Description
• Underlying rhythm is sinus or atrial.
• QRS complexes are of uniform shape, but irregular rate.
• P waves are irregular, with premature beat; may precede at less than 0.12 sec, be hidden within or follow QRS, and distort ST segment.

Junctional escape complexes

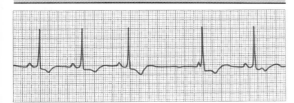

Causes
• Often follows pauses of nonconducted PACs, in second-degree heart block and in sinus bradycardia. Can be atrial or ventricular in origin.

Description
• Delayed arrival of the impulse from the prevailing rhythm occurs. (Tracing shows P wave distorting the T wave preceding the pause. QRS following the pause is junctional escape complex.)

Junctional (nodal) escape rhythms

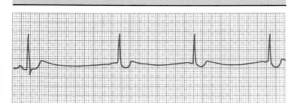

Causes
• Occurs to protect the heart whenever the sinus rhythm is too slow or in the presence of complete AV heart block.

Description
• Junctional escape rhythms may be accompanied by AV dissociation or complete heart block.

• P waves are either hidden in the QRS complex or missing because of retrograde block; may also precede at less than 0.12 sec or follow the QRS.

First-degree AV heart block

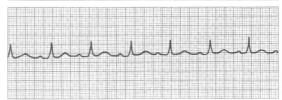

Causes
• Inferior myocardial ischemia or infarction, hypothyroidism, digitalis effect, potassium imbalance, rheumatic fever, coronary artery disease

Description
• PR interval is prolonged > 0.2 sec because of slowed AV node conduction.
• Normal rate, rhythm, QRS complex, and P wave occur.
• Usually no treatment is needed.

Second-degree AV heart block, Mobitz, Type I (Wenckebach)

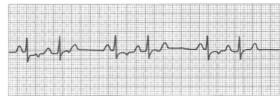

Causes
• Inferior wall myocardial infarction, digitalis or quinidine toxicity, vagal stimulation, and arteriosclerotic heart disease

Description
• Every second, third, or fourth impulse from the atria is fully blocked, creating a discrepancy between atrial and ventricular rates.
• PR interval becomes progressively longer with each cycle until QRS disappears (dropped beat). After a dropped beat, PR interval is shorter than preceding cycle.
• Ventricular rate is irregular; RR interval shortens.
• Atrial rhythm is regular.
• Second-degree may progress to third-degree heart block.

continued

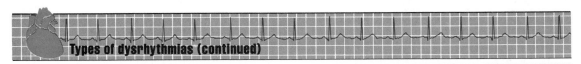

Types of dysrhythmias (continued)

Second-degree AV block, Mobitz, Type II

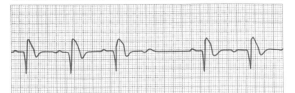

Causes
• Degenerative disease of conduction system, ischemia of AV node in anterior myocardial infarction, anteroseptal infarction, digitalis or quinidine toxicity

Description
• Every second, third, or fourth impulse from the atria is fully blocked, creating a discrepancy between atrial and ventricular rates.
• PR interval is constant, with QRS complex dropped at intervals.
• Ventricular rhythm may be irregular, with varying degrees of block.
• Second-degree may progress to third-degree heart block.
• Must have two or more conducted sinus impulses before the blocked P wave.

Third-degree AV block (complete heart block)

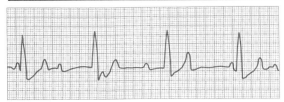

Causes
• Ischemic heart disease or infarction, postsurgical complications of mitral valve replacement, digitalis toxicity, hypoxia, congenital abnormalities, and infections, such as rheumatic fever

Description
• Atrial impulses are blocked at AV node; atrial and ventricular impulses dissociated; no relationship between P waves and QRS complexes.
• Atrial rate is regular; ventricular rate, slow and regular.
• No constant PR interval is present.
• QRS interval is normal (nodal pacemaker); wide (ventricular/infranodal pacemaker).
• Onset may initiate pause before ventricular pacemaker activates. During this pause, cardiac output decreases, causing syncope, or ventricular standstill (asystole) characterized by convulsions (Stokes-Adams syndrome). Sudden death will result if an artificial pacemaker is not used.

Atrioventricular dissociation

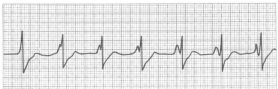

Causes
• Secondary to dysrhythmia from sinus slowing, AV junctional or ventricular acceleration, from sinoatrial or atrioventricular block, or combination of these conditions

Description
• Atria and ventricles are controlled by these inherent pacemakers; P rate $\simeq$ QRS rate.
• Changing relationship occurs between P waves and QRS complexes.

Preexcitation syndromes

Wolff-Parkinson-White syndrome (WPW)

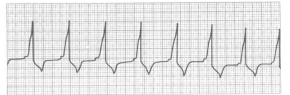

Causes
• Preexcitation of the ventricles because accessory conduction fiber (bundle of Kent) connects the atria and ventricles, bypassing the AV junction

Description
• Shortened PR interval (< 0.12 sec) occurs from ventricular preexcitation.
• Widened QRS complex gives superficial appearance of bundle branch block. QRS complex is as wide as PR interval is short.
• Delta wave—slurring or notching of QRS complex appears.
• Patient is prone to atrial dysrhythmias, particularly paroxysmal atrial tachycardia and atrial fibrillation.

Lown-Ganong-Levine syndrome (LGL)

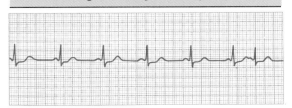

Causes
• Bypass tract (James fiber) connects the atria and AV junction

Description
• Short PR interval (< 0.12 sec) occurs with normal QRS (as shown by tracing). (Also shows PAC.)
• Patient may also have "reentrant" paroxysmal atrial tachycardia.

NURSE'S CLINICAL LIBRARY™
CARDIOVASCULAR DISORDERS

Cardiovascular Disorders gives you every bit of information you need to care for your cardiac patient with the utmost skill and confidence. No more will you have to go to one book for drug information, then another for current procedures, and still another for pathophysiology. Just open *Cardiovascular Disorders.* Everything you need is here:

- Assessment—you'll get valuable tips on history taking, inspection, palpation
- Symptoms—you'll get a comprehensive review of common signs, symptoms, and chief complaints
- Therapy—you'll learn the latest advances
- Drugs—you'll find all the drug information you need, *fast*
- Patient teaching—you'll get expert advice and illustrated aids you can photocopy
- And much more—nursing management, diagnostic tests, prognosis, anatomy, all in this one complete volume.

Send for this NURSE'S CLINICAL LIBRARY book now, then examine it for 10 days...FREE!

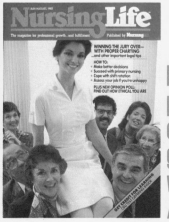

Keep your professional expertise growing with *NursingLife.*®

Mail the postage-paid card at right. ▶

Introduce yourself to the brand-new NURSE'S CLINICAL LIBRARY™ series.

NURSE'S CLINICAL LIBRARY gives you a single volume for disorders affecting each body system. No longer will you have to go to one book for drug information...then another for pathophysiology...then still another for the most current procedures. Everything you need to know to care for your renal, cardiac, cancer, or neurologic patients can be found in each separate volume of the NURSE'S CLINICAL LIBRARY. Each volume is about 190 pages long and brims with new and vital information on managing disorders. Almost every page has a clear, beautiful illustration amplifying important points for you. See the NURSE'S CLINICAL LIBRARY for yourself. Join this brand-new series today and examine each volume at your leisure for 10 days—*free!*

© 1983 Springhouse Corporation

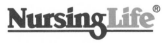
Mail the card at left to get your trial copy of *NursingLife.*

Send no money now. Just mail the card at left and we'll send you a trial copy of *NursingLife,* the fastest growing nursing journal in the world. You'll discover how to avoid malpractice suits, answer touchy ethical questions, get along better with doctors and other nurses, work better under pressure, and much more. Send for yours today!

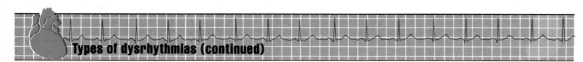

Types of dysrhythmias (continued)

Ventricular dysrhythmias

Premature ventricular contraction (PVC)

Interpolated PVCs

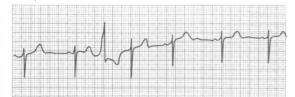

Multifocal PVCs

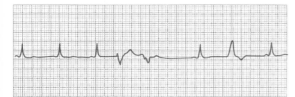

R-on-T phenomenon

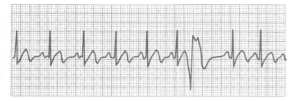

Causes
• Heart failure; old or acute myocardial infarction or contusion with trauma; myocardial irritation by ventricular catheter, such as a pacemaker or PA line; hypoxia, as in anemia and acute respiratory failure; drug toxicity (digitalis, aminophylline, tricyclic antidepressants, beta-adrenergics [isoproterenol or dopamine]); electrolyte imbalances (especially hypokalemia); and stress

Description
• Most common dysrhythmia
• PVC may be interpolated—falling exactly between two normal beats.
• Focus can be unifocal (same appearance in every lead) or multifocal (in serious organic heart disease).
• PVCs are most ominous when clustered, multifocal, with R wave on T pattern (may precipitate ventricular tachycardia or fibrillation).
• Beat occurs prematurely, usually followed by a complete compensatory pause after PVC; irregular pulse.
• QRS complex is wide (>0.14 sec) and distorted.
• Dysrhythmias can occur singly, in pairs, or in threes; and can alternate with normal beats as in ventricular bigeminy, one normal beat followed by a PVC, or trigeminy, two normal beats followed by PVC.
• Coupling interval—time between normal beat and PVC—is usually fixed, but may vary, especially if ectopic focus is "parasystolic."

Ventricular tachycardia

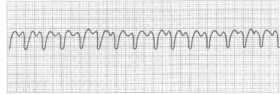

Causes
• Irritable ectopic focus in ventricles usurps pacemaker role because of myocardial ischemia, infarction; ventricular catheters, PA lines, or pacemaker catheters; digitalis or quinidine toxicity; hypokalemia; hypercalcemia; anxiety

Description
• Ventricular rate is 140 to 220 beats/minute; may be regular.
• QRS complexes are wide, bizarre, and independent of P waves. Rapidly occurring series of PVCs with no normal beats may have fusion beats in between.
• No visible P waves. (If visible, usually AV dissociation has occurred.)
• Because of dangerously low cardiac output, ventricular tachycardia can produce chest pain, anxiety, palpitations, dyspnea, shock, coma, and death; can lead to ventricular fibrillation.

Ventricular flutter

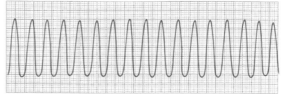

Causes
• Irritable ectopic focus in ventricles usurps pacemaker role because of myocardial ischemia, infarction, or aneurysm; ventricular catheters, PA lines, or pacemakers; digitalis or quinidine toxicity; hypokalemia; hypercalcemia; anxiety

Description
• Rapid ventricular tachycardia that gives a modified pattern in the EKG.
• QRS waves are continuous, in a regular zig-zag pattern; QRS cannot be distinguished from ST segment and T wave.

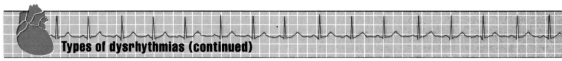

Types of dysrhythmias (continued)

Accelerated idioventricular rhythm (AIVR) or slow ventricular tachycardia

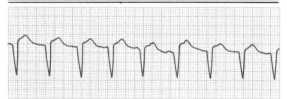

Causes
- Acute myocardial infarction
- Benign escape rhythm that competes with the underlying sinus mechanism (AIVR appears when sinus rate slows and disappears when sinus rate speeds up.)
- Very premature beats

Description
- Ventricular rate: 60 to 120 beats/minute.
- Wide QRS complexes occur without P waves.

Torsades de Pointes

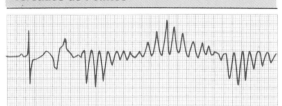

Causes
- Complete heart block, hereditary QT prolongation syndrome, low protein diets, myocardial ischemia, electrolyte imbalance (hypokalemia and hypomagnesemia prolong repolarization), drug toxicity (particularly quinidine, pronestyl, and related antiarrhythmics such as disopyramide), and psychotropic drugs (phenothiazines and tricyclic antidepressants)

Description
- Twisting of the points—QRS complexes appear to rotate cyclically in opposite directions across baseline. In the same row, complexes point downward for several beats and then turn upward for several beats.
- Associated delayed ventricular repolarization is shown by *prolonged QT interval* or prominent QT interval (tracing shows QT prolongation [0.52 sec]).

Ventricular fibrillation

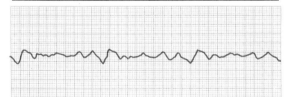

Causes
- Myocardial ischemia or infarction; untreated ventricular tachycardia; electrolyte imbalances (hypokalemia and alkalosis, hyperkalemia and hypercalcemia); digitalis (rarely), epinephrine, or quinidine toxicity; electric shock; hypothermia

Description
- Ventricular rhythm is rapid and chaotic.
- QRS complexes are not identifiable.

- Loss of consciousness, with no peripheral pulses, blood pressure, or respirations; possible seizures, and sudden death within minutes if treatment is unavailable.

Ventricular conduction dysrhythmias

Right bundle branch block (RBBB)

V₁   V₆

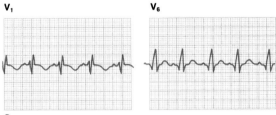

Causes
- Ischemia, hypokalemia, digitalis toxicity

Description
- After left ventricle depolarizes, right ventricle continues to depolarize, producing third phase of ventricular stimulation.
- Triphasic complexes seen in chest leads—lead V₁ shows an rSR¹ complex with a wide R¹ wave, and lead V₆ shows a QRS pattern with a wide S wave.
- Complete RBBB shows a QRS complex (rSR¹ complex in lead V₁ and QRS complex in lead V₆) of 0.12 sec or more in width.
- Incomplete RBBB shows QRS duration between 0.10 and 0.12 sec.

Left bundle branch block (LBBB)

V₁   V₆

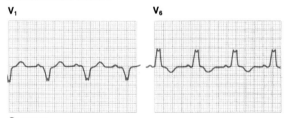

Causes
- Ischemia, infarction, hypokalemia, digitalis toxicity (rarely)

Description
- LBBB blocks the normal pattern of septal depolarization. Septum depolarizes from right to left instead of from left to right.
- Lead V₁ shows wide, entirely negative QS complex (rarely a wide rS complex).
- Lead V₆ shows wide, tall R wave without a Q wave.
- Complete LBBB shows QRS ≥ 0.12.
- Incomplete LBBB shows QRS varies between 0.10 to 0.12 sec.

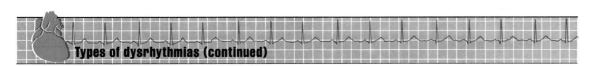

Types of dysrhythmias (continued)

Hemiblocks
(partial blocks in the left bundle system involving either the anterior or posterior fascicle)

Left anterior hemiblock

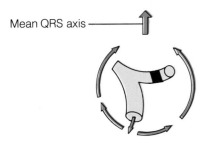

Mean QRS axis —

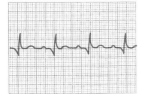 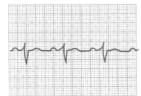

Lead I   **Lead III**

Causes
• Relatively common
• Ischemia, infarction, hypokalemia, degeneration of cardiac skeleton

Description
• Conduction through left anterior fascicle (left bundle divides into two fascicles) is blocked.
• Mean QRS axis $> -45°$ (left axis deviation).
• QRS width is normal or prolonged.
• Q wave occurs in lead I (QR pattern); RS pattern in lead III.

Left posterior hemiblock

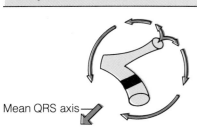

Mean QRS axis —

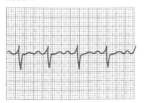 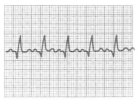

Lead I   **Lead III**

Causes
• Rare
• Sometimes a normal variant
• Ischemia, infarction, hypokalemia, degeneration of cardiac skeleton

Description
• Conduction through left posterior fascicle (left bundle divides into two fascicles) is blocked.
• Mean QRS axis $\geq +120°$ (right axis deviation).
• QRS width is normal or prolonged.
• Initial R wave and terminal S wave occur in lead I; initial Q wave in lead III.

Aberrant conduction

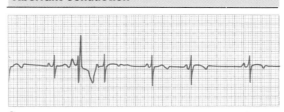

Causes
• Refractory period varies between two ventricles, so during rapid rates, or after premature beats, AV nodal stimulus carries from one ventricle to the other, with a change in the conduction pattern and a delay.

Description
• Temporary abnormal intraventricular conduction of supraventricular impulses occurs.
• Often associated with bundle branch block.

Pacemaker patterns

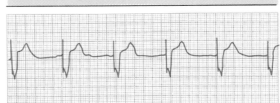

Causes
• Pacemaker delays activation of left ventricle, since electrode placed in right ventricle stimulates it (right ventricle) first.

Description
• Paced QRS complex resembles LBBB.
• Shows pacer spike.

Points to remember

• Dysrhythmias are becoming more common, possibly because improved monitoring techniques are detecting them more often.
• Dysrhythmias are generally classified according to their site of origin (ventricular or supraventricular). Ventricular dysrhythmias are potentially more life-threatening than supraventricular dysrhythmias.
• To manage dysrhythmia correctly, you must understand mechanisms of cardiac conduction and know how they are expressed in EKGs so you can identify dysrhythmias accurately.
• After recognizing dysrhythmia, you must accurately assess the patient's cardiac, electrolyte, and overall clinical status, noting especially whether the dysrhythmia is life-threatening.
• New advances in the treatment and detection of dysrhythmias—new antiarrhythmic drugs, cardiac pacemakers, electrical cardioversion, cardiopulmonary resuscitation, and endocardial stripping (for ventricular dysrhythmias)—offer a brighter outlook.

APPENDIX A

Common congenital heart defects

A congenital heart defect is an abnormality in the heart's structure. By the eighth week of embryonic development, the heart is well formed. Normally, the foramen ovale (opening between the atria) and ductus arteriosus (prenatal channel between the aorta and pulmonary artery) remain patent to shunt blood away from unexpanded fetal lungs. Soon after birth, these openings close and normal extrauterine circulation is achieved.

With normal cardiovascular development, the heart's low pressure right side receives unoxygenated blood from the body and delivers it to the lungs for reoxygenation; in turn, the heart's high pressure left side receives oxygenated blood from the lungs and delivers it to all body parts. But improper development can obstruct or alter this blood-flow pattern. The result? A congenital defect—either acyanotic or cyanotic. Acyanotic defects shunt oxygenated blood from the left to the right heart, but do not mix unoxygenated blood in the systemic circulation. Cyanotic defects shunt blood from the right to the left heart and permit unoxygenated blood to flow from the left ventricle to all parts of the body, resulting in cyanosis.

To identify a congenital heart defect, take a careful history and make a thorough assessment. Always be alert for signs of inadequate oxygenation, such as cyanosis, nail-bed clubbing, and labored breathing. Also, watch for inadequate cardiac output and CHF, murmurs, and easy fatigability. If a congenital heart defect has been diagnosed, help parents to understand and accept the condition and teach them to prevent complications.

Congenital defect	Assessment findings
Ventricular septal defect (VSD) Abnormal opening in the ventricular septum allows shunting of oxygenated blood from left ventricle to mix with unoxygenated blood in right ventricle. Results from inadequate development of septal tissue during fetal life. Defect varies from size of pinhole to absence of entire septum. Most defects are small and close spontaneously by ages 4 to 6. May cause pulmonary artery hypertension in sizable left-to-right shunts.	**History:** In small VSD, unremarkable. In medium-size VSD, increased susceptibility to respiratory infection and easy fatigability. In large VSD, feeding difficulty, poor weight gain, frequent respiratory infections, and markedly increased fatigability. **Inspection:** In large VSD, child is thin, small, and tachypneic, with prominent anterior chest wall and active precordium. **Palpation:** In small VSD, cardiac thrill at left sternal border. In medium-size VSD, possible liver enlargement from CHF; PMI displaced to left, with significant cardiomegaly. **Auscultation:** In small VSD, loud, harsh systolic murmur at left sternal border. In medium to large VSD, rumbling systolic murmur heard best at lower left sternal border; loud, widely split S_2. With pulmonary artery hypertension, quieter murmur but loud, booming pulmonic S_2.
Atrial septal defect (ASD) One or more openings between the atria (includes ostium secundum, ostium primum, and sinus venosus) allow blood to shunt from left to right. Condition caused by delayed or incomplete closure of foramen ovale or atrial septum. Results in right heart volume overload. Depending on size of the defect, it often goes undetected in preschoolers and may lead to CHF and pulmonary vascular disease in adults.	**History:** In child, usually good health and growth; at times, frequent respiratory tract infections and fatigability after extreme exertion. In child with ostium primum, feeding difficulty, dyspnea, frequent respiratory infections. In adult, pronounced fatigability and dyspnea on exertion (after age 40); syncope and hemoptysis in severe pulmonary vascular disease. **Inspection:** In child with ostium primum, growth retardation. In adult, cyanosis and clubbing of fingers. **Palpation:** Possible thrill accompanies murmur. **Auscultation:** In a child, soft early to mid-systolic murmur, heard at second or third left intercostal space; fixed and widely split S_2. In large shunts, low-pitched diastolic murmur heard at lower left sternal border. In older patients with large ASD and obstructive pulmonary vascular disease, right ventricular hypertrophy with accentuated S_2, and fixed wide splitting; possible pulmonary ejection click and audible S_4.
Patent ductus arteriosus (PDA) Patent duct between the descending aorta and pulmonary artery bifurcation allows left-to-right shunting of blood from aorta to pulmonary artery. Caused by failure of the ductus to close after birth. Results in recirculation of arterial blood through lungs and increased left-heart work load. In time, can precipitate pulmonary vascular disease and infective endocarditis.	**History:** In premature infant, frank CHF. In child, mild symptoms of heart disease, such as frequent respiratory tract infections, slow motor development, and fatigability. In adult, fatigability and dyspnea on exertion (by age 40). **Inspection:** In premature infant, signs of CHF. **Palpation:** In infant or child with large PDA, possible thrill at left sternal border and a prominent left ventricular impulse. **Auscultation:** Loud, continuous machinery murmur heard at left upper sternal border and under left clavicle that may obscure S_1; S_3 in CHF; widened pulse pressure.
Coarctation of aorta Constriction of the aorta near the site of the ligamentum arteriosum (remnant of the fetal ductus arteriosus). May be classified as preductal or postductal. It may result from spasm and constriction of smooth muscle in ductus arteriosus as it closes, or from abnormal development of aortic arch.	**History:** In infant with preductal coarctation: signs of CHF. In some infants with postductal coarctation: possible CHF in first few months of life. In others: normal growth and health. In some children: headaches, epistaxis, fatigue, or cold feet. In adult: dyspnea, syncope, claudication, headaches, and leg cramps. **Inspection:** Infant often displays signs of CHF; peripheral cyanosis in end stages of severe untreated coarctation. In adolescents, visible aortic pulsations in suprasternal notch due to collateral circulation. **Palpation:** Hepatomegaly in infant with CHF. Increased amplitude of peripheral pulses in arms; weak, absent, or delayed pulses in legs. **Auscultation:** In preductal coarctation, normal heart sounds and absence of murmurs. In CHF, S_3 or S_4. In postductal coarctation, continuous systolic murmur over back if collateral circulation is extensive. In severe coarctation, loud S_2.
Tetralogy of Fallot Four defects: ventricular septal defect (VSD), overriding aorta, pulmonary stenosis, right ventricular hypertrophy. Results from incomplete development of ventricular septum and pulmonic outflow tract. Coexisting VSD and obstructed blood flow from right ventricle cause unoxygenated blood to shunt right to left, and to mix with oxygenated blood, resulting in cyanosis.	**History:** After 3 to 6 months, cyanosis. In some infants: intense cyanotic "blue" spells (dyspnea, deep sighing respirations, bradycardia, fainting, seizures, loss of consciousness), precipitated by awakening, crying, straining, infection, or fever. In older child: decreased exercise tolerance, increased dyspnea on exertion, growth retardation, eating difficulties, squatting when short of breath. **Inspection:** Remarkable cyanosis, even during rest. Older child displays clubbing of fingers and toes. **Palpation:** Thrill along left sternal border. Prominent right ventricular impulse or heave at inferior septum. **Auscultation:** Loud systolic murmur along entire left sternal border, which may diminish or obscure pulmonic component of S_2. Possible continuous murmur over back if extensive pulmonary collateral circulation develops.
Transposition of the great arteries Great arteries are reversed: aorta leaves right ventricle and pulmonary artery leaves left ventricle, producing two noncommunicating circulatory systems. Unoxygenated blood flows through right atrium and ventricle and out the aorta to systemic circulation; oxygenated blood flows from lungs to left atrium and ventricle and out the pulmonary artery to lungs.	**History:** In infant, cyanosis. In older child, cyanosis, frequent respiratory infections, diminished exercise tolerance, fatigability. **Inspection:** In infant, cyanosis, tachypnea, dyspnea (worsens with crying); poor feeding. In older child, dyspnea and clubbing of fingers. **Palpation:** Hepatomegaly due to CHF. **Auscultation:** S_2 louder than normal, but no murmur during first days of life. Murmurs may later be associated with ASD, VSD, PDA, or pulmonary stenosis. Gallop rhythm possible with CHF.

Diagnostic tests

Chest X-ray: In small VSD, normal. In medium-size to large VSD, enlarged left atrium and left ventricle, prominent pulmonary vascular markings. With pulmonary artery hypertension, enlarged right atrium and ventricle and pulmonary artery.
EKG: In small VSD, normal. In medium-size to large VSD, left ventricular hypertrophy. With pulmonary artery hypertension, right ventricular hypertrophy.
Echocardiography: May detect VSD and its location, determine size of left-to-right shunt, and suggest pulmonary hypertension; more useful in identifying associated lesions and complications.
Cardiac catheterization: Confirms size of VSD; calculates degree of shunting; determines extent of pulmonary hypertension; detects associated defects.

Chest X-ray: Enlarged right atrium and right ventricle and prominent pulmonary artery, increased pulmonary vasculature, small aorta.
EKG: May be normal, but prolonged PR interval, right axis deviation, varying degrees of right bundle branch block, right ventricular hypertrophy, and, in ostium primum, left axis deviation. In adult, possible atrial fibrillation.
Echocardiography: Measures extent of right ventricular enlargement and may locate ASD.
Cardiac catheterization: Confirms ASD, determines volume of shunting, and detects pulmonary vascular disease.

Chest X-ray: Increased pulmonary vascular markings and prominent pulmonary arteries. If shunt is large, enlarged left atrium, left ventricle and aorta.
EKG: May be normal or show left ventricular hypertrophy.
Echocardiography: Detects PDA and reveals enlarged left atrium and left ventricle.
Cardiac catheterization: Shows PDA. Increased PA pressure indicates large shunt, or, if PA pressure exceeds systemic arterial pressure, severe pulmonary vascular disease. Allows calculation of blood volume crossing ductus.

Chest X-ray: In preductal coarctation, shows cardiomegaly. In postductal coarctation, shows enlarged left atrium and ventricle and dilated ascending aorta.
EKG: In preductal coarctation, shows right ventricular hypertrophy. In postductal coarctation, shows left ventricular hypertrophy.
Echocardiography: May show increased left ventricular muscle thickness, aortic valve abnormalities, site of defect, and associated defects.
Cardiac catheterization: Locates site of defect, evaluates collateral circulation, measures pressure in the left and right ventricles and in ascending and descending aortas, and detects associated defects.
Aortography: Locates site of defect.

Chest X-ray: Normal cardiac size, decreased pulmonary vascular markings, and a boot-shaped cardiac silhouette.
EKG: Shows right ventricular hypertrophy, right axis deviation, and, occasionally, right atrial hypertrophy.
Echocardiography: Identifies VSD and pulmonary stenosis. Detects enlarged right ventricle and displaced aorta.
Cardiac catheterization: Confirms diagnosis by detecting pulmonary stenosis and VSD, visualizing overriding aorta, and ruling out other cyanotic heart defects.

Chest X-ray: Often normal in first days of life. Within days or weeks, enlarged right atrium and right ventricle (oblong shape). Also shows increased pulmonary vascular markings.
EKG: May be normal in first days of life. Later, reveals right axis deviation, right ventricular hypertrophy, and possibly right atrial hypertrophy.
Echocardiography: Demonstrates reversed aorta and pulmonary artery, and records echoes from both semilunar valves simultaneously, because of aortic valve displacement.

Treatment

Medical: In small VSD, conservative management. In medium-size to large VSD, bed rest, oxygen, digoxin, diuretics, and fluid restrictions for acute CHF; prophylactic antibiotics to prevent infective endocarditis; monitoring to detect pulmonary artery hypertension.
Surgical: In medium-size to large VSD, closure or patch graft, using cardiopulmonary bypass and deep hypothermia, during preschool years.

Medical: Not usually necessary, except in ostium primum with accompanying CHF.
Surgical: Direct closure or patch graft recommended during preschool or early school-age years.

Medical: CHF regimen; cardiac catheterization deposits a plug in ductus to stop shunting; administration of indomethacin (a prostaglandin inhibitor) induces ductus spasm and closure.
Surgical: In infant with CHF who fails to respond to treatment, ductal ligation. After age 1, ligation and division of ductus.

Medical: In infant with preductal coarctation, CHF regimen. Balloon angioplasty shows promise in relieving this anomaly in infants. A balloon-tipped catheter is advanced through the femoral artery up the aorta to the area of coarctation. The balloon is rapidly inflated and deflated many times, forcing open the area of coarctation.
Surgical: Resection with anastomosis of aorta or insertion of prosthetic graft usually recommended between ages 4 and 8, unless unmanageable CHF develops in infant with preductal coarctation.

Medical: Avoidance of cyanosis is key objective. If it occurs, knee-chest position and administration of oxygen and morphine improve oxygenation. Administration of propranolol may relieve spasm of right ventricular outflow tract and improve oxygen saturation. Prophylactic antibiotics aim to prevent infective endocarditis. Continuous assessment aims to detect other serious bacterial infections and polycythemia.
Surgical: Palliative surgery, such as Blalock-Taussig, Potts-Smith-Gibson, or Waterston procedures, enhances blood flow to lungs to reduce hypoxia. Corrective surgery relieves pulmonary stenosis and closes VSD. Administration of prophylactic antibiotics continues after surgery.

Medical: Balloon septostomy enlarges foramen ovale and improves oxygenation; CHF regimen; administration of alprostadil maintains open ductus arteriosus in newborns.
Surgical: Recommended during first years of life, Mustard or Senny procedure redirects venous return to appropriate ventricle.

Ventricular septal defect

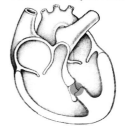

Atrial septal defect

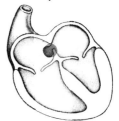

Patent ductus arteriosus

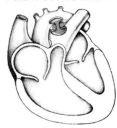

Coarctation of aorta

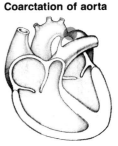

Tetralogy of Fallot

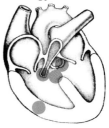

Transposition of great arteries

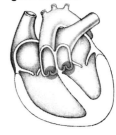

APPENDIX B

Cardiovascular drugs

Antianginals

Drug, dose, and route	Interactions	Side effects	Special considerations
diltiazem 30 to 60 mg P.O. q.i.d.	*Beta-adrenergic blockers:* increased risk of congestive heart failure.	Headache, fatigue, drowsiness, edema, dysrhythmias, nausea, skin rash.	If nitrate therapy is prescribed during titration of diltiazem dosage, urge patient to continue compliance. Sublingual nitroglycerin, especially, may be taken concomitantly as needed when anginal symptoms are acute.
isosorbide dinitrate 2.5 to 10 mg q 2 to 3 hours p.r.n. sublingual or chewable form; 5 to 30 mg P.O. q.i.d. for prophylaxis.	*Ergot alkaloids:* increased toxic effects.	Throbbing headache, dizziness, orthostatic hypotension, tachycardia, palpitations, ankle edema, flushing.	Monitor blood pressure, and intensity and duration of response to drug. Additional dose may be taken before anticipated stress or at bedtime if angina is nocturnal. Warn patient not to confuse sublingual with oral form. Advise him to avoid alcoholic beverages. 　Teach patient to take sublingual tablet at first sign of attack. He should wet the tablet with saliva, place it under the tongue until completely absorbed, and sit down and rest. Burning sensation indicates potency. Dose may be repeated every 10 to 15 minutes for a maximum of three doses. If no relief, patient should call doctor or go to hospital emergency room.
nadolol 80 to 240 mg P.O. once daily.	*Prazosin:* increased hypotension. *Lidocaine:* increased blood levels. *Theophyllines:* decreased therapeutic effect. *Indomethacin:* decreased therapeutic effect of nadolol.	Bradycardia, hypotension, congestive heart failure, increased airway resistance.	Always check apical pulse before giving drug. If slower than 60 beats/minute, hold drug and call doctor. Monitor blood pressure frequently. If patient develops severe hypotension, give a vasopressor, as ordered. 　Don't discontinue abruptly: can exacerbate angina and MI. This drug masks common signs of shock and hypoglycemia. May be given without regard to meals.
nifedipine 10 to 30 mg P.O. q.i.d.	*Beta-adrenergic blockers:* increased risk of congestive heart failure.	Dizziness, light-headedness, flushing, headache, nausea, heartburn.	Monitor blood pressure regularly, especially of patient who is also taking beta blockers or antihypertensives. Patient may briefly develop anginal exacerbation when beginning drug therapy or at times of dosage increase. Reassure him that this symptom is temporary. If patient is kept on nitrate therapy while drug dosage is being titrated, urge him to continue his compliance. Sublingual nitroglycerin, especially, may be taken as needed when anginal symptoms are acute. Instruct patient to swallow capsule whole without breaking, crushing, or chewing.
nitroglycerin 0.15 to 0.6 mg sublingually q 5 minutes p.r.n.; 1 to 2 inches ointment q 4 hours; 5 to 10 mg transdermal patch applied q 24 hours.	*Ergot alkaloids:* increased toxic effects.	Throbbing headache, dizziness, orthostatic hypotension, tachycardia, flushing, palpitations.	Monitor blood pressure, and intensity and duration of response to drug. Advise patient to avoid alcohol. Only sublingual form should be used in acute attack. Teach patient to take tablet at first sign of attack. If no relief, he should call doctor or go to emergency room. 　To apply ointment, spread in uniform thin layer on any nonhairy area. Do not rub in. Cover with plastic film to aid absorption and to protect clothing. 　Transdermal dosage forms can be applied to any hairless part of the skin except distal parts of the arms or legs, because absorption is poorer at these sites.
propranolol hydrochloride 80 to 160 mg P.O. daily in single dose (sustained-action capsule) or divided doses.	*Prazosin:* increased hypotension. *Lidocaine:* increased blood levels. Monitor for toxicity. *Theophyllines:* decreased therapeutic effect. *Barbiturates, indomethacin, rifampin, thyroid hormones:* decreased pharmacologic effect of propranolol. *Chlorpromazine, cimetidine, oral contraceptives:* increased pharmacologic effect of propranolol.	Fatigue, bradycardia, hypotension, congestive heart failure, increased airway resistance.	Always check patient's apical pulse rate before giving this drug. If you detect extremes in pulse rates, hold medication and call the doctor immediately. If patient develops hypotension, monitor blood pressure frequently. 　Don't discontinue abruptly; can exacerbate angina and MI. This drug masks common signs of shock and hypoglycemia. Food may increase the absorption of propranolol. Give consistently with meals.
verapamil 240 to 480 mg P.O. daily in divided doses.	*Beta-adrenergic blockers:* increased risk of congestive heart failure. Use together cautiously. *Digoxin:* elevated blood level. Monitor for toxicity. *Quinidine:* don't use together in cardiomyopathy. May cause hypotension.	Hypotension, heart failure, heart block, asystole.	Notify doctor if signs of CHF occur. If patient is kept on nitrate therapy while dosage of verapamil is being titrated, urge him to continue compliance. Sublingual nitroglycerin, especially, may be taken as needed when anginal symptoms are acute.

Antiarrhythmics

Drug, dose, and route	Interactions	Side effects	Special considerations
bretylium 5 to 10 mg/kg I.V. q 15 to 30 minutes to maximum of 30 mg/kg followed by maintenance dose of 5 to 10 mg/kg q 6 to 8 hours I.V. or I.M.	None significant.	Severe orthostatic hypotension and syncope, bradycardia, vertigo, dizziness.	Monitor blood pressure, heart rate, and rhythm frequently. Notify doctor immediately of significant changes. Keep patient supine until he develops tolerance to hypotension. Give I.V. injections for ventricular fibrillation as rapidly as possible; do not dilute. Rotate I.M. injection sites to prevent tissue damage, and don't exceed 5-ml volume in any one site.
disopyramide 4 mg/kg P.O. followed by maintenance dose of 100 to 200 mg q 6 hours.	*Ethotoin, mephenytoin, phenytoin, rifampin:* decreased disopyramide blood levels.	Anticholinergic effects, blurred vision; dry eyes, mouth, and nose; urinary retention; hypotension; heart failure; heart block.	Check apical pulse before administering drug. Notify doctor if pulse rate is slower than 60 beats/minute or faster than 120 beats/minute. Discontinue if heart block develops, if QRS complex widens by more than 25%, or if QT interval lengthens by more than 25%.
lidocaine 1 to 1.5 mg/kg I.V. bolus. Repeat q 3 to 5 minutes. Don't exceed 300 mg total bolus during 1-hour period. Follow with maintenance infusion of 1 to 4 mg/minute.	*Procainamide:* increased neurologic side effects. *Beta-adrenergic blockers, cimetidine:* increased pharmacologic effect of lidocaine. *Succinylcholine:* increased neuromuscular blocking effects.	Confusion, stupor, restlessness, light-headedness, convulsions, hypotension, tinnitus, blurred vision.	In severely ill patient, convulsions may be first toxic sign. If toxic signs occur, stop drug and notify doctor. During infusion, *always* remain with patient and check cardiac monitor. Use an infusion pump or a microdrip system and timer for monitoring precisely. Never exceed an infusion rate of 4 mg/minute, if possible. A faster rate greatly increases risk of toxicity. A bolus dose not followed by infusion will have a short-lived effect.
phenytoin 250 mg I.V. over 5 minutes until dysrhythmias subside (up to maximum dose of 1 g), or 1 g P.O. over 4 hours. Followed by maintenance dose of 200 to 400 mg I.V. or P.O. daily.	*Alcohol, barbiturates, folic acid, loxapine:* monitor for decreased phenytoin activity. *Oral anticoagulants, antihistamines, chloramphenicol, diazepam, diazoxide, disulfiram, isoniazid, phenylbutazone, salicylates, sulfonamides, cimetidine, trimethoprim, valproic acid:* monitor for increased phenytoin activity. *Corticosteroids:* may need higher dose. *Levodopa:* may need higher dose. *Primidone:* increased primidone toxicity. *Quinidine:* decreased pharmacologic action. *Theophyllines:* decreased pharmacologic effects of both drugs.	Ataxia, nystagmus, lethargy, blood dyscrasias, severe hypotension, and vascular collapse (if given too rapidly by I.V.).	Watch patients on phenytoin and other anti-arrhythmics (disopyramide, quinidine, procainamide, propranolol) closely for signs of additive cardiac depression. Phenytoin can be diluted in normal saline solution and infused without precipitation. Such infusions should not take longer than 1 hour. Don't mix with 5% dextrose I.V. fluids, as crystallization will occur. Flush I.V. line with saline solution before and after administration. Administer drug by slow I.V. push, not to exceed 50 mg/minute in adults.
procainamide 100 mg q 5 minutes by slow I.V. push to maximum of 1 g (or 1 to 1.25 g P.O.), followed by I.V. infusion of 2 to 6 mg/minute. Maintenance P.O. dose is 500 mg to 1 g q 4 to 6 hours.	None significant.	Lupus-like syndrome, blood dyscrasias, hypotension, nausea, vomiting, maculopapular rash.	Continuously observe patient. Use an infusion pump or a microdrip system and timer to monitor the infusion precisely. Monitor blood pressure and EKG continuously during I.V. administration. Watch for prolonged QT and QR intervals, heart block, or increased dysrhythmias. If these occur, withhold drug, obtain rhythm strip, and notify doctor immediately. Teach patient importance of taking drug exactly as prescribed.
propranolol hydrochloride 1 to 5 mg I.V. infused slowly, not to exceed 1 mg/minute. Oral maintenance dose is 10 to 80 mg t.i.d. or q.i.d.	*Prazosin:* increased hypotension. *Lidocaine:* increased pharmacologic effect. Monitor for toxicity. *Theophyllines:* decreased therapeutic effect. *Barbiturates, indomethacin, rifampin, thyroid hormones:* decreased pharmacologic effect of propranolol. *Chlorpromazine, cimetidine, oral contraceptives:* increased pharmacologic effect of propranolol.	Heart block, bradycardia, hypotension, heart failure, asthma, fatigue.	Check apical pulse and blood pressure before giving drug. If you detect extremes in pulse rate, withhold drug and notify doctor. Monitor patient daily for weight gain and peripheral edema. Auscultate for rales and S_3 or S_4. If these develop, notify doctor. Always withdraw drug slowly. Abrupt withdrawal might precipitate MI or aggravate angina, thyrotoxicosis or pheochromocytoma. Before any surgery, notify anesthesiologist that patient is receiving drug. Double-check dose and route. I.V. doses much smaller than P.O.
quinidine (all salts) 200 to 400 mg P.O. (quinidine sulfate or equivalent base) q 4 to 6 hours.	*Acetazolamide, antacids, sodium bicarbonate:* increased quinidine blood levels due to alkaline urine. *Barbiturates, phenytoin, rifampin:* antagonized quinidine activity. *Verapamil:* don't use together in cardiomyopathy. May cause hypotension. *Digoxin:* increased toxicity. *Oral anticoagulants:* increased pharmacologic effect. Monitor prothrombin time.	Diarrhea, nausea, vomiting, cinchonism, thrombocytopenia, hypertension, heart block, EKG changes.	Use with caution in digitalized patients. Monitor digitalis levels. GI side effects, especially diarrhea, indicate toxicity. Notify doctor if these occur. GI symptoms may be decreased by giving with meals. Instruct patient to notify doctor if skin rash, fever, unusual bleeding, bruising, tinnitus, or visual disturbance occurs.
verapamil 5 to 10 mg I.V. bolus over 2 to 3 minutes followed by a maintenance infusion.	*Quinidine:* don't use together in cardiomyopathy. May cause hypotension. *Digoxin:* increased blood levels. *Beta-adrenergic blockers:* increased risk of congestive heart failure.	Hypotension, heart failure, heart block, asystole.	Patient with severely compromised cardiac function or patient receiving beta blockers should receive lower doses of verapamil. Monitor these patients closely. In older patients, give I.V. doses over at least 3 minutes to minimize the risk of adverse effects. Notify doctor if signs of congestive heart failure occur.

Antihypertensives

Drug, dose, and route	Interactions	Side effects	Special considerations
atenolol 50 to 100 mg P.O. daily as a single dose.	*Prazosin:* increased hypotension. *Lidocaine:* increased blood levels. *Indomethacin:* decreased antihypertensive effect. Monitor blood pressure and adjust dosage. *Theophyllines:* decreased therapeutic effect.	Bradycardia, hypotension, congestive heart failure.	Always check patient's apical pulse before giving this drug; if slower than 60 beats/minute, hold drug and call doctor. Monitor blood pressure frequently. 　Explain importance of taking drug, even when patient feels well. Tell him not to discontinue drug suddenly, but to call doctor if unpleasant side effects develop. Counsel patient to take drug at regular time each day.
captopril 25 to 50 mg P.O. t.i.d.	None significant.	Leukopenia, hypotension, loss of taste, proteinuria, renal failure, skin rash.	Question patient about impaired taste sensation. Should be taken 1 hour before meals. Monitor blood pressure and pulse rate frequently.
clonidine hydrochloride 0.2 to 0.8 mg P.O. daily in divided doses.	*Tricyclic antidepressants:* decreased antihypertensive effect.	Drowsiness, mouth dryness, constipation, orthostatic hypotension.	Monitor blood pressure and pulse rate frequently. Dosage is usually adjusted to patient's blood pressure and tolerance. May be given to rapidly lower blood pressure in some hypertensive emergencies. Advise patient to avoid sudden position changes. Tell him to take last dose just before retiring.
diazoxide 300 mg I.V. bolus push, administered in 30 seconds or less into peripheral vein.	*Thiazide diuretics:* increased effects of diazoxide.	Sodium and water retention, orthostatic hypotension, nausea, vomiting, hyperglycemia, headaches.	Monitor blood pressure frequently. Notify doctor immediately if severe hypotension develops. Keep norepinephrine available. Monitor intake and output. Weigh patient daily and report any increase. Watch diabetics for severe hyperglycemia or hyperosmolar nonketotic coma.
guanabenz acetate 4 to 8 mg P.O. b.i.d.	*CNS depressants:* increased sedation.	Drowsiness, sedation, dizziness, weakness, mouth dryness.	Advise patient to drive a car or operate machinery cautiously until CNS effects are known. Warn that tolerance to alcohol or CNS depressants may decrease.
guanadrel sulfate 20 to 75 mg P.O. daily in divided doses.	*MAO inhibitors, sympathomimetics, methylphenidate, phenothiazines, tricyclic antidepressants:* decreased antihypertensive action.	Fatigue, dizziness, orthostatic hypotension.	Monitor supine and standing blood pressure, especially during dosage adjustment. Tell outpatient to avoid strenuous exercise and hot showers. Inform patient that orthostatic hypotension can be minimized by avoiding sudden position changes.
guanethidine sulfate 25 to 50 mg P.O. daily.	*MAO inhibitors, sympathomimetics, methylphenidate, phenothiazines, tricyclic antidepressants:* decreased antihypertensive action.	Dizziness, weakness, orthostatic hypotension, nasal stuffiness, diarrhea, edema, weight gain, inhibition of ejaculation.	Tell outpatient to avoid strenuous exercise, and warn that hot showers may cause hypotensive reaction. Inform patient that orthostatic hypotension can be minimized by rising slowly and avoiding sudden position changes. Give this drug with meals to increase absorption.
hydralazine hydrochloride 10 to 50 mg P.O. q.i.d. 10 to 20 mg I.M. or I.V. q 4 hours. Switch to oral administration.	None significant.	Sodium retention and weight gain, lupus erythematosus-like syndrome, headache, tachycardia, angina.	Monitor patient's blood pressure and pulse rate frequently. Watch closely for signs of lupus erythematosus-like syndrome (sore throat, fever, muscle and joint aches, skin rash). Call doctor immediately if any of these develop. Give this drug with meals to increase absorption.
methyldopa 500 mg to 2 g P.O. daily in divided doses; 500 mg to 1 g q 6 hours, diluted in D$_5$W, given I.V. over 30 to 60 minutes.	*Lithium:* increased toxicity. Lithium dose may have to be decreased.	Sedation, decreased metal acuity, hemolytic anemia, edema and weight gain, orthostatic hypotension, mouth dryness.	Weigh patient daily. Notify doctor of any weight increase. Inform patient that orthostatic hypotension can be minimized by rising slowly and avoiding sudden position changes.
metoprolol tartrate 50 to 100 mg P.O. daily in 2 or 3 divided doses.	*Prazosin:* increased hypotension. *Lidocaine:* increased blood levels. *Theophyllines:* decreased therapeutic effect. *Barbiturates, indomethacin, rifampin, thyroid hormones:* decreased pharmacologic effect of metoprolol. *Chlorpromazine, cimetidine, oral contraceptives:* increased pharmacologic effect of metoprolol.	Bradycardia, hypotension, congestive heart failure.	Monitor blood pressure frequently. If patient develops severe hypotension, notify doctor. Tell outpatient not to discontinue this drug suddenly; abrupt discontinuation can exacerbate angina and MI. Instruct patient to call doctor if unpleasant side effects develop. Food may increase absorption. Give consistently with meals.
minoxidil 10 to 40 mg P.O. daily.	None significant.	Edema, weight gain, hypertrichosis (elongation, thickening and enhanced pigmentation of fine body hair), tachycardia.	About 80% of patients experience hypertrichosis within 6 weeks of beginning treatment. Suggest a depilatory or shaving, and assure patient that extra hair will disappear within 1 to 6 months of stopping minoxidil. Advise patient not to discontinue drug without doctor's consent.
nadolol 80 to 240 mg P.O. once daily.	*Prazosin:* increased hypotension. *Lidocaine:* increased blood levels. *Theophyllines:* decreased therapeutic effect. *Indomethacin:* decreased therapeutic effect of nadolol.	Bradycardia, hypotension, congestive heart failure, increased airway resistance.	Always check patient's apical pulse before giving this drug. If slower than 60 beats/minute, hold drug and call doctor. Tell outpatient not to discontinue drug suddenly, but to call doctor if unpleasant side effects develop. This drug masks common signs of shock and hypoglycemia. May be given without regard to meals.

Antihypertensives (continued)

Drug, dose, and route	Interactions	Side effects	Special considerations
nitroprusside Infuse intravenously at 0.5 to 10 mcg/kg/minute. Average dose is 3 mcg/kg/min.	None significant.	Headache, dizziness, restlessness, muscle twitching, diaphoresis, nausea, vomiting.	Because of light sensitivity, wrap I.V. solution in foil. It's not necessary to wrap the tubing in foil. Fresh solution should have faint brownish tint. Discard after 24 hours. Obtain baseline vital signs before giving drug, and find out what parameters the doctor wants to achieve. Check blood pressure every 5 minutes at start of infusion and after every rate change. If severe hypotension occurs, turn off I.V. and notify doctor.
pindolol 10 to 20 mg P.O. b.i.d.	*Prazosin:* increased hypotension. *Theophyllines:* decreased therapeutic effect. *Indomethacin:* decreased therapeutic effect of pindolol.	Fatigue, lethargy, congestive heart failure, hypotension, increased airway resistance, muscle and joint pain.	Always check apical pulse rate before giving drug. If you detect extremes in pulse rates, hold and call doctor. Tell outpatient not to discontinue this drug suddenly to prevent exacerbation of angina and MI. Tell patient to call doctor if unpleasant side effects develop. This drug masks common signs of shock and hypoglycemia.
prazosin hydrochloride 3 to 20 mg P.O. daily in divided doses.	*Beta-adrenergic blockers:* increased hypotension.	Dizziness, "first-dose syncope," palpitations, nausea, orthostatic hypotension, dryness of mouth.	If first dose exceeds 1 mg, patient may develop severe syncope with loss of consciousness. Increase dose slowly. Instruct patient to sit or lie down if he feels dizzy. Inform him to avoid sudden position changes.
propranolol hydrochloride 160 to 480 mg daily.	*See* propranolol hydrochloride on page 182.	*See* propranolol hydrochloride on page 182.	*See* propranolol hydrochloride on page 182.
timolol maleate 10 to 20 mg P.O. b.i.d.	*Prazosin:* increased hypotension. *Lidocaine:* increased blood levels. *Theophyllines:* decreased therapeutic effect. *Indomethacin:* decreased therapeutic effect of pindolol.	Fatigue, lethargy, hypotension, congestive heart failure, bradycardia, increased airway resistance.	Always check apical pulse rate before giving drug. If you detect extremes in pulse rates, withhold drug and call doctor. Tell patient not to discontinue drug suddenly; abrupt discontinuation can exacerbate angina and MI. This drug masks common signs of shock and hypoglycemia.

Cardiac glycosides

Drug, dose, and route	Interactions	Side effects	Special considerations
digitoxin Loading dose 1.2 to 1.6 mg I.V. or P.O. in divided doses over 24 hours; maintenance dose 0.1 mg daily. **digoxin** Loading dose 0.5 to 1 mg I.V. or P.O. in divided doses over 24 hours; maintenance 0.125 mg to 0.5 mg I.V. or P.O. daily. Large doses often needed for arrhythmias.	*Antacids, cholestyramine, colestipol, kaolin-pectin, metoclopramide:* decreased absorption of cardiac glycosides. *Amphotericin B, bumetanide, carbenicillin, ticarcillin, corticosteroids, and diuretics:* hyokalemia may increase cardiac glycoside toxicity. *Parenteral calcium, thiazides:* hypercalcemia and hypomagnesemia may increase cardiac glycoside toxicity. *Thyroid hormones:* decreased therapeutic effectiveness of cardiac glycosides. *Phenylbutazone, phenobarbital, phenytoin, rifampin:* decreased digitoxin levels. *Quinidine, nifedipine, and verapamil:* increased digoxin blood levels. *Anticholinergics:* increased digoxin absorption of oral tablets. *Amiloride:* altered digoxin excretion.	Yellow-green halos around visual images, blurred vision, anorexia, nausea, vomiting, diarrhea, fatigue, generalized muscle weakness, agitation, hallucinations, increased severity of congestive heart failure, dysrhythmias.	Hypothyroid patients are very sensitive to glycosides; hyperthyroid patients may need larger doses. Obtain baseline data (heart rate and rhythm, blood pressure, electrolytes) before giving first dose. Take apical-radial pulse for a full minute. Record and report to doctor any significant changes (sudden increase or decrease in rate, pulse deficit, irregular beats, and particularly regularization of a previously irregular rhythm). Check blood pressure and obtain 12-lead EKG with these changes. Excessive slowing of pulse rate (60 beats/minute or less) may be a sign of toxicity. Hold drug and notify doctor. Observe eating pattern. Ask patient about symptoms of toxicity. Instruct patient and responsible family member about drug action, dosage regimen, how to take pulse, reportable signs, and follow-up plans.

Diuretics

Drug, dose, and route	Interactions	Side effects	Special considerations
amiloride 5 to 10 mg P.O. daily.	*Potassium preparations:* may result in hyperkalemia. Use together cautiously.	Headache, nausea, vomiting, anorexia, diarrhea, impotence, hyperkalemia.	Discontinue immediately if potassium level exceeds 6.5 mEq/liter. Warn patient to avoid excessive ingestion of potassium. Give amiloride with or after meals.
chlorothiazide 500 mg to 2 g P.O. or I.V. daily in 2 divided doses.	*Cardiac glycosides:* hypokalemia may increase digitalis toxicity. *Lithium:* may cause lithium toxicity. *Oral hypoglycemics:* hypoglycemic effect antagonized.	Volume depletion and dehydration, hypokalemia, hyperuricemia, hyperglycemia, rash.	Consult with doctor and dietitian to provide high-potassium diet. Patients on digitalis have increased risk of digitalis toxicity. May use with potassium-sparing diuretic to prevent potassium loss. Only injectable thiazide. For I.V. use only.
chlorthalidone 25 to 100 mg P.O. daily.	*Cardiac glycosides:* hypokalemia may increase digitalis toxicity. *Lithium:* may cause lithium toxicity. *Oral hypoglycemics:* hypoglycemic effect antagonized.	Volume depletion and dehydration, hypokalemia, hyperuricemia, hyperglycemia, rash.	Consult with doctor and dietitian to provide high-potassium diet. Watch for hypokalemia. Patients on digitalis have an increased risk of digitalis toxicity.
furosemide 40 to 160 mg P.O. or I.M. daily for maintenance therapy. 40 to over 200 mg I.V.	*Cardiac glycosides:* hypokalemia may increase digitalis toxicity. *Aminoglycoside antibiotics:* increased ototoxicity.	Volume depletion and dehydration, hypokalemia, hyperuricemia, hyperglycemia, fluid and electrolyte imbalances.	Potent loop diuretic; can lead to profound water and electrolyte depletion. Monitor blood pressure and pulse during rapid diuresis. Watch for hypokalemia. Give I.V. doses over 1 to 2 minutes. Give P.O. and I.M. preparations in a.m., second doses in early p.m.

Diuretics (continued)

Drug, dose, and route	Interactions	Side effects	Special considerations
hydrochlorothiazide 25 to 100 mg P.O. daily at once or in divided doses.	*Cardiac glycosides:* hypokalemia may increase digitalis toxicity. *Lithium:* may cause lithium toxicity. *Oral hypoglycemics:* hypoglycemic effect antagonized.	Volume depletion and dehydration, hypokalemia, hyperuricemia, hyperglycemia, rash.	Consult with doctor and dietitian to provide high-potassium diet. Watch for hypokalemia. Patients also on digitalis have an increased risk of digitalis toxicity.
metolazone 2.5 to 10 mg P.O. daily.	*Cardiac glycosides:* hypokalemia may increase digitalis toxicity. *Lithium:* may cause lithium toxicity. *Oral hypoglycemics:* hypoglycemic effect antagonized.	Volume depletion and dehydration, hypokalemia, hyperuricemia, hyperglycemia, rash.	Consult with doctor and dietitian to provide high-potassium diet. Watch for hypokalemia. Patients on digitalis may have an increased risk of digitalis toxicity. Give drug in a.m. Elderly patients are especially susceptible to excessive diuresis.
spironolactone 25 to 100 mg P.O. daily in divided doses.	*Potassium preparations:* may result in hyperkalemia. Use together cautiously.	Hyperkalemia, gynecomastia in males, menstrual disturbances.	Warn patient to avoid excessive ingestion of potassium-rich foods or potassium-containing salt substitutes. Give drug with meals. Elderly patients are especially susceptible to excessive diuresis.
triamterene 100 mg P.O. b.i.d.	*Potassium preparations:* may result in hyperkalemia. Use together cautiously.	Hyperkalemia, nausea, vomiting.	Warn patient to avoid excessive ingestion of potassium. Give drug after meals.

Miscellaneous cardiovascular drugs

Drug, dose, and route	Interactions	Side effects	Special considerations
atropine sulfate *For AV block, junctional or escape rhythms, severe nodal or sinus bradycardia:* 0.5 to 1.0 mg I.V. bolus.	None significant.	Dry mouth, mental confusion, palpitations, urinary retention, tachycardia.	Monitor heart rate and rhythm to determine the drug's effects. Doses lower than 0.5 mg can cause paradoxical bradycardia. Store drug in amber or light-resistant container. Dose may be repeated q 5 minutes up to 2 mg.
calcium chloride *For asystole:* 0.5 to 1 g I.V. bolus.	*Cardiac glycosides:* increased digitalis toxicity; administer calcium very cautiously, if at all, to digitalized patients.	Bradycardia, hypercalcemia, syncope, tingling sensations.	Monitor EKG when administering drug I.V. Don't confuse calcium chloride with calcium gluconate. Don't exceed rate of 1 ml/minute.
dobutamine *For refractory congestive heart failure:* 2.5 to 10 mcg/kg/minute as I.V. infusion. Increase rate to 40 mcg/kg/minute.	*Beta-adrenergic blockers:* may decrease dobutamine's effectiveness. Use together cautiously.	Tachycardia, hypertension, premature ventricular beats.	Monitor EKG, blood pressure, PCWP, and cardiac output continuously. Also monitor urinary output. Incompatible with alkaline solutions. Oxidation of drug may slightly discolor admixtures. This does not indicate a significant loss of potency. I.V. solutions remain stable for 24 hours.
dopamine *For cardiogenic shock, hypotension, and hypovolemic shock:* 5 to 20 mcg/kg/minute as I.V. infusion.	*Ergot alkaloids, tricyclics:* extreme elevations in blood pressure. *Phenytoin:* may lower blood pressure of dopamine-stabilized patients.	Hypotension, ectopic beats, nausea, vomiting, palpitations.	Mix with D_5W, saline, or combination just before use. Use large vein to minimize risk of extravasation. If extravasation occurs, stop infusion and call doctor. Check blood pressure, pulse, urinary output, and extremity color and temperature often during infusion. Titrate infusion rate according to findings, using doctor's guidelines.
epinephrine hydrochloride *For cardiac and circulatory failure:* 0.5 to 1 mg I.V. bolus or 4 mg/500 ml of I.V. solution at 1 to 8 mcg/minute; 0.1 to 0.2 mg intracardiac.	*Beta-adrenergic blockers:* increased blood pressure and decreased heart rate. *Guanethidine:* decreased antihypertensive action. *Tricyclic antidepressants:* may increase epinephrine's effects.	Nervousness, palpitations, ventricular fibrillation, tachycardia.	If drug is given I.V., record baseline blood pressure and pulse before beginning therapy. Monitor patient closely until desired effect is obtained, then every 5 minutes until stable. After the patient's condition stabilizes, monitor blood pressure every 15 minutes. If blood pressure rises sharply, reduce I.V. flow rate and alert doctor.
isoproterenol hydrochloride *For asystole and bradyarrhythmia:* 0.02 to 0.06 mg I.V., then 0.01 to 0.2 mg I.V. or 5 mcg/minute I.V. *For shock:* 0.5 to 5 mcg/minute by infusion.	None significant.	Palpitations, tremors, tachycardia.	Closely monitor vital signs and urinary output. If heart rate exceeds 110 beats/minute (BPM) slow or discontinue the infusion. Heart rate over 60 BPM can trigger ventricular dysrhythmia in complete heart block. Draw blood to obtain arterial blood gas values. When drug is given for shock, monitor blood pressure, central venous pressure, and EKG. Measure hourly urinary output, and adjust infusion rate accordingly.
norepinephrine hydrochloride *For hypotension:* 8 to 12 mcg/min. I.V. infusion.	*Guanethidine:* decreased antihypertensive action. Monitor blood pressure. *Tricyclic antidepressants:* may increase norepinephrine's effects.	Decreased urinary output, headache, ventricular fibrillation, tachycardia, severe hypertension.	Report decreased urinary output to the doctor immediately. If prolonged I.V. therapy is necessary, change injection site frequently.
sodium bicarbonate *For cardiac arrest:* 1 to 3 mEq/kg of body weight I.V. bolus. Further dose based on ABGs.	*Ephedrine, pseudoephedrine:* increased pharmacologic effect. Monitor for toxicity. *Quinidine:* increased blood levels due to alkaline urine. Monitor for increased effect.	Alkalosis, hypernatremia.	Drug may be added to I.V. solution unless solution contains dopamine, epinephrine, or norepinephrine injection. Don't infuse through I.V. line containing calcium. During administration, draw blood for ABG values and electrolyte measurements.

Selected References

Anthony, Catherine P., and Gary A. Thibodeau. *Textbook of Anatomy and Physiology,* 10th ed. St. Louis: C.V. Mosby Co., 1978.

"A Balloon to Block an Aneurysm." *Emergency Medicine,* September 15, 1982, 140-145.

Barry, John, and Dieter W. Gump. "Endocarditis: An Overview." *Heart & Lung* 11 (March-April 1982): 138-143.

Brunner, Lillian S. *The Lippincott Manual of Nursing Practice,* 3d ed. Philadelphia: J.B. Lippincott Co., 1982.

Brunner, Lillian S., and Doris S. Suddarth. *Textbook of Medical-Surgical Nursing,* 4th ed. New York: Harper & Row, 1980.

Campbell, Claire. *Nursing Diagnosis and Intervention in Nursing Practice.* New York: John Wiley & Sons, 1978.

Chaffee, Ellen E., I.M. Lytle, et al. *Basic Physiology and Anatomy,* 4th ed. Philadelphia: J.B. Lippincott Co., 1980.

Cohen, Judith A., Nancy Pantaleo, and William E. Shell. "A Message from the Heart: What Isoenzymes Can Tell You About Your Cardiac Patient." *Nursing82* 12 (April 1982): 47-49.

Conn, Howard F., and Rex B. Conn, Jr. *Current Diagnosis Six.* Philadelphia: W.B. Saunders Co., 1980.

Conover, Mary B. *Understanding Electrocardiography: Physiological and Interpretive Concepts,* 3d ed. St. Louis: C.V. Mosby Co., 1980.

Dossey, Barbara, and Cathie E. Guzzetta. "Nursing Diagnosis." *Nursing81* 11 (June 1981): 34-38.

Dracup, Kathleen A. "Unraveling the Mysteries of Cardiomyopathy." *Nursing79* 9 (May 1979): 84-87.

Dracup, Kathleen A. "Managing and Understanding the Patient with Ineffective Endocarditis." *Nursing80* 10 (May 1980): 44-50.

Egoville, Barbara Boyd. "IHSS: What to Teach the Patient Who Has It." *Nursing80* 10 (April 1980): 50-55.

Ekers, Mitzi A., and Bhagwan Satiani. "EAB: A New Route for Vascular Rehabilitation." *Nursing82* 12 (November 1982): 34-41.

Fowler, Noble O. *Cardiac Diagnosis and Treatment,* 3d ed. Philadelphia: Harper & Row, 1980.

Giblin, E.C., et al. "Guidelines for Educating Nurses in High Blood Pressure Control." *Report of the Task Force on the Role of Nursing in High Blood Pressure Control.* Bethesda, Md.: National Institutes of Health. NIH Pub. No. 80-1241, March 1980.

Guyton, Arthur C. *Basic Human Physiology: Normal Function and Mechanisms of Disease,* 3d ed. Philadelphia: W.B. Saunders Co., 1982.

Guyton, Arthur C. *Textbook of Medical Physiology,* 6th ed. Philadelphia: W.B. Saunders Co., 1981.

Harvey, A.M., ed. *The Principles and Practice of Medicine,* 20th ed. New York: Appleton-Century-Crofts, 1980.

Heart Facts 1983. Dallas, Tex.: American Heart Association, 1983.

Hill, Martha, and Janis W. Fink. "In Hypertensive Emergencies, Act Quickly but Also Act Cautiously." *Nursing83* 13 (February 1983): 34-41.

Hook, Edward W. "The War Against Endocarditis." *Emergency Medicine* 14 (October 30, 1982): 29-50.

Hurst, J.W., ed. *The Heart,* 5th ed. New York: McGraw-Hill Book Co., 1980.

Isselbacher, Kurt, et al. *Harrison's Principles and Practices of Medicine.* New York: McGraw-Hill Book Co., 1981.

Johanson, Brenda, et al. *Standards for Critical Care.* St. Louis: C.V. Mosby Co., 1980.

Kern, Leslie S., and Anna Gawlinski. "Stage-Managing Coronary Artery Disease." *Nursing83* 13 (April 1983): 34-40.

Luckmann, Joan, and Karen C. Sorensen. *Medical-Surgical Nursing: A Psychophysiologic Approach,* 2d ed. Philadelphia: W.B. Saunders Co., 1980.

McCarthy, Claire. "PTCA: Therapeutic Intervention in the Cardiac Catheterization Laboratory." *Heart & Lung* 11 (November-December 1982): 499-504.

McCauley, Kathleen. "Probing the In's and Out's of Congestive Heart Failure." *Nursing82* 12 (November 1982): 60-65.

Matheny, Leona. "Emergency! First Aid for Cardiopulmonary Arrest." *Nursing82* 12 (June 1982): 34-45.

Muir, Bernice L. *Pathophysiology: An Introduction to the Mechanisms of Disease.* New York: John Wiley and Sons, 1980.

The 1980 Report of the Joint National Committee on Detection, Evaluation, and Treatment of High Blood Pressure. Bethesda, Md.: National Institutes of Health. NIH Pub. No. 81-1088, December 1980.

"Patient Behavior for Blood Pressure Control." *Journal of the American Medical Association* 241:2534-2537.

Price, Sylvia, and Lorraine M. Wilson. *Pathophysiology: Clinical Concepts of Disease Processes.* New York: McGraw-Hill Book Co., 1978.

Report of the Working Group on Critical Patient Behaviors in the Dietary Management of High Blood Pressure. Bethesda, Md.: National Institutes of Health. NIH Pub. No. 81-2269, 1981.

Sana, Josephine M., and Richard P. Judge. *Physical Assessment Skills for Nursing Practice,* 2d ed. Boston: Little, Brown, 1982.

Scordo, Kristine Ann. "This Procedure Called PTCA: Your Patient's CABG Substitute?" *Nursing82* 12 (February 1982): 50-55.

Smith, Janis B., M.H. Giblin, and J.A. Koehler. "The Cardiovascular System," in *Pediatric Critical Care.* New York: John Wiley and Sons, 1983.

Smith, Lloyd H., Jr., and James B. Wyngaarden, eds. *Cecil Textbook of Medicine.* Philadelphia: W.B. Saunders Co., 1982.

Underhill, Sandra, et al. *Cardiac Nursing.* Philadelphia: J.B. Lippincott Co., 1982.

Wadsworth, Linda, Sheila Goodwin, Chris Dragoo, et al. "Intracoronary Streptokinase Infusion." *Nursing82* 12 (May 1982): 58-65.

Wenger, Nannette K., J.W. Hurst, and M.C. McIntyre. *Cardiology for Nurses.* New York: McGraw-Hill Book Co., 1980.

INDEX

i = illustration; t = table

i = illustration; t = table

in CAD, 94-95
in cardiomyopathy, 137
Raynaud's disease, 115.
  diagnosis, 119
    nursing, 124t
  nursing goals, 124t
  treatment, 119, 125
Raynaud's phenomenon, 115
Rehabilitation program
  for angina patient, 111
  for MI patient, 111
Renal arterial stenosis
  DSA and, 52
  in hypertension, 67
Renal failure
  complication of septal my-
    otomy-myectomy, 142
  in hypertension, 59
Renal function, in CHF, 77
Renin-angiotensin-aldosterone
    system
  blood pressure regulation
    and, 13-14
  in CHF, 19
  in hypertension, 58-59i
Renovascular hypertension,
    58, 60
Reserpine, 119
Respiratory alkalosis, in CHF,
    77
Respiratory failure, 142
Retinopathy, hypertension and,
    56i, 57, 64i, 68i
Rheumatic fever
  causes, 145
  effect on heart wall, 146
  pathophysiology, 144i, 146,
    152i
  signs, 146, 148
  treatment, 147
Romano-Ward syndrome, 161
Roth's spots, in endocarditis,
    148

S

Salbutamol (albuterol), 80
Salicylates
  in pericarditis, 147
  in rheumatic fever, 147
Secondary hypertension, 57,
    58, 60
Septal myotomy-myectomy
  complications, 142
  in IHSS, 138
Sexual dysfunction, drug-re-
    lated, 72
SGOT. See Glutamic-oxaloac-
    etic   transaminase,
    serum.
Shock, carotid pulse and, 28-
    29
Sick sinus syndrome, 159-160,
    172
Sinoatrial block, second-de-
    gree, Type II, 173
Sinoatrial exit block, second-
    degree, Type I, 173
Sinoatrial node dysrhythmias,
    172-173. See also spe-
    cific dysrhythmias.
  EKG in, 159
  pathophysiology, 159-160
Sinus arrest, 172
Sinus arrhythmia, 172
Sinus bradycardia, 172
Sinus exit block, 173
Sinus tachycardia, 172

Skin assessment
  CAD and, 104
  cardiac output and, 21
  peripheral circulation and,
    21, 23, 25
  tissue perfusion and, 21
Smoking
  in arterial occlusive disease,
    117
  in hypertension, 69
  in vascular disorders, 129
Sodium bicarbonate, 186
Sodium-potassium pump, 16
Spironolactone, 80, 186
Starling's law, 16, 18i
  in CHF, 19
  in MI, 92
Stepped-care approach, 65,
    66i
Sternal notch, 29i, 31
Stethoscope, 21, 32i
Streptokinase therapy, 9, 101-
    102, 107i
  contraindications, 106
  patient education, 106, 107i
  post-therapy care, 106
  in thrombophlebitis, 121
Streptomycin, in endocarditis,
    147
Stress, hypertension and, 69
Stress-relaxation, blood pres-
    sure regulation and, 14
Stroke volume, 18
  in CHF, 19
Sudden death
  complication of MI, 92
  dysrhythmias and, 163
  in IHSS, 136
Summation gallop, 33
Suprasternal notch, 29
Supraventricular dysrhythmias.
    See Atrial dysrhyth-
    mias, junctional node
    dysrhythmias, and si-
    noatrial node dysrhyth-
    mias.
Swan-Ganz catheterization.
    See Pulmonary artery
    catheterization.
Sydenham's chorea, in rheu-
    matic fever, 148
Syncope, in IHSS, 142-143
Systemic hypertension, 31, 33
  heart sound in, 34t

T

Tachycardia
  atrial, 160
  in CHF, 75, 77, 82
  in dilated congestive cardio-
    myopathy, 133-134
  EPS in, 53
  heart sounds in, 33
  in IHSS, 136
  in MI, 92
  in preexcitation syndromes,
    161
  ventricular, 161, 163
Technetium pyrophosphate
    scanning, 50
  in MI, 94-95
Temperature extremes, vascu-
    lar disorders and, 129
Teprotide, 80
Tetralogy of Fallot, 180-181t
  cardiac catheterization in, 47
Thallium imaging, 50

antianginal therapy and, 50
CABG and, 50
in CAD, 94, 94i, 137
in MI, 50, 94
PTCA and, 50, 109
Thiazide diuretics, 80, 185, 186
Thrill, 29, 31
Thrombectomy, in thrombo-
    phlebitis, 121
Thromboembolism
  in CHF, 85
  complication of
    EPS, 53
    MI, 93
  treatment, 95-96
Thromboendarterectomy
  in aortic arch syndrome, 119
  in arterial occlusive disease,
    118
Thrombolytics, in thrombo-
    phlebitis, 121
Thrombophlebitis, 116-117
  complication of cardiac
    catheterization, 49t
  diagnosis, 119, 121
    nursing, 124t
  nursing goals, 124t
  pulmonary emboli, preven-
    tion of, 127
  signs, 25, 116-117
  treatment, 121
Thromboxane, 91
Thrombus. See also Thrombo-
    phlebitis.
  mural, 113, 115i
  treatment, 121
TIAs. See Transient ischemic
    attacks.
Timolol maleate, 96, 185
Tocainide, 163
Tolazoline, 125
Tomography, computerized ax-
    ial
  in arterial occlusive disease,
    117
  in pericarditis, 146
Torsades de Pointes, 161, 178
Transient ischemic attacks, 59
Transplantation, heart, 100i
Transposition of great arteries,
    180-181t
Trendelenburg test, in varicose
    veins, 119
Triamterene, 80, 186
Tricuspid regurgitation, 154-
    155t
  heart murmur, 35t
  in inflammatory disorders,
    potential for, 153
Tricuspid stenosis, 154-155t
  a wave in, 27
  heart murmur in, 35t
Tricuspid valve disease, car-
    diac radiography in, 42
Trimethaphan camsylate, 71
Tumors
  DSA and, 52
  in hypertension, 66
  NMR and, 52

U

Ulcers
  arterial, 125t
  patient-teaching aid, 126
  prevention, 127
  venous, 125t
Ultrasonography, Doppler, 51t

in aneurysms, 117
in arterial occlusive disease,
    117
in thrombophlebitis, 119
Urinalysis, in hypertension, 60,
    65
Urokinase, 121

V

Vagal response, complication
    of cardiac catheteriza-
    tion, 49t
Valsalva maneuver, 163
  contraindication, 29, 106,
    163
  in dysrhythmia, 163
  in IHSS, 136
Valvular disorders. See also
    specific valvular disor-
    ders.
  cardiac catheterization in,
    37, 47
  cardiac output and, 47
  echocardiography in, 37, 47
  inflammatory disorders, 144-
    153
Varicose veins, 115-116
  diagnosis, 119
    nursing, 124t
  nursing goals, 124t
  treatment, 119
Vascular disorders, 112-129.
    See also specific disor-
    ders.
  assessment, 121-123
  circulation in, 128-129
  complications, prevention of,
    127-128
  management
    medical, 117-119, 121
    nursing, 121-125, 127-129
  nursing diagnoses, 124t
  pathophysiology, 113-117
  patient education, 123-127,
    129
  postoperative care, 127-128
Vascular resistance, 12i, 13.
    See also Hemodynamic
    regulation.
Vasoconstrictors, 136, 138, 142
Vasodilators
  in arterial occlusive disease,
    117
  in CAD, 95, 96
  in CHF, 80
  in dilated congestive cardio-
    myopathy, 138, 141
  in IHSS, 136, 138, 140i, 142
Vasopressin. See Antidiuretic
    hormone.
Vectorcardiography, 51t
Venography, in thrombophle-
    bitis, 119
Venous insufficiency
  in hypertension, 65
  signs, 25
Venous pressure, 27-28, 29i
Ventilation, ineffective, in car-
    diomyopathy, 141-142
Ventricle(s)
  assessment, 27-28, 30, 43,
    53
  location, 10i
Ventricular aneurysm
  aneurysmectomy and, 165
  cardiac catheterization in, 47
  complication of MI, 93, 161

Ventricular assist pump, 100i
Ventricular conduction dysrhyth-
    mias, 161-162, 178-179
Ventricular dilatation, in dilated
    congestive cardiomy-
    opathy, 133-134, 135i,
    138i
Ventricular dysrhythmias, 161-
    162, 177-178. See also
    specific dysrhythmias.
  in IHSS, 136
  treatment, 138
Ventricular failure. See also
    Heart failure, conges-
    tive.
  left
    carotid pulse and, 28-29
    in CHF, 75, 76-77, 80i
    in dilated congestive car-
      diomyopathy, 134
    heart sound, 33, 34t
    treatment, 95
  right
    in CHF, 75
    in dilated congestive car-
      diomyopathy, 134
    jugular pulse and, 27-28
    pulmonary artery cathe-
      terization in, 44
    systolic impulse and, 31
    venous pressure and, 29i
Ventricular fibrillation, 178
  in preexcitation syndromes,
    161
Ventricular flutter, 177
Ventricular gallop. See Heart
    sounds, S3.
Ventricular heave, in CHF, 82-
    83
Ventricular hypertrophy
  decompensated heart failure
    and, 19
  left, 30, 74i
    heart sound in, 34t
    hypertension and, 65
    PMI and, 31
  right, 27, 30, 31
    cor pulmonale, 79
Ventricular infarction, pulmo-
    nary artery catheteriza-
    tion in, 44
Ventricular septal defect, 180-
    181t
  cardiac radiography in, 43
  complication of MI, 93
  heart murmur, 35t
  pulmonary artery catheter-
    ization in, 44
Ventricular tachycardia, 177
Ventriculography, contrast, 137
Verapamil, 96, 182
  in dysrhythmia, 163, 183
  in IHSS, 136, 138, 142

W

Warfarin, 121
Weight control, in hyperten-
    sion, 68-69
Weight gain, in CHF, 77
Wolff-Parkinson-White syn-
    drome, 161, 176
  EKG in, 136, 161
  EPS in, 53, 163

X

X-rays. See Cardiac radiogra-
    phy, chest X-ray.

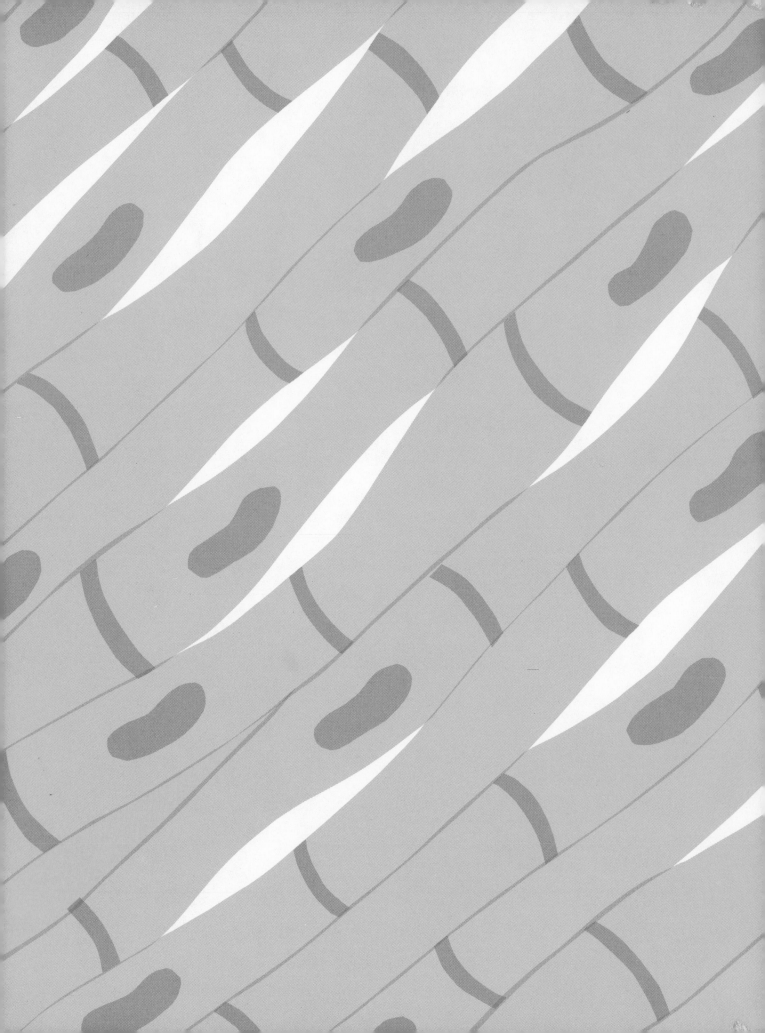